A *Jerry Baker* Good Health Book

AMAZING

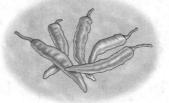

ANTIDOTES

www.jerrybaker.com

AMAZING

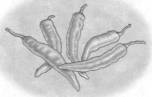

ANTIDOTES

976 NIFTY NEW WAYS TO STAY HAPPY AND HEALTHY

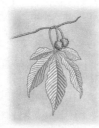
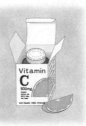
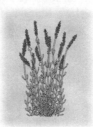
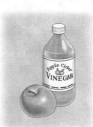

MARCIA HOLMAN

Published by American Master Products, Inc./Jerry Baker
Kim Adam Gasior, Publisher

A Jerry Baker Good Health Book and a Blackberry Cottage Production
Editorial: Ellen Michaud, Blackberry Cottage Productions
Design: Nest Publishing Resources

Editor: Megan Othersen
Book Composition: Wayne F. Michaud
Illustrator: Wayne F. Michaud
Researcher: Anita Small
Copy Editor: Jane Sherman

Printed in the United States of America

Illustrations copyright © 2004 by Wayne F. Michaud

Publisher's Cataloging-in-Publication
(Provided by Quality Books, Inc.)

Holman, Marcia.
    Jerry Baker's amazing antidotes : 976 nifty new ways to stay happy and healthy / Marcia Holman.
        p. cm. — (Jerry Baker's good health series)
    Includes index.
    ISBN 0–922433–52–6

    1. Traditional medicine.   2. Medicine, Popular.
    3. Naturopathy.   4. Self-care, Health.   I. Baker, Jerry.
    II. Title.   III. Title: Amazing antidotes

RC81.H713 2004   615.8'8
                           QB104-200091

2 4 6 8 10 9 7 5 3 hardcover

CONTENTS

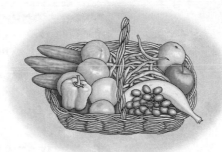

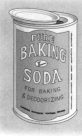

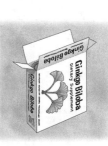

Lavender

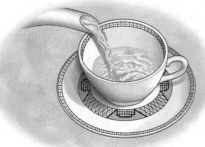

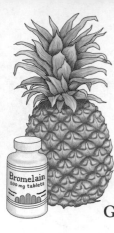

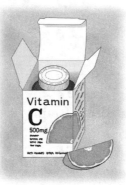

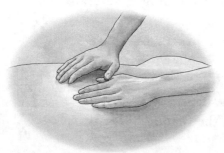

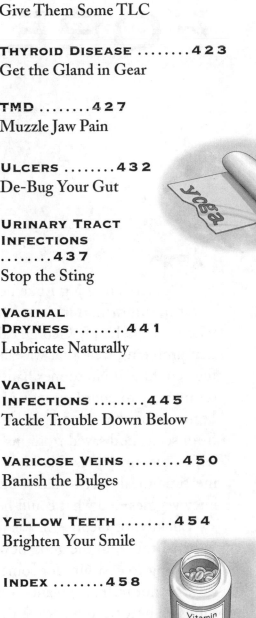

FOREWORD

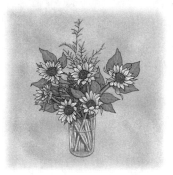

There's nothing I like better than the thought of spending a warm, sunny morning out in my yard putterin' around, so when my old buddy George called me in a lather about his garden problems, well, that was about the best invitation this old fella could get! No sooner had I hung up the phone than I was on my way to poor George's place. And what a sight it was! His beans, cucumbers, and even his prized tomato plants—grown from seeds he'd saved from his family's heirloom variety—had white, blotchy leaves that looked downright sad. George's summertime meals just wouldn't be the same without those fresh, juicy veggies—so what could he do?

Luckily for George, it was just a case of powdery mildew. When I told him the good news, he grumbled about the $20 it was going to cost him for some Miracle-Kill-Everything chemical whatnot to fix his plants. I told George he already had everything he needed to massacre the mildew right in his kitchen. No sooner had I given him the lowdown than he was hightailing it inside to whip up my Magic Mildew Mix.

While George was fixing up the concoction, I sat out on his

porch to take in some of the morning sunshine. It was then that I noticed several red blotches on my hands. Good grief! The last thing I wanted to do was spend $45 at the doctor's office to take care of a little post-gardening rash. And that's not even taking into account what it would cost me in time and aggravation spent in the waiting room!

While the blotches were probably nothing major, what if they got worse? Why wasn't there some easy way to tell how serious the rash was and to learn, step by step, what I could do about it?

Just then, George bounded out onto the porch with his homemade cure-all spray and darted off to save his prized plants. I soon left, and just as I walked up my front steps, it hit me: *If there are simple, commonsense antidotes for a whole host of garden problems, then there darn well ought to be some of the same for health problems, too!*

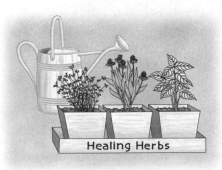

I decided to call my friend Marcia Holman—a former health editor at a major publishing company—and ask her to check into it. Now, I'm happy to report that with help from her team of researchers, Marcia uncovered hundreds of great home remedies and quick-and-easy treatments for oodles and oodles of ailments. Why, I couldn't believe some of the things she came up with, like an onion poultice to battle bronchitis, a potato juice constipation cure, and a dandelion tea to bust high blood pressure! And you know me—I just couldn't keep all these terrific tips to myself.

So we've crammed them all into this new book: *Amazing Antidotes*. Whether you're looking for the best exercise to relieve back pain, a fruity feast to flatten arthritis, or even a

Healing Herbs

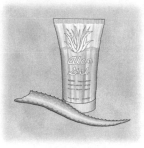

quick citrus drink to ease your worst stom-achache—we've discovered hundreds of timely tips, remarkable remedies, and super solutions for some of your most bothersome health problems. If you want to save money, get instant relief, or find a do-it-yourself treatment, this book is a dream come true.

Amazing Antidotes offers 976 grab-you-by-the-tonsils reme-dies that'll save you tons of time, money, and aggravation. You'll discover loads of great features to help keep those greenbacks in your wallet—the "Save Your Money" tips will give you the relief you need for just pennies! Or, if you need instant help for a troublesome problem, check out the remedies in "On-the-Spot Relief." "When to Dial the Doc" tells you when you really need expert attention fast, and our "Homegrown Solutions" show you how to whip up a miracle mix from items growing right in your own garden!

If it's amazing relief you need, it's amazing antidotes you

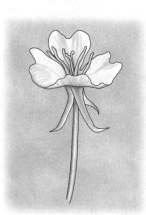

get—from salves and lotions to teas and tinc-tures, along with massage, acupuncture, and herbal treatments—as well as the telltale signs of a serious condition. And the antidotes are fast, easy, and cheap! So save your hard-earned cash for those serious medical problems that fall from the sky. With this book, you'll learn how to save money with do-it-yourself remedies for 159 common health problems—and gain a life-time of good health in the process!

Jerry Baker

ADULT ACNE

No More Breakouts

———◆◆◆———

Pimples are a pain in the fanny no matter what your age. As teens, we could cover the angry bumps—those on our fore-heads, anyway—with a fringe of bangs. Adult acne, though, which typically crops up on the chin, isn't so easily hidden. It's bangs-proof, and it's possibly even more vexing than the teenage variety because it's so unexpected—and so totally unfair.

"It feels like you have a neon arrow on your face pointing to your zit," gripes my neighbor Kris, a newspaper photographer who gets "really bugged" when blemishes pop

SHOULD YOU POP IT?

We know it's oh-so-tempting to squeeze, but curb the urge—it's counterproductive. When you press on a zit, you can inadvertently push pus and bacteria farther into the pore, causing deeper, more serious inflammation. Instead, apply a warm washcloth to it several times daily. This will coax the bacteria to the surface so the blemish bursts naturally.

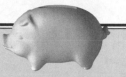
out right before she has to shoot photos of a VIP.

WHY ME?

When we get pimples as adults, they tend to appear right before our periods, during pregnancy, in the years just prior to menopause, and anytime we're stressed out. Not coincidentally, these are all times when our hormones are raging.

Just before menstruation and during pregnancy, our bodies pump out more of the hormone progesterone. Progesterone in turn triggers the production of more sebum, a waxy, oily material excreted through the hair follicles that keeps the skin supple and moist. When we're under stress or approaching menopause, our bodies pump out more of another sebum-producing hormone called androgen.

"This excess oil can clog your pores, trapping dead skin cells there, and bacteria can multiply like fish behind a dam," says Phillip Shenefelt, M.D., associate professor in the division of dermatology at the University of South Florida in Tampa. The result is an infected, inflamed pore, better known as a pimple. If the blockage is really deep, it can create lumps (cysts) beneath the skin surface—the most severe form of acne.

BANISH THE BUMPS

While some breakouts require a heavy-duty prescription treatment such as tretinoin (Retin-A, a drug derived from vitamin A that speeds up cell turnover and the elimination of sebum from hair follicles, so pores can't become blocked), the occasional pesky pimple outbreak usually doesn't require any medication—prescription or over the counter. It doesn't even necessitate wearing bangs. What it does call for are just a few of these milder zit-zapping tricks.

CLEANSE WITH CALENDULA. Using your fingers, not a washcloth, cleanse with warm water and a mild herbal soap such as calendula (which you can find at health food stores). The herb is a mild but potent natural astringent that will gently strip your skin of oils. Finish with a splash of cold water to close the pores.

SHOWER WITH SALICYLIC ACID. If your chest or back looks like a connect-the-dots game, check your health food store for Sal-Ac, a commercial shower rinse that contains salicylic acid. Not only is it a gentle de-oiler, it can also act as a mild peel and help open clogged pores, says Dr. Shenefelt. Limit cleansing to twice a day, and use warm water.

TRY TEA TREE OIL. This herbal oil, which you can find at the health food store, battles acne as well as medicines like Clearasil, but with much less irritation, says Scott M. Dinehart, M.D., professor of dermatology at the University of Arkansas in Little Rock. The drawback: It works more slowly, has an unpleasant odor, and may sting a bit. Dilute it with water before applying it to your skin, and don't use it more than twice daily.

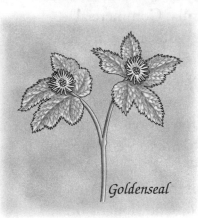
Goldenseal

GRAB SOME GOLDENSEAL. Don't leave your health food store without picking up powdered goldenseal root—a mild but effective disinfectant. Add 1/2 teaspoon to 12 drops of tea tree oil and dab the resulting paste onto your blem-

Whip Up a Skin "Smoothie"

You can blend sugar, fruit, and milk into a "smoothie" that can discourage blemishes as well as delight your taste buds. The ingredients are packed with alpha hydroxy acids, which help unclog pores by dissolving the "glue" that holds dead skin cells together. The best dissolver is glycolic acid (which is made from sugar cane) because its small molecules penetrate the walls of skin cells. To make the mixture, combine 1 teaspoon of sugar, a few tablespoons of milk (for lactic acid), 5 grapes (for tartaric acid), a kiwi (for citric acid), and an apple (for malic acid) in a blender. Apply some to each blemish, leave it on for 10 minutes, and rinse with warm water.

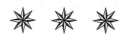

ishes. Rinse after about 20 minutes. Apply the paste twice a day, and your pimple will vanish, promises Jeanette Jacknin, M.D., a dermatologist in Scottsdale, Arizona.

Go nuts. Add some almonds to your skin "smoothie" (see box at left). These nuts contain mandelic acid, which dermatologists have found to be useful in treating women who have sun-damaged skin and acne, says Mark B. Taylor, M.D., a dermatologist in Salt Lake City.

Wash with witch hazel. Sweaty workouts are great for your body, but they increase sebum production—which is not so great for your face. To get rid of the extra oil gently, swab your face with the tannin-packed herb witch hazel, suggests Kathlyn Quatrochi, N.D., a naturopathic physician in Oak Glen, California. Commercial witch hazel products contain few tannins, so it's best to whip up your own. Simply pick up 5 to 10 grams of witch hazel bark at a health food store, then steep it 1 cup of boiling water for 10 to 15 minutes. Strain, let cool, and pour into a plastic bottle for spot treating pimples after exercise.

Dab on zee clay. French women often use clay as a cleansing mask because it soaks up excess oil and sloughs off dead skin cells without irritation, says Dr. Quatrochi. Simply add a little water to a teaspoon of green clay (available at health food stores), then mix a few drops of lavender oil into the paste. The oil's antibacterial and anti-inflammatory properties will help your acne heal faster, and its lovely aroma should lower your stress level. Leave the mask on for 15 minutes, then rinse it off.

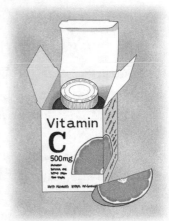

TAKE ANTIOXIDANTS. Vitamins A, C, and E are collectively referred to as antioxidants because they protect the body from oxygen-related free radicals that damage skin cells and promote inflammation, which can lead to blocked pores. Make sure your daily multivitamin/mineral tablet provides all three.

ZAP ZITS WITH ZINC. This mineral helps your oil-producing glands work properly, so you might try taking 15 milligrams of zinc along with 1 milligram of copper once a day with food.

TRY A CAL-MAG CALMER. Calcium and magnesium can help relax a stressed nervous system and nip sugar cravings in the bud. Since both of these factors contribute to blemishes, some doctors suggest popping 750 milligrams of calcium and 375 milligrams of magnesium once a day with food.

GET YOUR Bs. The B vitamins—particularly B_6—help regulate those pesky hormones that set the stage for adult acne, especially breakouts triggered by hormonal changes during menstruation and menopause, says Dr. Shenefelt. Try a B-complex supplement (with your doctor's approval, of course).

TRY VITEX. Also known as chasteberry, this herb (which you can find in tablet form at health food stores) is a mild anti-

Egg-xactly!

It sounds like a tabloid headline—Whipped Egg White Shrinks Pores!—but it's true, swears Kathlyn Quatrochi, N.D. Simply dab a bit of whipped egg white on each pimple, let it dry, rinse off the excess, then cover with a flesh-colored acne lotion—not regular makeup.

androgen and may also help regulate progesterone levels and squelch premenstrual breakouts. The recommended dose is 40 milligrams a day, but talk to your doctor before taking it—especially if you're on prescription hormone drugs of any kind.

GET YOUR EFAs. Taking 2 tablespoons of flaxseed oil or evening primrose oil daily could make up for a deficiency of essential fatty acids (EFAs), says Dr. Jacknin. Both oils are excellent sources of gamma-linolenic acid (GLA), a type of EFA that spurs production of an anti-inflammatory prostaglandin known to promote healing. Check your health food store for both.

AGE SPOTS

Watch Them Fade

———◆◇◈◇◆———

Like a lot of young women, I once took sunning nearly as seriously as studying for spring finals. I'd tote my trusty, foil-covered reflecting board to the roof of my dorm, where I'd place it under my chin to catch the best of the day's rays. I really "went for the bronze" back then. And to remind me of it now, I have a smattering of "the brown"—a bunch of flat, freckle-like age spots, which are technically called lentigines and sometimes dubbed (wrongly) liver spots.

WHY ME?

While lentigines usually debut—often on the hands, face, or shoulders—around age 40, they are years in the making. Back when I sat in the sun and baked on a regular basis, my body tried to protect my skin from solar damage by producing an excess of protective melanin. Over time, however, the

WHEN TO DIAL THE DOC

• • • • • • • • • • • •

While age spots are harmless, precancerous lesions may not be. Consult a dermatologist immediately if one of your "age spots" suddenly darkens to a deep brown or black, changes shape, becomes raised, or bleeds.

SHOWER YOUR SKIN WITH 'SHROOMS

Mushroom juice contains kojic acid, a lightening agent derived from Japanese mushrooms that has been found to block the over-production of melanin. "It's just as effective as hydroquinone for fading age spots without over-lightening or irritating skin," says Jeanette Jacknin, M.D.

Mind you, juice from your portobello burger probably won't do the trick, but any over-the-counter skin lotion that contains kojic acid will. Simply apply it twice daily, and your age spots may fade significantly in less than two months.

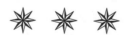

melanin turned to cellular debris that bunched up in irregular patches. And voilà—age spots! While they're completely harmless (much like freckles), they're rarely, if ever, considered cute.

If you want to fade your spots, your doctor is likely to suggest that you try one of the many vitamin A skin creams, called retinoids, that peel off the top layer of skin and along with it—possibly—those vexing spots.

If over-the-counter retinol products don't do the job, you may need to up the ante to a prescription-strength retinoid such as tretinoin (Retin-A). These drugs slough off old age spots and stop new ones from forming. Their only drawback is that they can be quite harsh, especially if you're very fair-skinned. In fact, if you use a prescription-strength retinoid, you may trade age spots for a nasty sunburn with the slightest exposure to sunlight, warns Jeanette Jacknin, M.D., a dermatologist in Scottsdale, Arizona. And isn't that what sent you scurrying for the stuff in the first place?

If, despite your best efforts, you find yourself applying your foundation with a putty knife, you may want to consider pulling out all the stops with one or more skin-stripping medical procedures. Your doctor may suggest removing your spots with a chemical peel, which uses strong acids to dissolve the skin surface; a liquid nitrogen peel, which "freezes" spots for easier removal; or a laser peel, in which your doctor actually lifts off age spots using a high-intensity light. All of these methods can erase age spots as completely as paint stripper peels off unwanted varnish—but they're pricey, and recovery can be painful.

GET THE BROWN OUT

Sometimes the very best remedies are the most basic. Here are some low-tech but highly effective ways to coax pesky age spots into the background. Just remember, though, no matter how you attack them, your age spots will reappear with sun exposure. So never go outside without sunscreen.

ATTACK WITH ACID. One tried-and-true spot-reducing substance—available in most commercial fading creams—is hydroquinone, an acid that slows the production of brown skin cell patches and helps them fade. Over-the-counter formulations, such as Porcelana, may do the trick. Just follow the package directions.

MIX UP LEMON AID. Lemon is a mild bleaching aid that works as well on lentigines as it does on stains on fabrics. Mix equal parts of lemon juice and water and apply to each spot. Leave on for 5 minutes before rinsing. Repeat three times a week, and the brown spots may fade to taupe, says Dr. Jacknin. Add more lemon juice and less water as your skin gets used to the preparation. Your goal is to be able to apply the juice "straight up."

ADD ELDERFLOWERS. Boost

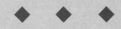

HOMEGROWN SOLUTION

◆ ◆ ◆

Gel Rx

Best known for its ability to heal burns, aloe gel may help fade skin spots by boosting cell turnover so the pigmented cells eventually slough off. Apply the gel directly to the spots twice a day for a month or two. The smell's a bit pungent, but the results are well worth it.

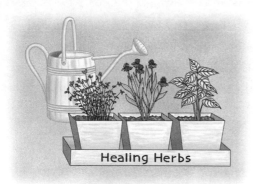
Healing Herbs

your lemon aid by adding equal parts of dried elderflowers, which you can find in health food stores. The denser mixture will act as a safe, natural acid peel, stripping away the top layer of skin and leaving you with the fresh, less spotty layer beneath.

HORSE AROUND WITH STRONGER STUFF. For darker spots, combine 1 teaspoon of grated horseradish, 1 teaspoon of lemon juice, and 1 teaspoon of vinegar with 3 drops of rosemary oil. It has a strong odor, but it will make spots fade swiftly, says Dr. Jacknin.

SMEAR ON SOME VITAMIN C. Topical vitamin C penetrates the outer layers of the skin and encourages shedding of old skin cells, including those that contain melanin. Plus, it reduces what's called free radical damage—one of the consequences of too much sun exposure.

Why not just drink a glass of O.J.? Because you can find vitamin C in cream and lotion forms that provide a whopping 30 times more C than oral forms, explains Dr. Jacknin. Plus, it's available without a prescription from dermatologists, plastic surgeons, and licensed aestheticians. Start by applying topical C to spots every other day, but never use it more than twice a day. The higher the concentration of vitamin C, the better the lightening power.

CONSIDER KINERASE PRODUCTS. Kinerase is a plant growth hormone that stops leaves from turning brown—and it may help diminish brown spots on your skin with little or no irritation, notes Phillip Shenefelt, M.D., associate professor of dermatology at the University of South Florida in Tampa. Look for it in over-the-counter lotions, then use it twice a day.

ALLERGIES

Tamp Down the Triggers

I can barely look at my cherry tree bursting with buds or my sycamore dropping moldy leaves without exploding into ferocious sneezing fits. It makes me wish my supermarket stocked bottles of pristine ocean air, so I could uncap one and breathe without sniffling, snuffling, or wanting desperately to doze off at my desk.

For me and all the other people who have allergic rhinitis (hay fever), normally harmless pollen, mold spores, animal dander, dust mites, and other airborne molecules spur the immune system to defend itself by producing what are called IgE (immunoglobulin E) antibodies. These antibodies glom onto mast cells, which release histamines (nasty inflammatory substances) into the bloodstream. As a result, mucus flows, tissues swell,

If you have throat tightening, tingling or swelling of the lips or mouth, shortness of breath, wheezing, hives, or lightheadedness, head for the hospital immediately. You're having an anaphylactic reaction—a potentially fatal, whole-body allergic response in which histamines flood your mucous membranes with fluid that can swell your throat and airways, shut off your breathing, and even stop your heart.

In 1 to 15 percent of allergy sufferers, anaphylaxis occurs when the body is overwhelmed by an allergen—typically fish, peanuts, bee or wasp venom, contact with latex (gloves or balloons), or drugs such as penicillin and aspirin. If you know you're allergic to any of these substances, always carry self-injectable epinephrine (such as EpiPen), which can stave off the allergic response until you can get to the hospital for further treatment to reduce the swelling and relax your airways.

and sneezing begins, all in an effort to evict the offending irritants.

WHY ME?

Genes are at least partly to blame for allergies. My daughter inherited hers from both parents, which made her immune system 70 percent more likely to overreact to a slew of triggers, from soaps to shellfish. But lifestyle plays a role, too.

"The simple truth is, if you overtax your system with too many stimulating substances, from harsh chemicals to stress to certain foods, anyone, no matter what their genetic makeup, can develop allergies," says Glen Rothfeld, M.D., clinical assistant professor of medicine at Tufts University School of Medicine in Boston.

That cheesy pizza or the wine you love? Both are fermented foods that trigger histamines. That yummy omelet or milkshake? They're high-protein foods that pack arachidonic acid (AA), which produces inflammatory prostaglandins. And bagels? They're carbohydrates that feed yeast (known as candida), which normally lives in your gut but can proliferate to such an extent that it overwhelms your immune system.

"The bombardment from these substances continually stimulates your immune system, keeping it in 'react mode,'" explains Dr. Rothfeld. Over time, your immune system reacts to more and more offenders, from car fumes to perfume.

TACKLE THE TROUBLEMAKERS

One simple but surefire way to calm your overreacting immune system and control your allergies is to limit your exposure to irritants. To squelch severe reactions, however, you may need to go a step further, using prescription antihistamines, corticosteroid nasal sprays, and/or cromolyn sodium, an anti-inflammatory nasal spray that keeps mast cells from bursting with histamines. For people with airborne allergies, the best defense may be "allergy shots"—injections that contain increasing doses of allergens to help keep antibodies from going ballistic around every dust bunny.

For many people, these interventions can be lifesavers, but they come with a price, often making you drowsy and jittery and suppressing your immune system so much that it can't rally against infection. You can minimize these side effects, assures Dr. Rothfeld, by working hard to control your triggers so you can reduce your dosages. Here are some ways to do exactly that.

ON-THE-SPOT RELIEF

Move Over, Gatorade!

All you sneezers and wheezers may soon be carrying a new beverage to the grassy playing fields—iced green tea. Green tea contains epigallocatechin gallate (EGCG), a compound that studies show blocks the allergic response in human cells. While researchers don't know how much you need to drink to stop the reaction, you might try downing a glassful even before heading outside.

FISH FOR RELIEF. Tuna, salmon, and other cold-water fish contain omega-3 essential fatty acids (EFAs), which inhibit inflammation, notes Richard N. Firshein, D.O., medical director of the Firshein Center for Comprehensive Medicine in New York City.

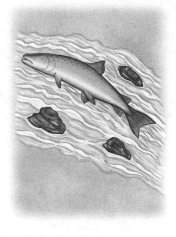

Fish also provide vitamin A, which boosts IgA, a "good guy" antibody that's released in saliva and attaches to allergens to keep them from invading your system. For allergy relief, the recommended dose of fish oil (available at any health food store) is 1 to 3 grams (1,000 to 3,000 milligrams) daily if you eat fish regularly. If you'd rather avoid fish, you can take 3 tablespoons of flaxseed oil daily. This oil, also sold at health food stores, is another excellent source of EFAs. Both oils can thin your blood, so avoid them if you take aspirin, other NSAIDs, or prescription blood thinners.

OIL UP. Borage and evening primrose oils come from plants and seeds and

---

DON'T GIVE BOOTS THE BOOT!

New baby on the way? If you have a cat and are worried about allergies, you may not need to give up your precious puss, as was once widely recommended. Studies reveal that early exposure to a cat, and therefore its dander, may protect children from developing a cat allergy.

"The dander may work like a vaccine, helping the immune system build up resistance so it's less likely to react to the allergen," says Thomas A. E. Platt-Mills, M.D., Ph.D., professor of medicine and microbiology at the University of Virginia Medical Center in Charlottesville.

What if *you're* allergic to Boots? Bathe him weekly; remove any wall-to-wall carpeting in your home, which can trap cat dander; use HEPA air cleaners; and seal mattresses in plastic covers. Odds are, you'll reduce your symptoms by 95 percent.

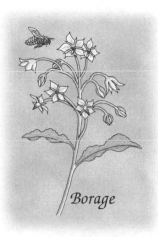
Borage

provide gamma-linolenic acid (GLA), which your body converts to beneficial EFAs. Both are available at health food stores, but borage oil packs four times more GLA than primrose oil, notes Dr. Firshein. He suggests taking 1 gram (1,000 milligrams) three times a day.

MAKE YOUR BODY BERRY HAPPY. Blueberries, blackberries, and cherries are bursting with substances called bioflavonoids that keep mast cells from releasing troublemaking histamines. They also boost cell levels of vitamin C, an anti-inflammatory/antihistamine powerhouse that targets the sinus passages. As long as you don't have stomach or kidney problems, Dr. Firshein recommends taking 1,000 milligrams of vitamin C three times a day at the height of pollen or mold season.

MIX THINGS UP. Eating some foods day after day may set you up for allergies and sensitivities because you're continually exposing your body to what it may see as a potential enemy. For instance, rice is a common allergen in Japan, while in the United States, the most common allergens are wheat, corn, fermented foods, sugar, and dairy foods—all foods we eat every day. In fact, studies show that rotating foods on a four-day schedule can help reduce

SAVE YOUR MONEY!

Hold the Mold Check

After hearing the hype about toxic black mold—ghastly-looking indoor mold with unproven links to serious health problems—you may be tempted to hire an air-sampling service to test your abode for mold spores. Don't bother, say experts from the Centers for Disease Control and Prevention in Atlanta: Mold concentrations in the air can vary dramatically within a house, and there are no standards for acceptable mold levels. Plus, airsampling services can charge upwards of $100 a sample.

food allergies. You might begin by alternating your usual wheat cereal with a bowl of oatmeal and stewed fruit, then return to wheat again.

DITCH THE OFFENDERS. Try eliminating foods (including milk, eggs, peanuts, wheat, and soy) that typically prompt inflammatory reactions in the body. You can get lists of foods to avoid as well as allergen-free recipes from organizations such as the American Academy of Allergy, Asthma, and Immunology (www.aaaai.org).

GO FOR CANOLA. Soybean, corn, cottonseed, safflower, and sunflower oils contain omega-6 fatty acids, which can encourage hay fever symptoms such as sneezing and congestion. Canola oil, on the other hand, contains omega-3's, which may decrease the IgE response so your body doesn't erupt with "ah-choos," says Michael D. Seidman, M.D., director of neurotologic surgery at Henry Ford Hospital in Detroit.

EAT AN APPLE A DAY. Apples—as well as tomatoes, onions, and the Indian spice turmeric—contain quercetin, a potent bioflavonoid-antihistamine combo that "works as well as cromolyn to make mast cells less reac-

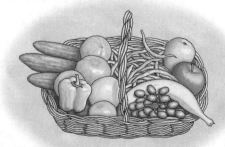

tive," says Connie Cantellani, M.D., an internist who specializes in integrative medicine in Skokie, Illinois.

If you have airborne allergies, the best way to get ample quercetin is from capsules, which you can find at health food stores. To get a jump on hay fever, take four 200- to 250-milligram capsules a day between meals, beginning in February. For food allergies, try taking quercetin a half-hour before eating, along with 250 to 500 milligrams of bromelain. This anti-inflammatory enzyme (also available in health food stores) found in pineapple increases the absorption and effectiveness of quercetin, says Skye Weintraub, N.D., a naturopathic physician in Eugene, Oregon. Don't take bromelain if you take aspirin or prescription blood thinners.

FIGHT BACK WITH A B. The most important B vitamin for folks with allergies is pantothenic acid. It works like an antihistamine and reduces levels of cortisol, the stress hormone that can spark or worsen allergy attacks. For relief from sneezing and congestion, Dr. Weintraub advises taking 100 milligrams of pantothenic acid three times a day after meals.

OPT FOR HARDWOOD FLOORS. Wall-to-wall carpeting can harbor dust mites, dander, and pollen and release toxic formaldehyde gas. Plus, carpeting laid over concrete provides a perfect residence for mold, warns Dr. Firshein. Whenever possible, choose hardwood or laminate flooring, use washable area rugs, and dust with electrostatic floor cloths such as Swiffer or Grab-It brands. Studies show the cloths can snatch up nearly 95 percent of cat and dog dander.

ANEMIA

Beef Up Wimpy Blood Cells

When I watch my 80-year-old mother wield a giant tree trimmer with ease or my teenage daughter jump a horse over a 3-foot fence, I can scarcely believe they once had a problem most people associate with being weak. I'm talking about anemia, a condition caused by runty red blood cells.

Red blood cells contain hemoglobin, the protein that ferries life-giving oxygen to cells throughout the body. If you don't have enough red blood cells, or if they become small or even wimpy, your organs don't get enough oxygen, and you're left feeling weak as a newborn kitten, overtired, short of breath, and prone to thumping heartbeats and ringing in your ears. Like my daughter, you may also become as

HAD YOUR PIPES CHECKED LATELY?

If you happen to have a colon polyp that's bleeding, your iron supply may be in jeopardy. "Everyone over age 40 who has iron-deficiency anemia should have a colonoscopy," says Connie Cantellani, M.D. If the test shows you have polyps, removing them can slash your risk of colon cancer and stop the iron drain.

pale as skim milk (her only symptom), since red blood cells keep skin, lips, and nail beds in the pink.

Even if you have all the classic signs, however, you should never try to diagnose or treat anemia on your own. "Anemia is always due to some other condition—anything from an iron deficiency to bleeding hemorrhoids to kidney failure," says Joe Lamb, M.D., an internist who specializes in mind-body medicine in Alexandria, Virginia. "You need a doctor's help to find out exactly why you're anemic."

WHY ME?

Most women who have anemia—my mom and daughter included—have iron-deficiency anemia. As the name suggests, it's caused by a lack of iron, which your blood cells need to make oxygen-carrying hemoglobin. Normally, the body holds on to iron in the liver, but iron levels can gradually fall if you have slow bleeding from ulcers, colon polyps, or digestive cancer, or if you regularly use nonsteroidal anti-inflammatory drugs (NSAIDs) such as ibuprofen.

You don't have to be sick to become anemic. Women especially don't need a serious illness to develop iron-deficiency anemia, since many of us don't get enough iron in our diets (women who menstruate need about 15 milligrams a day; pregnant women require up to twice as much)—and we lose iron all the time when we menstruate. In fact, women who bleed very heavi-

HOMEGROWN SOLUTION

◆ ◆ ◆

Dandy Dandelions

Lawn lovers may despise pesky dandelions, but they're super sources of iron and are gentle to the liver, points out Ryan Drum, Ph.D. Plus, they taste great—a little like arugula, a nutty, spiky-leaved salad green. It's the leaves at the crown of the dandelion plant that you want. Just be sure to pick them from an area that you're sure is free of pesticides and lawn chemicals—then rinse them thoroughly and toss 'em into salads.

SUSHI CAN PUMP YOU UP

Forget the avocado and other enticing ingredients inside that little roll. Nori, the black, paper-thin seaweed that holds the roll together, contains more iron than any land plant, says Ryan Drum, Ph.D. If sushi isn't your style, simply pick up some dried nori in a health food store and crumble it into your favorite salad.

ly during their periods are at greater risk of developing iron-deficiency anemia than women who simply spot or have very light flow.

In addition, pregnancy can make us more susceptible. When you're pregnant, the number of red blood cells in your body rises, but the volume of fluid containing those cells goes up even more. Thus, the level of red blood cells relative to the amount of blood coursing through your veins decreases. What's more, your developing baby can siphon off some of your iron supply.

While iron-deficiency anemia is by far the most common type in women, there are others, including:

• Anemia associated with chronic diseases such as liver problems, rheumatoid arthritis, inflammatory bowel disease, and lupus.

• Folate-deficiency anemia, which tends to affect moms-to-be and women who are breastfeeding. The B vitamin folate (the natural form of folic acid) is a red cell builder that comes from whole grain products; dark, leafy greens; citrus fruits; and beans. Unlike iron, it isn't stored in your body, so you need to replenish your supply daily. Check with your doctor for the correct amount.

• Pernicious anemia, which can plague women over age 50 (when nutrient absorption begins to be a problem) and strict vegetarians, who often come up short on vitamin B_{12}. Besides making red blood cells, this B vitamin, which is found in meat, dairy foods, and eggs, preserves nerve function and keeps memory sharp.

IRON IT OUT

The trick in treating anemia is to pinpoint the reason behind it with a simple blood test, called a serum ferritin test. If you have iron-deficiency anemia, which is most likely, your doctor may prescribe iron supplements—but only with great care. "Iron, great as it is, can speed hardening of the arteries, and too much of it can prompt heart attacks," warns Connie Cantellani, M.D., an internist who specializes in integrative medicine in Skokie, Illinois. "In general, no one should get more than 20 milligrams of iron a day in supplemental form"—and no one should take iron supplements unless they've been diagnosed with an iron deficiency. Even that much can cause bothersome side effects, such as constipation.

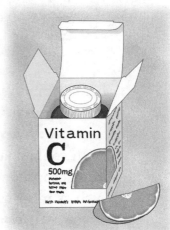

If your doctor recommends that you take supplemental iron, ask if you can take it in syrup form, which tends to be less binding. Take it on a full stomach with 250 milligrams of vitamin C to boost absorption. Plus, take the following steps to safely pump up your iron—and your energy level—on your own.

SIMMER SAUCE IN A BLACK POT. Acidic foods, such as tomato-based sauces, leach iron out of cast-iron pots, and every little bit counts when you tally your iron gains for the day. So whether you're making spaghetti, bowties, rotini, or shells, cook the sauce in an iron pot.

IMPROVE ON POPEYE. We hate to break it to you, but spinach isn't the absolute best source of iron out there. Whenever you can, try to chow down on foods that are really rich in iron, such as meat, poultry, salmon, broccoli, asparagus, brussels sprouts, and dried beans like black-eyed peas and lentils.

TURN OVER A NEW LEAF. As many as one-fifth of all vegetarian women are anemic. If you don't eat meat, try your best not to be one of them by loading up on salads made with iron-rich kale, beet greens, collard greens, chard, and parsley.

EAT YOUR VEGGIES RAW. Heat destroys the protein atom around ferritin, or iron, points out Ryan Drum, Ph.D., a medical herbalist in Washington state. Eat produce in its natural, fresh form whenever you can.

GO FOR YOGURT AND SAUERKRAUT. Both contain lactic acid, which promotes iron absorption. Fermented soy foods, such as miso, can help, too.

REACH FOR WRINKLED FRUIT. Figs, dates, prunes, raisins, and especially dried peaches and apricots are rich in iron.

SWEETEN UP WITH MOLASSES. A teaspoon of blackstrap molasses twice daily provides iron as well as essential B vitamins.

DOWN YELLOW DOCK. This herb, available in capsules or tincture form at health food stores, helps your body absorb iron from your diet and is especially recommended for moms-to-be, says Dr. Drum. If you're pregnant, be sure to check with your obstetrician before taking it.

LIMIT IRON ROBBERS. Tannins in black tea inhibit iron absorption. Other thieves include antacids, the food additive EDTA (look for it on food labels), and phosphates in soft drinks and ice cream.

ANGINA

Shove That Boulder Off Your Chest

———◆◇◆———

Maybe you've just had a shouting match with your spouse, a four-course meal at your mom's, or an arduous Saturday morning spent hauling bags of gravel to build a serpentine garden path. Suddenly, you feel as if someone has rolled a giant boulder onto your chest. It weighs heavily on your lungs, making it difficult to breathe. You stop what you're doing and take stock, but after a few minutes, the boulder disappears. The pressure eases. You're fine.

But are you really?

WHY ME?

Sudden, heavy chest pressure is a hallmark of angina—chest pain that occurs when your heart can't get enough oxygen because the arteries that deliver blood to it have narrowed. This occurs either

---

HOMEGROWN SOLUTION

◆ ◆ ◆

"Beet" Fatigue!

If you can muster the energy to plant just one packet of seeds, make them beet seeds. Betacyanin, the compound that gives beets their rich color, may help cells take in more oxygen, so eating fresh beets or freshly grated beetroot in salads could give your heart a breath of fresh air!

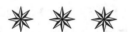
because fatty deposits have accumulated on the insides of the artery walls (coronary artery disease) or, much more rarely, because the arteries are simply in spasm. But angina takes many forms: Sometimes it can be a shooting pain up your arm and at other times, a sharp, squeezing sensation near your shoulders. In women especially, it can even be super-subtle—say, a tiny twinge that radiates toward your neck—and therefore super-scary.

"Angina is the heart's distress call, but it's not an early warning system," says Peter Brunschwig, M.D., director of Helios Integrated Medicine in Boulder, Colorado. "By the time a person gets angina, his arteries have probably already become narrow and weak from a slow buildup of cholesterol-laden plaque." Anyone with angina, no matter how infrequent or fleeting, should consult a doctor immediately to rule out serious heart disease.

NITRO ISN'T ENOUGH

If you've been diagnosed with angina due to coronary heart disease, odds are that you also have nitroglycerin, the drug equivalent of an American Express card—you simply don't leave home without it. Taking nitroglycerin during an angina attack quickly relaxes the arteries, opening them so oxygen-rich blood can flow easily to your heart—and that breath-sucking boulder can slip easily away. Beta-blockers and calcium channel blockers do essentially the same thing.

If your angina persists, and your physician finds that the arteries to your heart are very nearly closed due to a pileup of plaque there, she may recommend angioplasty—a surgical procedure that involves inflating a balloon to force open blocked vessels—or bypass surgery to shunt blood flow around the narrowed arteries.

These treatments work in the sense that they increase blood flow to the heart, possibly preventing a heart attack. And while that's hugely significant, it's not a cure. "The very best way to control your angina," explains Dr. Brunschwig, "is to adopt a comprehensive program aimed at lowering plaque." Here are several ways to do that.

DO AS DEAN DOES. It's been more than 10 years since studies by renowned heart guru Dean Ornish, M.D., showed that people who eat a low-fat diet loaded with fruits and veggies, exercise regularly, maintain a healthy weight, and manage stress are less likely to be ambushed by angina than sedentary, overweight, stressed-out types. In fact, Dr. Ornish's regimen proved even better for reducing angina than taking cholesterol-lowering drugs. "And the evidence still holds," says Gerdi Weidner, Ph.D., director of research at Dr. Ornish's Preventive

CAN MARRIAGE COUNSELING SAVE YOUR HEART?

It just might. If you're a husband who feels your wife doesn't show her love, studies show you're twice as likely as husbands with more demonstrative wives to have angina. Likewise, if you're the withholding wife, anger, depression, or even garden-variety stress may have left you feeling stingy with your emotions—and predisposed to your own chest pain. Let a counselor help you sort out the affairs of the heart, and you may ease pain in your life in more ways than one.

Medicine Research Institute in Sausalito, California. "Our studies show that people who follow our program cut their angina episodes in half."

LOAD UP ON LEAFY GREENS. Spinach, kale, mustard greens, and turnip greens are all loaded with magnesium, a mineral that relaxes the body's smooth muscles, including those that encircle blood vessels.

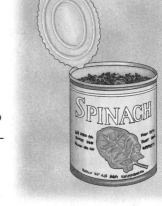

"Magnesium is critical for keeping blood vessels toned so they're less likely to seize up with exertion," says Robert Bonakdar, M.D., director of pain management and heart health at the Scripps Center for Integrative Medicine in La Jolla, California. Since magnesium can cause loose stools in some people, Dr. Bonakdar suggests starting with 200 milligrams daily, taken between meals, then slowly building up to 400 milligrams twice a day if your bowels can tolerate it. Just be sure to talk to your doctor beforehand.

ADD AMINOS. The mighty amino acid arginine, much like nitroglycerin, helps relax artery walls and keep the vessels open. In fact, supplemental arginine has been shown to prolong the time people can exercise before chest

WHEN TO DIAL THE DOC

• • • • • • • • • • • •

Angina and a heart attack differ in two very significant ways: While both signal that the heart isn't receiving enough oxygen, the oxygen deprivation and pain associated with angina are temporary and don't damage the heart. The pain of a heart attack, on the other hand, doesn't go away, and the oxygen deprivation can be permanent—or lethal. Be alert to changes in your angina pattern that may signal a heart attack. Call 911 if you have chest pressure, squeezing, fullness, or pain in the center of your chest, or pain in your neck, jaw, shoulders, or arms, that lasts longer than 5 minutes, even if you take nitroglycerin.

pain kicks in, which is significant because exercise reduces cholesterol, blood pressure, stress, and weight—all risk factors for heart disease.

Arginine's cousin, carnitine, is an amino acid abundant in red meat that may help strengthen the heart muscle. Dr. Bonakdar recommends that people with angina take 500 milligrams of carnitine a day, but since there's no exact dose for arginine, he suggests asking a doctor about a combination formula that's tailored to specific conditions.

FISH FOR HEART ATTACK PREVENTION. According to the American Heart Association, people with heart disease should take at least 1 gram of fish oil a day, for two reasons. First, the oil that comes from tuna, salmon, and other cold-water fish is packed

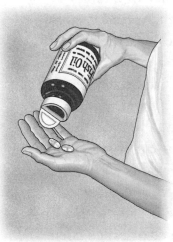

with omega-3 essential fatty acids (EFAs), which can make red blood cells more slippery and improve their flow, even in tiny capillaries. Second, fish oil helps lower trigclyerides—other blood fats that can clog arteries—and stabilize insulin resistance, a major factor in heart disease. Not much of a fish lover? Take 1 to 3 grams (1,000 to 3,000 milligrams) of fish oil in capsule form (available at health food stores) a day—but talk to your doctor first, especially if you're taking aspirin or prescription

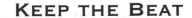

KEEP THE BEAT

Beat a drum. Blow a horn. Even pound the ivories. "Music therapy is one of the best outlets there is for stress and aggression," notes Robert Bonakdar, M.D. The physical work of making music releases pent-up energy and emotions. Plus, it improves heart rate, blood pressure, and the ability to sleep soundly—all of which lessen the demands on your heart. Your neighbors may not love your new drum set, but your heart certainly will.

blood-thinning medication.

GET AN OIL CHANGE. "Flaxseed, borage, and walnut oils all contain an omega-3 that gets converted to EFAs in the body," says Dr. Bonakdar, "so they're the next best thing to fish oil." Pour the oils over some magnesium-packed leafy greens. Just be sure to use a liberal amount; you need 1 tablespoon a day to get any benefit.

SPREAD IT ON. Some margarine-like spreads, such as Benecol, contain plant stanols that block the absorption of cholesterol in the intestines, forcing your liver to snatch it from your

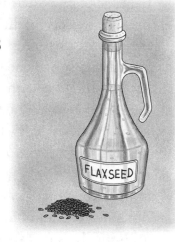

bloodstream—and keep it away from your heart. In fact, studies show that people who add plant stanols to a low-fat diet can reduce plaque-building cholesterol by 10 to 24 percent. To get the benefits, you'll need three servings a day of 2 tablespoons each. Spread it on toast at breakfast, crackers at lunch, and a dinner roll at supper. But don't go overboard—these spreads still contain fat.

MUNCH ON NUTS. Soy nuts and peanuts—as well as fish, spinach, and organ meats—are packed with a little miracle elixir called coen-

HEARTBAR, ANYONE?

Energy bars aren't just for scarfing on the trail anymore—instead, they may help you get on the trail in the first place. A Stanford University cardiologist has developed a first-of-its-kind energy bar called HeartBar, which contains such heart-healthful (and angina-reducing) ingredients as arginine, antioxidants, oat fiber, and fruit pectins. And studies with heart patients have shown that the bar increases the ability to exercise without angina. While HeartBar isn't yet available in stores, you can get it from the Internet at www.HeartBar.net.

zyme Q_{10} (CoQ_{10}). "This antioxidant appears to bring oxygen to the heart and may even help curb the damage caused by a lack of oxygen," says Dr. Brunschwig, who recommends taking 100 milligrams a day. You can find CoQ_{10} supplements at health food stores and drugstores.

SPRINKLE YOUR WHEATIES WITH WHEAT GERM. The idea is to pad your diet with vitamin E, which is also found in nuts, seeds, olives, spinach, and other green, leafy veggies. Vitamin E is an antioxidant, meaning it prevents what's called oxidative damage in cells—including those in the arteries. As a result, low blood levels of vitamin E are associated with higher rates of angina.

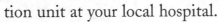

MANAGE YOUR ANGER. "People who have angina tend to be hostile," notes Dr. Bonakdar. Anger releases adrenalin, the "fight or flight" hormone that signals a bump up in blood pressure, heart rate, and blood flow away from the heart and to the muscles (so we can fight or flee). All of these physiologic responses can precipitate angina. To help you manage your anger and sidestep angina, you might seek the help of a support group. To locate one in your area, contact the cardiac rehabilitation unit at your local hospital.

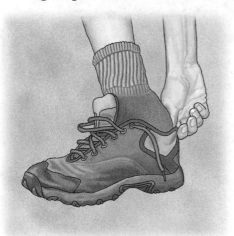

PICK UP THE PACE. "With your doctor's guidance, you should not be afraid to exercise, as long as it's not an activity where you suddenly break into a sprint," says Dr. Brunschwig. The best way to start is with slow walking. "It reduces cholesterol, blood pressure, stress, and weight," he notes. In fact, if you're overweight, daily walks combined with a low-fat diet could help you lose a pound a week, which studies show can help reduce chest pain.

JUST SAY NO. "The behavior that seems to make the most difference in reducing heart disease is managing stress," notes Dr. Bonakdar. "The outside pressure to, say, head another church committee is absolutely matched by the pressure inside your arteries." The best way to minimize that internal pressure? "Say no to mounting demands," he says. As a bonus, once you're not quite so overcommitted, you'll have the time for yoga, deep breathing, or other calming techniques proven to help keep a lid on angina.

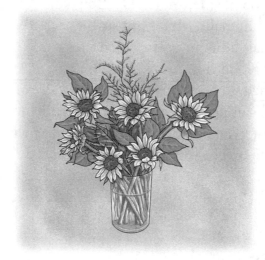

ANXIETY

Find Some Peace of Mind

It's one thing to worry when you're driving in a snowstorm or facing a mammogram. It's quite another to feel distressed or edgy from day to day with no single, discernable trigger.

My friend Jill's worries spiral out of control when she feels what she describes as a "sense of compressed time" in her busy life. "My anxiety builds to a crescendo," she explains, "until I lie awake, literally counting my worries: 'What if I miss my deadline?' 'What if my son hates his new teacher?' You name it, I obsess about it."

On the other hand, my pal Melissa's anxiety takes a different form—out-of-the-blue, out-of-her-mind panic. "I had a panic attack on a bus one time that scared me so much I pulled my

---

TURN OFF THE TALK

Whether you regularly listen to NPR's Dr. Dan Gottleib or to Dr. Laura, you may want to turn off the docs every once in a while and either slip in a Brahms CD or turn the dial to a classical station. According to one study, 30 minutes of classical music can be as calming as 10 milligrams of Valium.

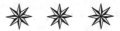

---

sweater collar over my head," she says.

Whether you're nagged by niggling worries or chased by heart-pounding panic, you've got plenty of company. "Anxiety is a soaring trend," notes Paul Foxman, Ph.D., director of the Center for Anxiety Disorders in Burlington, Vermont. "And given our jam-packed lifestyles, uncertain economy, and shaky world politics, some worrying is understandable and quite healthy. But when your anxiety is unexplained or overwhelming, you can literally become worried sick."

WHY ME?

In a true high-threat situation, anxiety can be a lifesaver. If, say, you're skidding on a rain-slicked road, you naturally become distressed. Your anxiety signals your brain to direct your adrenal glands to release a flood of "fight or flight" hormones, some of which prime your muscles for quick action while another (cortisol) sends sugar, or glucose, through your system to amp up your energy. As a result, you're alert and responsive. You remember to take your foot off the accelerator. You fight the urge to yank the steering wheel. In short, you survive the skid—thanks in no small part to your body's hyper-alert state. The danger passes, and you chill out.

When you have chronic anxiety, however, you never chill

out—your muscles and mind remain on high alert and ready to fight or flee, even when you're safe and sound. Your level of "feel good" hormones remains low, which makes you feel jittery, achy, and constantly vigilant. Your immune system becomes depleted, and you're more likely to get sick, says Dr. Foxman.

In fact, anxiety can give rise to everything from headaches to high blood pressure. But that's not all: Untreated anxiety can spiral into full-blown panic attacks that frighten you so much you may start to avoid the places and situations in which they initially occurred.

WORRY NOT

If chronic anxiety is seriously limiting the way you live your life, seek help from a mental health professional. You may need a prescription medication such as alprazolam (Xanax) to block the fight-or-flight response and calm your mind and body, cognitive therapy to give you a different way to think about things that happen, and talk therapy to address the question of why you're panicking in the first place.

Whether you have major panic or minor worries, however, you can take steps on your own to overcome chronic fretting and dis-

ON-THE-SPOT RELIEF

Naturally Sweet!

When panic rises in the midst of a crowd, concentrate on something else: Wiggle your toes in your shoes. Read a nearby sign. Fumble for your keys. Ask someone for directions. Focusing on concrete, familiar objects and activities keeps your anxiety from commandeering your thoughts—and building to all-out panic. Heidi Weinhold, N.D., also suggests whispering "soft belly." Saying the words will shift your focus and remind you to take a deep breath, which will instantly diffuse the fight-or-flight hormones, she says.

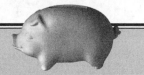

SAVE YOUR MONEY!

Junk the Junk

In the habit of quaffing passionflower soda to calm your racing heart? Well, you can save your money—and the calories! This product doesn't contain enough of the active ingredients to help.

charge those arousal hormones. Here's what to do.

IXNAY THE WHAT IF'S. Let's say you worry, "What if the bus crashes?" To nip your anxiety in the bud, simply counteract your concern with hard facts. Ask yourself, "What's the probability of being in a bus crash?" Then answer, "Unless I'm an extra in the next *Speed* sequel, it has to be pretty low." In other words, talk yourself free of your spiraling emotions. "Talking back to negative chatter is just as effective as taking anti-anxiety drugs," says Dr. Foxman.

BREATHE FROM YOUR BELLY. When you're worrying about your deadline or how the dinner party will go, you're taking quick, shallow breaths high up in your chest, which signals the brain to release anxiety-producing chemicals. "Breathing slowly and fully from your lower abdomen is the best way to calm your body and mind," says Joan Borysenko, Ph.D., director of Mind/Body Health Sciences in Boulder, Colorado. Keep your shoulders still and expand your lungs fully so your belly bulges out. Then exhale slowly. Your heart rate will slow, and your anxiety will fade.

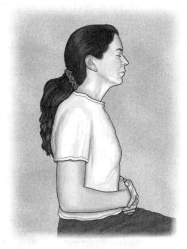

MIND THE MOMENT. Mindfulness—the practice of being fully absorbed in what you're doing, while you're doing it—anchors you in the present, slowing your breathing and quieting your mind, says Dr. Borysenko. For instance, try eating an orange mindfully: Peel it slowly and deliberately. Notice its nubby feel, garish color, and tangy scent. Savor the sweet-sour juice in your mouth. Linger there, in the moment. If any thoughts—say, of your coming day—intrude, gently turn your attention back to the orange. When you practice mindfulness in everything you do, you're less likely to be led astray by worries.

DON'T MIND THE MESS. Perfectionism pulls you out of the present and out of reality, explains Dr. Borysenko. On hectic days, for instance, a perfectionist might whip herself into a frenzy, rushing to the grocery store, rushing home, and rushing some more to prepare a nutritious sit-down dinner, despite the fact that simply sharing a plate of cheese and fruit could be a calmer, equally healthful—albeit less "perfect"—alternative. Recognize your limits and bend to them. Otherwise, you give them the power to break you.

LOSE THE LATTES. Drinking more than five caffeinated beverages a day boosts lactate, a substance that can induce anxiety in people who are panic-prone. Caffeine also influences noradrenaline, a chemical messenger that induces arousal. Sinus medicine, cold medication, and asthma drugs also contain adrenaline-like ingredients that may induce panic attacks in some people.

FISH FOR SERENITY. Salmon, tuna, and sardines are filled to the gills with omega-3 essential fatty acids (EFAs), which can powerfully improve your mood, says Hyla Cass, M.D., assistant clinical professor of psychiatry at the University of California, Los Angeles, School of Medicine. For the EFAs to have any effect, however, you'll need to eat fish three times a week. If this exceeds your taste for tuna, you can take 1 gram (1,000 milligrams) of fish oil in capsule form (available at health

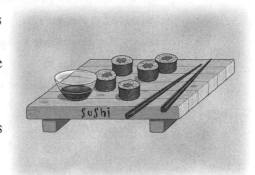

food stores) a day. Or you can get your EFAs from flaxseed. Take 1,000 milligrams a day, or check your health food store for flaxseed oil to use in place of salad dressing, for instance. Both oils can thin your blood, so avoid them if you take aspirin, other NSAIDs, or prescription blood thinners.

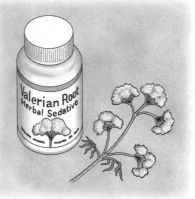

GET TO THE ROOT OF IT. "Valerian root is a great wind-down herb that relieves tension without dulling the mind," says Heidi Weinhold, N.D., a naturopathic physician in Pittsburgh. "If you aren't already taking anti-anxiety medication or prescription sleeping pills (if you are, you shouldn't take anything else), I suggest taking two 200- to 300-milligram tablets before bedtime."

SAVOR OATSTRAW. Sipped as a tea, the herb oatstraw (which you can find at a health food store) is both calming and energizing and is "awesome" if you're trying to cut back on caffeine, says Dr. Weinhold. Another plus: Oatstraw is packed with B vitamins, which soothe jangled nerves. Buy the herb in tea bags or add 20 to 60 drops of tincture to a glass of water and take it up to four times a day.

SOOTHE PALPITATIONS WITH PASSIONFLOWER. This herb is tailor-made for hyped-up people with thumping hearts, says Dr. Weinhold. Add 20 to 40 drops of passionflower extract (available at health food stores) to a glass of water and drink four or five glasses a day. Don't use it if you're pregnant, though.

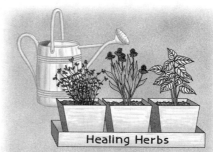

Healing Herbs

GO GA-GA OVER GABA. "Gamma-amino butyric acid (GABA) is the calming chemical in your brain that regulates all of your feel-good hormones," explains Dr. Cass, who says that supplementing with GABA (available at health food stores) reduces overall tension. She suggests taking 250 milligrams twice daily after meals. As always, however, you should consult with your doctor before trying it, and you should avoid GABA altogether if you take other anti-anxiety or antidepressant medications.

GET YOUR EAR NEEDLED. In Chinese medicine, it's believed that illnesses—including emotional disturbances—arise from blockages of energy, which flows along set pathways in the body. To promote healing, the Chinese use acupuncture, inserting hair-thin needles at points along the pathways to release the blocked energy. In fact, some Western studies indicate that needles inserted at points along your outer ear or lower arm or between your eyebrows may produce a sedating effect more powerful than that of anti-anxiety drugs. Interested in giving it a try? Ask your doctor to recommend a reputable acupuncturist near you.

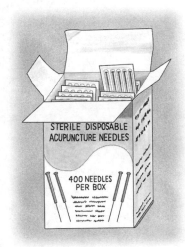

CONFRONT YOUR FEARS. Each time you leave an event in a panic or avoid a situation altogether because you're anxious about it, it becomes that much easier to let your fears run your life, says Jerilyn Ross, director of the Ross Center for Anxiety and Related Disorders in Washington, D.C. But the opposite is also true: Each time you confront your fears, it becomes easier to marginalize them—to strip them of their power. The next time you're anxious, assure yourself, "I may be frightened, but I'm not in any danger. I'm not having a heart attack; my heart is simply beating fast."

USE "OUTS," NOT CRUTCHES. An "out" is an escape clause that helps you remain in a fearful situation, explains Dr. Ross. Let's say you normally get panicky while driving. Don't ask someone else to drive—that's a crutch. Instead, take the wheel, but plan to pull over to the side of the road and take several deep, calming breaths if you become anxious.

PRAY. Close your eyes, take a deep breath, and admit that it's all just too much. Then ask that all the anxiety and fear be lifted from your shoulders. It will be.

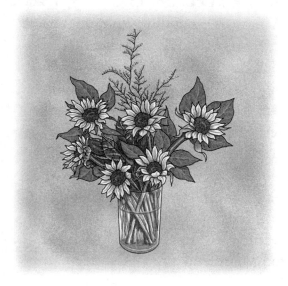

ARTHRITIS

Smooth Moves to Kill the Pain

———————◆◦◦◦◆———————

I have an intricate lace tablecloth that never ceases to amaze me—not simply because it's so lovely but also because my grandmother somehow managed to stitch it when her fingers were stiff and sore from osteoarthritis (OA). So far, my own fingers are pliable and able to pound like pistons on my keyboard, but my neck often gets so stiff that I wish I could drip some WD-40 into its joints.

There are a lot of us working stiffs out there. In fact, OA is the most common form of arthritis (there are more than 100 different types) and affects a third of all adults, most of them women.

WHY ME?

By age 40 or 50, many of us begin to notice some tightness in the hinges of our fingers, necks, hips, or knees because the spongy

---

TIMING IS EVERYTHING

The best time to take a pain reliever for osteoarthritis is before noon. The pain and inflammation tend to be worse in the late afternoon and evening, so start your treatment in the morning or at midday.

✳ ✳ ✳

cartilage that covers and protects the bones of our joints becomes thinner due to age and daily wear and tear. At the same time, our cartilage-rebuilding cells start to slack off.

Without their protective cushioning, bones may start to grind against each other, which can damage the tissue surrounding the joint. The immune system attempts to come to the rescue, but instead, the white blood cells overreact and release inflammatory proteins. The proteins cause swelling, pain, and further damage to the tissue. Joints become stiff and sore, although not all of them at once, and maybe never more than a few. But the diagnosis is still the same: osteoarthritis.

MEASURE THOSE HIGH HEELS

Skinny stilettos are murder on your knees—but they're not the only culprits. In fact, high, wide-heeled pumps may predispose you to osteoarthritis (OA) of the knee, too. The problem, it seems, isn't the stability of the platform but the height of the heel. Any woman who regularly wears heels higher than 2 inches is twice as likely to develop OA as women who don't, says Michael Weinblatt, M.D. Heels shift your body weight away from your ankles and onto your hips and the inner part of the knee joints, and arthritis of the knee is often the result.

HOW TO GLIDE THROUGH LIFE

If your joints are so swollen and painfully stiff you can barely climb out of your car, and you're popping aspirin or ibuprofen tablets as if they were breath mints, it's time for a doctor visit. Standard treatments for OA include rofecoxib (Vioxx) and celecoxib (Celebrex), both COX-2 (short for cyclooxygenase-2) inhibitor drugs that work by blocking the pain-prompting enzyme; antibiotics to slow the erosion of cartilage; and injections to reduce the swelling. These treatments can be expensive, but they all work well—actually, sometimes too well. A corticosteroid shot, for instance, can mask discomfort so effectively that you keep doing the very activities that injured your joints in the first place.

That's the problem with OA medication: It tackles the pain, but not the reasons behind it. As Todd Nelson, N.D., a naturopathic physician in Denver, puts it, your joints will respond if you "shift away from the things that promote inflammation and tear down cartilage and move toward things that shore up cartilage." Try these drug-free ways to do that—with your physician's permission, of course.

GRAB SOME GLUCOSAMINE. One of the most effective treatments for OA is glucosamine sulfate, a naturally occurring amino sugar that, in supplement form, is produced from shellfish. Not only does it provide pain relief equal to or better than that of nonsteroidal anti-inflammatory drugs (NSAIDs) such as aspirin without the pesky side effects, it also combats cartilage-destroying enzymes and halts cartilage loss in the knee and hip. What's more, it's sold over the counter, so you can find it in any drugstore. Sounds way too good to be true, right? It's not—but it's also not very fast.

"You start with 500 milligrams three times a day, and it takes two to four weeks to get relief from pain—and twice that long to ease functioning in your joint," says Dr. Nelson. Since glucosamine is made from shellfish, you should avoid it if you have a seafood allergy.

PAIR IT WITH CHONDROITIN. Glucosamine works best when combined with chondroitin, a cartilage component that acts like a sponge to soak up vital fluids so your joints glide without a hitch. Check your drugstore for a glucosamine-chondroitin combo and take a capsule that provides roughly 500 to 1,000 milligrams of glucosamine sulfate and 400 milligrams of chondroitin with each meal. If you don't get relief within four weeks, try another brand, because quality may vary.

LUBE UP. Trout, salmon, and other cold-water fish contain an abundance of omega-3 essential fatty acids (EFAs), which ease swollen, stiff joints by reducing both inflammation and cartilage destruction, says Michael E. Weinblatt, M.D., codirector of clinical rheumatology at Harvard's Brigham and Women's Hospital in Boston. Not a fish fan? Just pop three 1-gram (1,000-milligram) fish-oil capsules twice a day with meals. If you'd rather avoid fish altogether, try flaxseed oil, which also contains EFAs. You can mix 1 to 3 tablespoons with maple syrup to drizzle over waffles, or use it in place of butter on your steamed veggies. Both oils can thin your blood, so avoid them if you take

CUT PAIN IN HALF!

The next time your bathroom scale sneaks up a hair, don't fret about your fanny—it's your knees that deserve your pity! Every time you gain a single pound of body fat, experts say it'll feel like four times as much on your knees. The strain is especially hard on your muscles and tendons—your built-in shock absorbers. The good news is that studies show that if you lose 11 pounds, you can reduce stiffness and pain in your knees by half.

aspirin, other NSAIDs, or prescription blood thinners.

FLATTEN PAIN WITH FRUIT. Raisins, pears, apples, and other fruits, as well as nuts and beans, all contain the trace element boron, which can relieve pain and joint stiffness and actually appears to protect against arthritis, says Dr. Weinblatt. If you don't eat fruit on a regular basis or don't live in a particularly arid area, where concentrations of boron in the soil and water are highest, consider taking a daily multivitamin supplement that provides 1 to 3 milligrams of boron.

TRY WILLOW. White willow bark contains salicin, which the body converts to salicylic acid to relieve pain. Comb your health food store for capsules and take two 200- to 400-milligram capsules three times a day between meals, says Dr. Nelson. Just one caveat: This is the same substance found in aspirin, so check with your doctor first if you're already taking aspirin or other blood thinners.

BRING ON THE HEAT. The hot ingredient in red pepper is capsaicin, which helps stop the production of substance P, an inflammatory prostaglandin that's present in arthritic joints. Check your supermarket or drugstore for capsaicin cream and apply it directly to inflamed joints three or four times a day for a week. Be careful not to get it in your eyes or on any areas of broken skin, and wash your hands after using it.

LAY OFF THE LATTES. If you drink more than four cups of coffee a day, you're doubling your risk of developing arthritis, warns Dr. Nelson. Caffeine not only alters the mineral balance that's needed to make cartilage, it can also dry up the fluid required to keep cartilage and joints lubricated. So instead of a mocha cappuccino, reach for a mug of water—or many, as the case may be. You need to drink 1/2 ounce of water per pound of body weight per day (and double that when you're exercising). If you weigh 150 pounds, that's nearly 10 cups of water a day!

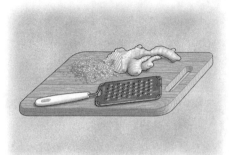

SIP GINGER TEA. Like some arthritis drugs, ginger is a natural COX-2 inhibitor, says Dr. Nelson. Stir 1 teaspoon of grated ginger into a cup of boiling water, steep for 10 to 15 minutes, and strain. Sweeten with honey and down two cups a day. Your knees may soon begin to feel as nimble as that other famous Ginger's.

WARM UP

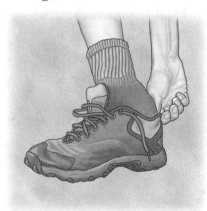

WITH A WALK. When you sit still, the synovial fluid between your joints can become as stiff as molasses in a Maine winter. Although you may not feel like walking when your joints are stiff, it's actually the ideal way to keep the synovial fluid warm and flowing—and your weight in check so you don't overload your joints.

DUST OFF YOUR OLD SCHWINN. "Strengthening the thigh muscles that support the knee is one of the best ways to control the progression of OA there," says Dr. Weinblatt. And one of the best non-weight-bearing ways to build your thigh muscles is to bicycle regularly. Bike buried too deeply in the basement to retrieve? Try squats: Simply stand with your legs apart and your knees slightly bent. Slowly lower your butt as if you're about to sit on a chair. Pause when your thighs are parallel (or nearly parallel) to the floor, then slowly straighten up. Repeat three to five times a day.

GET KNEE-DLED. Research directed by the National Institutes of Health indicates that people with OA of the knee who receive acupuncture have less pain and better function than people receiving standard care—even weeks after the treatment. Ask your doctor to recommend a reputable acupuncturist near you.

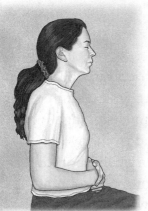

USE YOUR HEAD. The next time hip pain flares, sit comfortably, close your eyes, and slow your breathing. Imagine you're running a marathon or doing the rumba with pain-free, swaying hips. Note the expression on your face and the flower in your hair. Take the time to fully conjure the vision and savor the sensations it creates in your mind. Do it again the next day, and the next. "Repeatedly visualizing such scenarios can help reduce discomfort and may even improve mobility," explains Dr. Weinblatt.

ASTHMA

Relief Is Just a Breath Away

During a recent overnight visit with a friend in San Francisco, my sleep was disturbed by a noise I recognized immediately as the dry hack of asthma. For 15 years, my listening radar has been tuned to pick up the telltale sound from my daughter, who inherited this chronic inflammatory condition of the airways from me. And now this coughing was coming from my friend's room.

Sure enough, the next morning, she revealed to me that she sometimes uses an inhaler to open her airways and relieve some of the tightness in her chest, which worsens when she exerts herself. "It can feel as though I have an elastic bandage wound around my chest when I walk up hills," she told me.

SLEEP UP TOP

Heading to a dude ranch or rustic retreat anytime soon? Be sure to get dibs on the upper bunk. It's well worth the climb, say researchers in Spain. When you sleep in the bottom bunk, you're showered with dust bunnies and dust mites that fall from the bedding above when the sleeper tosses and turns—which makes your asthma more likely to flare up.

WHY ME?

The symptoms can be terrifying and confounding, especially if you're diagnosed with asthma (which many people think of as a childhood disease) in adulthood. Yet more and more adults—and more women than men—are developing it. Researchers aren't sure of the exact reason. They suspect that along with the usual triggers (such as pollen, dust, and frigid air) that can inflame airways and cause them to fill with mucus, both increased body weight (which can literally weigh on the chest wall, making it more difficult to breathe) and the surges and drops in hormones that are associated with menstruation and menopause may play a role.

BREATHE EASIER

A doctor who specializes in allergies and asthma can help you ferret out your triggers and treat your symptoms with a customized medication plan. For instance, if your asthma is mild or sparked by exercise, you may need a cromolyn sodium medication to help reduce airway tightness. If you have moderate to severe asthma, your doctor may recommend an oral leukotriene blocker and/or inhaled corticosteroid drugs to help control the disease by attacking its cause—inflammation that constricts the airways.

THE PERFECT ASTHMA EXERCISE

Preliminary research from the University of Colorado indicates that people with asthma who practice yoga poses that involve slow breathing and meditation may be less likely to need inhalers. In fact, I've found the "fish pose" eases my own breathing. To try it, lie flat on your back on an exercise mat and tuck your fists under your butt. Lift your chest as high as you can and tilt your head backward so your jaw is pointing toward the ceiling. Breathe deeply and see if you can feel, as I do, the coiled muscles across your chest loosening and your lungs opening up.

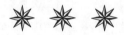

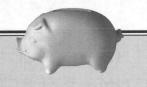

As powerful as these medications are, however, they often need your help in staying on top of asthma. "Your aim as an asthmatic," explains Richard N. Firshein, D.O., medical director of the Firshein Center for Comprehensive Medicine in New York City, "is, on your own, to curb your inflammation, open your airways, and repair any damaged tissue there." Sounds like a big job, doesn't it? But in addition to taking your medication on schedule, there are drug-free ways to tackle it.

MAXIMIZE MAGNESIUM. Think of magnesium, a mineral found in dark leafy greens, whole grains, nuts, and fish, as "a sedative for your bronchial tubes," suggests Anna Szpindor, M.D., director of Allergy and Asthma Care in Oak Park, Illinois. Studies show that if

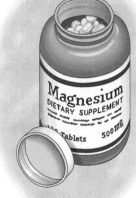

your diet is deficient in magnesium, your asthma may be more severe and flare up more frequently than it otherwise would. If you go the supplement route, take 400 milligrams each of magnesium gluconate and calcium citrate (which can guard against the bone thinning that may result from long-term use of steroids, as in corticosteroids) twice a day, suggests Dr. Szpindor.

You can find this duo in combination supplements at most health food stores and some drugstores.

EAT AN APPLE A DAY. Apples (as well as tomatoes, onions, and the Indian spice turmeric) contain quercetin, a potent bioflavonoid that may help keep your airways clear. Or you can take 500 to 1,000 milligrams of quercetin in capsule form along with 100 to 200 milligrams of bromelain, a pineapple-derived enzyme that will boost its absorption. You can find both at any health food store, but don't take bromelain if you take aspirin or prescription blood thinners.

FISH FOR OMEGA-3'S. Tuna, salmon, trout, and other cold-water fish contain loads of omega-3 essential fatty acids (EFAs), which not only inhibit inflammation but may also repair airway damage. If you eat fish regularly, take 1 to 3 grams (1,000 to 3,000 milligrams) of fish oil daily to minimize asthma symptoms. If you don't eat fish regularly or are sensitive to it, as many people with asthma are, down 3 tablespoons of flaxseed oil (another omega-3 source) a day. Try drizzling it on salads. You can find both oils at health food stores and drugstores, but don't use them if you take aspirin,

WHEN TO DIAL THE DOC

Even very mild asthma can flare up as instantly and seriously as severe asthma—and prove just as fatal. Whether you typically have mild, moderate, or severe asthma, if you have wheezing, shortness of breath, or tightness in your chest that doesn't respond to inhaled or oral medications, head to the hospital immediately. Other serious signs include difficulty talking, rapid or shallow breathing, enlarged nostrils, tightly stretched skin on your neck and/or around your ribcage with each breath, and gray or bluish skin around your mouth or under your fingernails.

other NSAIDs, or prescription blood thinners.

OIL UP WITH BORAGE. The star-shaped flowers of the borage plant are packed with an EFA called gamma-linolenic acid (GLA) that can be your best friend, since GLA fights asthma inflammation. Check your health food store for either borage or primrose oil (also packed with GLA), and take 3 grams (3,000 milligrams) daily, suggests Dr. Szpindor. If you're pollen-sensitive, however, check with your doctor first.

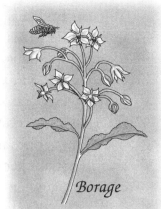

Borage

"B" GOOD TO YOUR LUNGS. "You can undo inflammatory damage in your airways by taking a daily supplement that contains vitamins A, C, and E," says Dr. Szpindor. "But the supplement will work even better if it also contains some Bs"—specifically vitamin B_6, because it relaxes the airways and is often deficient in people with asthma. Look for formulas that contain A, C, and E as well as each of the B vitamins, then take the supplements as directed on the package.

DROP A FEW POUNDS. Harvard researchers have

RED CLOVER, RED CLOVER...

If you're menopausal, bring it right over!

Much has been made in the news about the increased risk of heart attack, stroke, and breast cancer associated with hormone replacement therapy (HRT). But studies have also shown that HRT, with its supplemental estrogen, can double your risk of developing asthma. If the very prospect has you hyperventilating, ask your doctor about this lung-friendlier alternative. "Red clover in over-the-counter Promensil is an herbal estrogen that helps reduce hot flashes without causing asthma," says Richard N. Firshein, D.O. Simply follow the dosage directions on the package.

found that women who are 30 percent over their normal weight for their height are more than twice as likely to develop adult asthma as women who are not overweight. Aim to lose no more than a pound a week through healthful eating and regular exercise, and in less than four months, you may be using your inhaler less frequently.

AX THE ACID. "An asthmatic's breath is a thousand times more acidic than it should be," says Dr. Firshein. "One theory is that acid backwash in the mouth [from heartburn] inflames the lung tissues and constricts the airways."

To limit both the backwash and the constriction, avoid peppermint, tomatoes, coffee, and chocolate, all of which trigger reflux. Also, check your health food store for deglycyrrhizinated (DGL) licorice root, which helps reduce stomach acid. Either sip DGL extract (add about 40 drops of tincture to a cup of hot water) or chew a 200- to 500-milligram DGL wafer before meals, suggests Todd Nelson, N.D., a naturopathic physician in Denver.

GET IT OUT. Emotional stress doesn't cause asthma, but it can aggravate it, says Jack Routes, M.D., associate professor of medicine and immunology at the

TAP YOUR CHEST, THEN BLOW!

If you were to visit me at my home one fine spring day when the air is thick with pollen, you might catch me beating my chest. It's not because I'm angry at the airways I was given, mind you, but because beating my chest actually helps my asthma. At the first hint of chest tightening, I don't always need to puff on my inhaler if I cup my hands and tap rapidly on my chest to loosen the mucus plugs from my airways. If possible, I then get someone to tap rapidly on my back while I'm bending over from the waist. I inhale slowly and expand my belly like a balloon. Then I purse my lips and exhale very forcefully, as though I'm trying to blow out every last one of my birthday candles—and that's a lot of forceful air! It works almost every time.

University of Colorado Health Sciences Center in Denver. To reduce your anxiety and perhaps improve your breathing, take 20 minutes a day to write nonstop (don't edit yourself, just get it out) about what's stressing you. After about four months, studies show that you may be breathing easier—which is less stressful by itself!

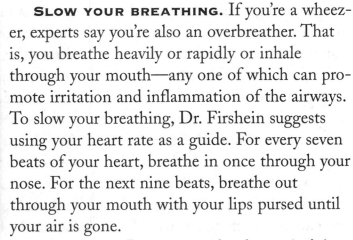

SLOW YOUR BREATHING. If you're a wheezer, experts say you're also an overbreather. That is, you breathe heavily or rapidly or inhale through your mouth—any one of which can promote irritation and inflammation of the airways. To slow your breathing, Dr. Firshein suggests using your heart rate as a guide. For every seven beats of your heart, breathe in once through your nose. For the next nine beats, breathe out through your mouth with your lips pursed until your air is gone.

KICK BUTT. It turns out that karate isn't just an excellent way to ward off bad guys—it's also a solid defense against asthma attacks. "The exclamation that accompanies the forceful kicks forces you to exhale quickly and deeply, so you draw in a deep breath before you continue," says Dr. Firshein. And deep, full-lunged breathing (also required when you're walking, running, or swimming) opens airways.

PASS A PERSONAL CLEAN AIR ACT. Because my asthma is triggered by airborne allergens, I've made my bedroom a no-allergen zone. It's easy: Simply keep the door and windows shut at all times. Never allow your beloved terrier or tabby to enter. Remove all carpet and throw rugs. Get rid of dust-collecting knickknacks. And use an air cleaner with a HEPA filter (a high-efficiency particulate air filter, which can trap nearly 100 percent of all airborne particles) continuously.

ATHLETE'S FOOT

Foil the Fungus

———⟨○○○○⟩———

I love the look of high suede boots. I'd wear them all winter long if my feet would allow it—but being so enclosed for prolonged periods makes them downright angry. Once, when they were trapped in sneakers on a steamy tennis court for hours, they had a major meltdown. They became so sweaty, and then inflamed and itchy, that I had to rip off my sneaks and rub a rough washcloth between my toes for relief. I may not be Serena Williams, but I did have a serious case of athlete's foot.

The nasty fungus, known as *Tinea pedis*, behind athlete's foot thrives in the warmth and dampness that are created by

---

LICK YOUR FUNGUS— WITH LICORICE!

Licorice contains a whopping total of 25 fungicidal substances, enthuses Jeanette Jacknin, M.D. Too bad munching on licorice whips won't do the trick. What you need to do is add 6 teaspoons of powdered licorice to a cup of boiling water and simmer for 20 minutes. Strain out any residue, let the tea cool, and apply it to your inflamed toes three times a day.

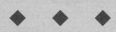

HOMEGROWN SOLUTION

◆ ◆ ◆

Season Your Feet

Mama mia! Garlic is such a potent topical antifungal that Daniel DeLapp, N.D., instructor in dermatology at the National College of Naturopathic Medicine in Portland, Oregon, suggests applying a film of olive oil to the foot, then placing a clove of raw, peeled garlic between each of your toes every night for a week. Be careful not to bruise or break open the clove, because garlic juice can burn the skin. You'll need to wear a pair of all-cotton socks to bed, then wash and dry your feet each morning. Although you may need to sleep in the guest bedroom (the garlic will stink up your room, your skin, and even your breath!), this treatment should stop the itch in its tracks.

the sauna inside airtight shoes or snug socks. It usually settles in the moist area between your fourth and fifth piggies and feeds off the dead skin cells. And as I know much too well, the webs of your toes become cracked and fire-engine red, and they itch like the devil.

WHY ME?

Because tinea is a fungus—an invader, if you will—it tends to gain a foothold in folks with weakened immune systems and those who have recently used antibiotics. Those drugs kill off all bacteria—including the beneficial types that keep fungi in check, explains Mike Cronin, N.D., a naturopathic physician in Scottsdale, Arizona. People with diabetes are also at increased risk because they tend to have more sugar—a yummy feast for fungi—in their systems. But you don't have to be sick to get athlete's foot. Fungal infections thrive in alkaline environments, so if your diet is high in sugar, yeast, and other alkaline foods, you can get the itch whether you're sick or not.

SOOTHING DA AGONY OF DA FEET

If the fungus has spread to the arches of your feet, or your feet are fiery red, swollen, and covered with blisters, contact your doctor—pronto. If you're on the ball (as quick as, say, Serena Williams might be), though, and you catch your infection in the early stages of itching, you can fight the fungus with an over-the-counter antifungal agent—or better yet, a nondrug substance found in your kitchen or a health food store. Your symptoms should clear up within a week. Here's what to try.

MAKE LIKE AN EASTER EGG. Fungi hate acids, and apple cider vinegar is one of the best acid soaks there is, says Lisa Murray-Doran, N.D., a naturopathic physician in Whitby, Ontario. Here's what you do: Simply fill a basin with equal parts of vinegar and warm, soothing water, then soak your feet for 10 minutes daily. Dry each toe and the area between your toes thoroughly when you're done.

PLUNGE YOUR PIGGIES. Place your feet in a basin of warm water spiked with 2 to 3 teaspoons of tea tree oil and soak for 15 minutes twice daily. This oil, from the Australian malaluca tree, is one of nature's best antifungals.

TREAD GENTLY. Since tea tree may sting when applied topically, Dr. Cronin suggests first trying one of the gentler antifungal herbs, such as

That great pair of heels you found at a flea market is no bargain if they contain a little surprise, such as athlete's foot fungus. Boxes of cast-off shoes are often kept in musty, moist basements, providing the perfect breeding ground for bugs. Other shoes to avoid include new vinyl sneakers, shoes with "vinyl uppers," and any shoes that are too snug. None of them can "breathe," so you're more likely to sweat in them—and invite moisture-lovin' fungi to come calling.

✳ ✳ ✳

goldenseal, chamomile, or calendula. You can even look for over-the-counter antifungal creams that pack all three for more healing punch.

SIP FOR THE ITCH. "Tea made from fresh ginger simmered in boiling water provides more than 20 antifungal compounds," says Jeanette Jacknin, M.D., a dermatologist in Scottsdale, Arizona. To make the tea, add 1 teaspoon of grated ginger to a cup of boiling water, steep for 10 to 15 minutes, and strain. Sweeten with honey and drink a cup three times

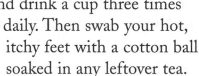

daily. Then swab your hot, itchy feet with a cotton ball soaked in any leftover tea.

LOAD UP ON BENEFICIAL BUGS. *Lactobacillus acidophilus*, which is found in some yogurts, is one of the "good" bacteria that your body needs to keep fungi in check, says Dr. Jacknin. Check yogurt labels to find a brand that contains live cultures (sorry, but frozen yogurt and yogurt-dipped raisins or nuts don't have them), then make a point of including it in your breakfast or lunch menu. Or look at a health food store for acidophilus powder or capsules, then follow the package directions.

YOU CAN BRAVE THE LOCKER ROOM

Despite what you may have heard, you're much less likely to get athlete's foot simply from going barefoot in public locker rooms or saunas than you are to, say, land an unused top locker—and you know how rare that is! In fact, your worst enemy in locker rooms is probably you—if you're in a rush and leave some moisture between your toes when slipping on your shoes, that is. Michael Cronin, N.D., suggests taking a moment while you're drying your hair to aim the hair dryer between your toes. Dry toes means no fungus grows—no matter where you've been!

GOBBLE LOTS OF BERRIES. Strawberries and blueberries are packed with vitamin C, which will help fight your athlete's foot infection from the inside. When fruit's out of season, and if you don't have kidney or stomach problems, take 1,000 milligrams of vitamin C in supplement form twice a day, suggests Dr. Cronin.

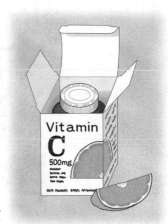

GET ZINC. Not only will zinc increase immunity (and thereby squash fungi), it will also help broken skin heal faster. Dr. Jacknin suggests taking 50 milligrams of supplemental zinc daily, with food, for as long as the fungus persists.

QUIT CORNSTARCH. This popular ingredient has replaced talc in many powdered anti-sweat products, but it can actually encourage fungal growth, warns Dr. Cronin. You're better off using a medicated antifungal powder or a foot spray that combines calendula and witch hazel, an astringent herb that reduces moisture.

WEAR ALL COTTON, ALL THE TIME. While you're treating your athlete's foot, avoid wearing pantyhose, and stick to socks made of 100 percent cotton. Wash and dry your feet twice daily, slipping into a fresh pair of all-cotton socks sprinkled with antifungal powder each time. "You don't want to give these nasty beasts room to grow in even a drop of moisture," reminds Dr. Murray-Doran.

ATTENTION DEFICIT DISORDER

Get Your Brain in Gear

⚬⚬⚬⚬⚬

Almost everyone feels scattered when juggling a jillion responsibilities, as most adults in this day and age must. But when your brain lacks the wiring for a "focus" button, as my friend Elana's does, it's, well, a jillion times worse.

The mother of two and owner of a home-based business, Elana's free-roaming attention flits from a half-finished conversation with a client to partial instructions to her assistant to frantically searching for car keys and a mad dash to a nearly forgotten school recital. Whew! "I feel like I'm playing 20 instruments without a conductor," she sighs.

WHY ME?

If, like Elana, your attention is harder to corral than a roomful of cats, you may have attention deficit disorder (ADD)—a condition that isn't just for kids. People with ADD lack sufficient dopamine, a chemical messenger in the brain, says Sari Solden, a psychotherapist in Ann Arbor, Michigan. "They don't really have a deficiency of attention but rather a deficiency of the brain's biochemical that helps them organize, sort, shift, and even stop attention."

Some people with ADD—many of them women—slip under the radar when they're young, often because they don't act out or seem hyperactive, as boys with ADD often do. Perhaps you were one of them: More inattentive than disruptive, you were labeled a daydreamer by your teachers and called "spacey" by your peers. Maybe you believed the label, and your self-image suffered. You think of yourself as a space cadet, stupid, or a slob. Or, like many women with ADD, you believe your life would improve if you could just make yourself get organized. Believe me, it wouldn't.

"ADD can't be cured by working harder or the power of the will," explains psychotherapist Edward M. Hallowell, M.D., founder of the Hallowell Center for Cognitive and Emotional Health in Sudbury, Massachusetts. "The trick to living successfully with ADD isn't to focus on your weaknesses but rather to work with your brain chemistry to maximize your strengths."

TRAIN YOUR BRAIN

If you take up one of the martial arts, such as aikido, karate, or tai chi, you may improve your concentration even as you master the moves. According to John Ratey, M.D., professor of psychiatry at Harvard Medical School, the martial arts demand a special kind of concentration that forces coordination of the attention centers in the brain—that is, the frontal cortex, the cerebellum, and the limbic system. If you have ADD, your ability to coordinate these centers is naturally erratic. With training in the martial arts—particularly tai chi, which is slow, healing, and often called "moving meditation"—you can improve it.

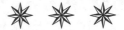

A mental health professional who specializes in ADD can help you do exactly that, possibly recommending a prescription medication, such as methylphenidate (Ritalin) or atomoxetine (Strattera), that boosts dopamine. These drugs may help keep you on task, reduce distraction, and curb impulsive reactions. But there isn't a "cookbook" recipe that will automatically rewire your brain, warns Dr. Hallowell. Whether or not you go the medication route, you'll still need to change your behavior.

"Medication can be the fuel that gets you going," echoes Solden, "but you must also learn how to drive your own car."

STAYING ON TRACK

To maximize your attention, you need to minimize your "deficit" and, to use Solden's analogy, get behind the wheel of the brain you were given and drive it in the direction you want to go. To do so, try these tips.

GET B ON BOARD. Everyone with ADD should take a daily vitamin B-complex capsule, stresses Robert Hedaya, M.D., clinical professor of psychiatry at Georgetown University Hospital

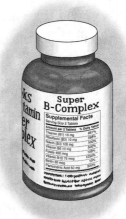

in Washington, D.C. The most important of the Bs is vitamin B_6, because it aids brain functioning. In fact, studies show it may be as effective as Ritalin for improving focus. Just be sure to ask your doctor for guidance in supplementing with B_6, since it can be toxic in high doses.

FOCUS ON PROTEIN. "A higher-protein, lower-carbohydrate diet will actually promote concentration," says psychiatrist Daniel Amen, M.D., medical director of the Amen Clinics in southern California and Washington state. While carbohydrates cause your energy levels and focus to soar, then quickly crash, protein helps make the neurotransmitter dopamine, which aids focus. Keep protein-packed munchies—such as string cheese, protein bars, or celery sticks filled with peanut butter—on hand.

"You'll be surprised at how just a few high-protein morsels can really stimulate your focus," says Judy E. Peabody, N.D., a naturopathic physician in Portland, Oregon.

MUNCH ON A MIX. If your problem isn't an inability to focus but rather a tendency to focus to the point of overabsorption in tasks (also a hallmark of ADD), your aim should be to boost brain levels of the calming neurotransmitter serotonin (by eating carbs) as well as dopamine (by downing protein), says Dr. Amen. To get both, toss your pasta with chunks of cheese or meat or go for thin-crust, meat-topped pizza.

GARNISH YOUR MEMORY. Regularly eating tuna, walnuts, Brazil nuts, soybeans, and flaxseed is a great way to enrich your diet with omega-3 essential fatty acids (EFAs), which reduce the inflammation that can impair focus and memory. In fact, to make sure you get enough, Dr. Amen recommends taking about 2 grams (2,000 milligrams) of omega-3 supplements (available at health food stores) a day. If you're taking blood

Focus Finder

The simplest way to stay focused? Breathe like a puppy! That's right: When you breathe by fully expanding your belly, you increase the oxygen content in your brain, says Daniel Amen, M.D. Even a slight increase in available oxygen can help you stick to a task and control impulsive behavior. To get the hang of breathing Fido-style, lie on your back with a small book on your belly. Breathe in so the book rises, then breathe out so it falls. Within minutes, you'll feel more focused.

thinners, check with your doctor first.

NUDGE BLOOD TO YOUR BRAIN. The antioxidant vitamins A, C, and E help increase concentration by boosting blood flow to the brain. Pick up a prepackaged antioxidant formula, then follow the dosage directions on the label. To up the ante, you might also try Pycnogenol, a very potent antioxidant derived from grapeseed and pine bark that also aids the ability to focus, says Dr. Amen. Check your health food store for either product, then follow the label directions.

EAT YOUR PEAs. If you have trouble focusing—and have a hankering for chocolate—chances are that your body needs the brain chemical phenylethylamine (PEA), which boosts energy and concentration and is also found in chocolate. PEA is made in the brain with the amino acid tyrosine, so taking 500 to 1,500 milligrams of supplemental tyrosine (available at health food stores) two or three times a day could help keep you on task, says Dr. Amen.

PUT BLINDERS ON YOUR MIND. At work or at home, position your desk so that you're facing away from any traffic visible through windows or a door. Use white noise (the kind produced by machines often used as sleep aids) to block out conversation in the next cubicle or the dialogue from a TV show in the family room. Ask your boss for flex time (so that, say, you arrive an hour earlier than most of your coworkers and leave an hour before they do) to have less time for distractions at work. And when intrusive thoughts pop into your head, write them down so you can give them their due after you finish the task at hand.

STAMP OUT ANTs. Automatic negative thoughts, or ANTs, as Dr. Amen calls them, invade your mind like real ants invade a picnic. Unlike the real pesky critters, though, ANTs lose their power if you talk back to them. Let's say, for instance, one of your ANTs is the nagging belief: "I'm an unfit mom because I don't do domestic things well." The next time it creeps into your head, says Dr. Amen, squash it by immediately telling yourself, "I help my kids decorate their rooms creatively, and their friends flock to our home because of my generosity and humor."

GET PLENTY OF EXERCISE. Intense aerobic exercise—a brisk 3-mile walk as opposed to a 2-block stroll—is absolutely one of the best ways to combat ADD because it stimulates the release of endorphins (brain chemicals that lift your mood and turn down the noisy static in your brain) and bumps up brain levels of the calming neurotransmitters tryptophan and serotonin, says Dr. Amen. There's just one catch: You have to exercise hard enough to quicken your heart rate and breathing for 30 to 45 minutes at least five times a week.

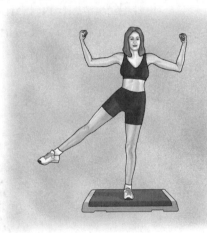

TRY POWERFUL POSES. Yoga can be a great way to rein in attention and maintain focus, but its deliberately slow pace may be too pokey for you—unless, suggests Carol Watkins,

M.D., director of Northern County Psychiatric Associates in Baltimore, you try power yoga, a faster-paced version during which the postures flow rapidly into one another. "Power yoga can be a good way to help center people with ADD," she says.

SPICE UP YOUR LIFE. Women with ADD who crave stimulation (when you don't have enough dopamine, you feel less fully alive) often satisfy it in passive ways, such as watching soaps, trolling the mall, or snacking, says Kathryn Nadeau, Ph.D., director of Chesapeake Psychological Services in Bethesda, Maryland. Whenever you get a craving for, say, an entire bag of sour cream and onion potato chips, think of it as a need for stimulation rather than for salt, then ask yourself, "What can I do that will make me feel interested and fully alive right this moment?" Then do exactly that: Plant an herb garden, leaf through travel brochures, head out on a challenging hike, or even just call a friend to chat.

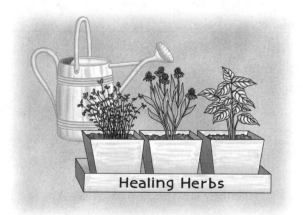

Healing Herbs

BACK PAIN

Beat It for Good

———◆———

I have one friend who can't drive for longer than 10 minutes unless her car seat is padded with specially shaped pillows to coddle her always-aching back. Another chum joined my yoga class specifically because she twisted her back with a decidedly un-Tiger-like golf swing. Does everybody have back pain?

Just about. "Back pain is the leading disability for folks under age 45," says Jacob Schorr, N.D., a Denver-based naturopathic physician and president of the Colorado Association of Naturopathic Doctors. "And it isn't just the freight lifters among us who are getting nailed." Sure, you can injure your back on the job or in a car crash, but far and away, the most frequent cause isn't catastrophic—it's everyday weakness and inflex-

DRIVE AWAY PAIN

If you have a long commute and a chronically tender back, you may want to look into purchasing a car with a massaging lumbar support system. Studies show that 1 minute of lumbar massage every 5 minutes can help reduce lower-back pain. And you thought leather seats were as good as it gets!

Consult a doctor if you have back pain that persists without abating for more than three days; it's accompanied by a fever, pain at night or when resting, or bowel or bladder changes; or you are weak or can't stand on your tiptoes, which may indicate nerve damage. You should see a doctor immediately if you have back pain as well as a history of cancer or diabetes, since it may indicate a tumor or nerve damage. Start with your primary physician, who can refer you to a specialist such as an orthopedist if necessary.

ibility in the muscles that support the back.

WHY ME?

The weaker your muscles (especially those in your upper back and hips and your hamstrings—the muscles at the backs of your thighs), the more apt you are to strain your back. A sudden, uncharacteristic movement—such as swinging a golf club—strains the stiff muscles, tendons, and ligaments, damaging tissue and causing swelling and intense aching. Your muscles may even spasm to protect your back from additional movement and injury.

You can develop another type of back pain—called sciatica—simply by sitting on a wallet stuffed in your rear pocket. While the stabbing pain can start in your buttocks and radiate down the back of your leg all the way to your foot, its origin is in your back, where the shock-absorbing disks between the vertebrae in your spine can press on or irritate the sciatic nerve.

Sometimes you don't even have to do anything to strain your back. Simply living under the burden of chronic emotional stress can create muscle tension, says John Sarno, M.D., professor of clinical rehabilitation medicine at New York University School of Medicine in New York City. That tension in turn can block blood flow to the muscles and create more spasms and pain. "The more pain, the more stress," he says. "It becomes a vicious cycle."

BANISH BACK PAIN

The good news is, as debilitating as back pain can be, it's rarely serious and usually temporary. In fact, in most cases, people recover from episodes of acute lower-back pain within three weeks to three months without a single treatment—and fully a third of all people with lower-back pain significantly improve within just a week.

That said, you don't have to twiddle your thumbs waiting for Father Time to cure your achy back—you can nudge him along. In fact, you should, because if you treat back pain in the acute phase, you may reduce the likelihood of long-term pain and disability. Here are several ways to ease both sudden and chronic back pain.

KEEP ON TRUCKIN'. "The worst thing anyone with an achy back can do is to sit still," says Carol Hartigan, M.D., assistant clinical professor of physical medicine and rehabilitation at Harvard Medical School. In fact, resting for more than a day or two reduces muscle flexibility and strength and can lead to further disability. On the other hand, movement keeps blood flowing into the site, waste products flowing out of it, and muscle spasms to a minimum. "Let your pain be your guide," says Dr. Hartigan. "You may not want to move your piano, but it's really okay to lift a bag of groceries. My advice is to do everyday activities as you can tolerate them."

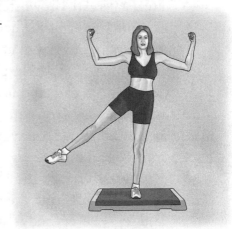

HIT THE GYM. That's right—just limit what you do while you're there. For instance, if you usually walk 3 miles on the treadmill, cruise through 2 miles at a slower speed than you normally stride. "Moving is the very best anti-inflammatory," explains Dr. Hartigan, "since it speeds removal of inflammation-causing

Sweep Up Spasms!

You can do it with a plain old broomstick. Here's how: First, roll the broom handle in a towel to pad it, then lie on your back on top of it, lining up your spine along the broomstick. Stay there for 5 minutes. Gravity will help pull your shoulders down and stretch out the muscles around your spine.

prostaglandins from the painful site."

PLAY BALL. The more you work certain back muscles, says Dr. Hartigan, the faster you can return to normal activities. Grab an oversize exercise ball and give this mini-workout a try: Lie face down across the ball with your hands and feet on the floor. Lift one arm and then the other as high as you can, raising your torso from the ball. Pause for a count of 10, then return both hands to the floor. Next, place both hands behind your head and lift your torso as high as you can. Hold for 5 counts, then release. Repeat this routine as many times as you can without causing discomfort.

S-T-R-E-T-C-H. Even if your back pain has you lying on the floor, you can stretch your arms and legs, elongating the tissues in your back and drawing healing blood and oxygen to the area, says Art Brownstein, M.D., clinical instructor of medicine at the University of Hawaii at Manoa. Just remember to stay relaxed, cushion your back with a pad, and use slow, gentle movements as you extend your arms over your head and stretch out your legs along the floor. Hold each stretch for about a minute, then relax.

SWIM WITH FINS. Swimming helps boost overall back health by targeting the muscles in the lower back, hips, buttocks, and legs—everybody's weak spots, notes Dr. Brownstein. He suggests donning swim fins and treading water for several minutes, or as long as you can. Since the exercise isn't weight-bearing, you'll place little or no strain on your back even as you build up your muscles.

FREEZE IT. "Ice is a great analgesic and is preferable to aspirin or other nonsteroidal anti-inflammatory drugs like ibuprofen, which, in large doses, can cause stomach upset," says Dr. Hartigan. Simply fill a paper or Styrofoam cup with water and freeze it, then peel away the rim to expose the ice surface. Grasping the cup, lie on your side and apply the ice directly to the painful area in a circular motion. Limit the massage to about 5 minutes, and don't place the ice directly on the bony portion of your spine.

SAVE HEAT FOR THE MORNING. Some doctors suggest alternating ice with heat to boost blood flow to the back and reduce inflammation, but you should use heat only in the morning, when you're sure to be active afterward. "If you use a heating pad just before sleeping, blood may pool in your back," warns Dr. Hartigan. A hot shower in the morning is also ideal.

TRY HERBAL ASPIRIN. Willow bark is a natural source of aspirin-like salicylates, which ease pain. But unlike aspirin or ibuprofen, it won't irritate your stomach while it's easing your back pain, notes Glen Rothfeld, M.D., clinical assistant pro-

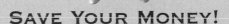

SAVE YOUR MONEY!

Go Sans a Belt

Have you got your eye on one of those supportive belts, braces, or corsets purported to protect your back muscles during lifting? Look elsewhere. All those belts do is put pressure on your back, says Jacob Schorr, N.D. To truly stabilize your back, you have to tighten the muscles inside your body—not a piece of material around the outside.

fessor of medicine at Tufts University School of Medicine in Boston. To make a tea, pick up some willow bark from a health food store and steep 2 teaspoons in a cup of boiling water, then strain and sip. You can also take capsules or apply willow bark ointment directly to your back. Don't use it in any form, however, if you take aspirin; the double dose of salicylates may be too much for your system.

RELAX NATURALLY. Scour your health food store for herbal pain formulas that contain cramp bark, black cohosh, and oatstraw in capsule form, suggests Dr. Schorr. These herbs are all excellent antispasmodics and muscle relaxants. If valerian, which is a sedative, is also among the ingredients, the capsules will make a great nightcap for a bad back. Follow the dosage directions on the label. Don't use a formula with valerian if you're taking other medications, however.

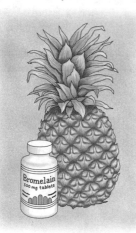

BABY IT WITH BROMELAIN. This anti-inflammatory enzyme, derived from pineapple, may be especially helpful for relieving painful inflammation or soft-tissue problems caused by sports injuries. "I like to use formulas that include bromelain, papain, and trypsin—all enzymes that help calm the chemical pathways that cause pain," says Tanya Baldwin, N.D., a naturopathic physician in Los Gatos, California. Check at a health food store for supplements that contain bromelain, then follow the label directions. Don't take bromelain if you take aspirin or prescription blood thinners.

BET ON BORON. This trace mineral boosts calcium absorption in bones, which may reduce bone thinning and the chronic discomfort that it can cause, says Dr. Rothfeld. Studies show that taking 10 to 20 milligrams of boron—which you can find at health food stores—with meals can reduce ongoing back pain.

POP ANTI-LOCK MINERALS. If your back tends to lock up

at the slightest movement, you need to beef up your intake of magnesium, potassium, and calcium—the kings of the natural muscle relaxants, says Dr. Schorr. Check a health food store or drugstore for "cal-mag" formulas that pack 200 to 300 milligrams of each mineral. Follow the package directions for use, and at the same time, limit your intake of coffee and soft drinks. Compounds in java increase the loss of calcium in urine, and the phosphoric acid in sodas inhibits calcium absorption by the bones.

RUB IN RELIEF. According to studies from the Group Health Cooperative in Seattle, weekly massages can cut the need for pain medication for back spasms and tight muscles in half. As a general rule, a muscle spasm should relax when the therapist massages it. If it persists, you probably have some inflammation, too, and massage may not be the best therapy for you, notes Beth Mueller, a massage therapist in Appleton, Wisconsin. Count on at least four massage treatments to smooth out spasms.

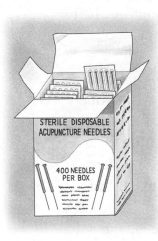

STICK IT TO SPASMS. If your back muscles tend to spasm and lock up suddenly, try acupuncture, which may ease the spasms and the pain—perhaps because those hair-thin needles stimulate the release of feel-good brain chemicals called endorphins. "While acupuncture isn't as effective at easing pain from chronically tensed muscles," notes Dr. Schorr, "it's great at opening up muscles that suddenly snap in spasm." Want to give it a try? Ask your physician to recommend a reputable acupuncturist near you.

BAD HAIR

Tame Your Tresses

———————◆◇◇◇◆———————

With the possible exception of Christie Brinkley, most women have some complaint with their hair. Mine becomes so brittle and flyaway in cold, dry air that I look as if I sleep in a wind tunnel for most of the winter! Maybe yours is similar—or perhaps it's too curly or too straight. Too fine or too coarse. Too limp or too unruly. You know the classic laments, and you've no doubt voiced them more than once. According to the experts, though, it's not us who should be complaining about our hair—it's our hair that should be complaining about us!

WHY ME?

"The high heat and harsh chemicals to which we routinely subject our hair actually alter its physical structure," says Zoe Draelos, M.D, clinical associate professor of dermatology at Wake Forest University Medical Center in Winston-Salem, North Carolina. "The hair shaft is roughed up, nicked, and sometimes even stripped of its protective outer cuticle, exposing it to further damage." As a result, smoothness, sheen, and softness disappear.

Unfortunately, chemicals are only half the problem. A dearth of adequate proteins and minerals and an overabundance of sugar can also boost the output of sebum, the fatty oil produced by the skin to keep your scalp from drying out. When there's too much sebum, though, your hair becomes flat and greasy and sprinkled with dandruff. Also, in one of nature's catch-22s, stress can boost the output of sebum. When you're weighed down with worry, your hair may become weighed down with oil—just to give you something more to worry about!

NO MORE BAD HAIR DAYS

To minimize your complaints with your mane—and its complaints with you—you don't have to resort to pricey hair repair appointments or prescription dandruff-control products (which contain potent antibiotics). All you have to do is feed your hair the nutrients it needs and revamp your hasty "wash, blow, and go" routine to include a few intensive repair sessions. Here's how to get started.

GET AMPLE NUTRIENTS. "Hair that's brittle and breaks when you brush it could indicate that you're not absorbing the minerals you need from your diet," says Kathleen Flewelling, N.D., a naturopathic physician in Seaside, Oregon. Try taking

DIP YOUR HEAD IN AVOCADO

Rich in vitamins, essential fatty acids, and minerals, avocados do more than just make excellent dip—they'll also restore luster to your hair, says Dee Anna Glaser, M.D., associate professor of dermatology at St. Louis University School of Medicine in Missouri. Simply remove the pit from a very ripe avocado and mash the flesh well. Then, after shampooing and rinsing, massage the pulp into your wet hair for about 5 minutes. Cover your hair with plastic wrap and leave it on for an hour, if you can. Rinse thoroughly, then shampoo and condition as usual.

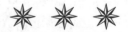

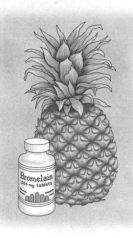

digestive enzyme supplements to aid absorption. Check your health food store for formulas that include hydrochloric acid to help break down minerals, plus protein and bromelain for better carbohydrate absorption.

GET TO THE ROOT OF IT. If your hair has suddenly become extremely oily or startlingly dry, it probably means that your levels of androgen hormones, which have an effect on sweating and oil production, have either soared or taken a nosedive, says Dr. Flewelling. One way to help your liver rebalance the hormones is to take milk thistle or dandelion root capsules, she says. "I suggest taking 20 milligrams a day of milk thistle or 150 milligrams of dandelion root twice daily." Look for both herbs at health food stores. Check with your doctor about using dandelion if you take diuretics or potassium supplements.

TURN DOWN THE HEAT. "Whether it's shampooing with hot water or drying with great blasts of hot hair, heat lifts up the cuticle scales on the hair's surface, just as wind raises shingles on a roof," says Bernard Cohen, M.D., professor of dermatology at the University of Miami School of Medicine in Tampa. "This prompts water loss from the hair shaft, and the lifted cuticles catch onto each other." The result is tangled, dull hair. To smooth down cuticles and bring up shine, wash your hair with warm water and rinse with cold, then dry your hair using a two-phase, heat-cool dryer. Use the heat phase for 75 percent of the drying, then press the cool-air button to dry the rest.

RECOAT YOUR LOCKS. Stressed-out hair is simply hair that has been stripped (usually by heat and chemicals) of its protective coating, or cuticle. To restore the coating—and manageability—use shampoos, conditioners, hair sprays, and styling aids that contain panthenol, suggests Dr. Draelos. Derived from vitamin B_5 (pantothenate), panthenol both recoats the hair and penetrates the hair shaft so each hair can hold more water, making it stronger and softer.

FLUFF IT UP. If you have baby-fine hair, you have more strands per square inch of scalp than average. The more hair, the more oil glands—and the greasier your hair will look even just a couple of hours after shampooing, says Thomas Goodman Jr., M.D., assistant professor of dermatology at the University of Tennessee Center for Health Sciences in Memphis. To outpace your oil glands, Dr. Goodman suggests using "clarifying" shampoos—preferably those containing rosemary or sage, which are astringent and help minimize oil buildup. Also, skip the conditioner or apply it only to the ends.

A TV STYLIST'S TOP FIVE TRICKS

A friend invites you on a spur-of-the moment outing, your hair looks like a rat's nest, and you literally don't have time to jump in the shower—much less get highlights! This is a job for Kristi "I've Seen It All" Fuhrmann, TV studio stylist to the stars. Here are her five best rescue remedies.

FLAT HAIR: Rub shaving cream into the roots to give it texture and lift.

OILY HAIR: Sprinkle cornstarch powder onto your scalp to absorb the oil, then brush your hair thoroughly. To sop up grease on the run, soak a cotton pad in mouthwash or witch hazel (they're both astringents) and dab your scalp.

GRAY ROOTS: Cover them with either brown or black mascara—whichever best matches your hair color. Simply stroke on the mascara with the wand.

DARK ROOTS WITH BLONDE HAIR: Replace your straight part with one that zigzags to make your roots less noticeable.

SPLIT ENDS: Curl your hair under using a curling iron or a hair dryer and a round brush.

WANT BRECK-GIRL HAIR?

You may want to lay off the Breck—or any other shampoo you've been using for a zillion years. "The buildup of shampoos, conditioners, sprays, gels, and other alkaline-based hair products can smother the life out of your hair," points out Kathleen Flewelling, N.D., "leaving it dull and flat."

To strip away the gunk and bring back the shine, Dr. Flewelling suggests tossing some acid on your tresses. Mix 2 parts apple cider vinegar or lemon juice and 1 part warm water. Pour most of the solution onto your scalp and cover it with a towel. Leave it on for 30 minutes, then shampoo and rinse with the remaining solution. Your hair will literally be squeaky clean—and look dazzlingly shiny.

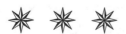

SIDESTEP STATIC. If your hair frequently looks as if you stuck your finger into a light socket, try using a conditioner that contains quaternary ammonium; its positively charged ions remove static electricity. Then, after towel drying, use a spray-on detangling conditioner. "This will further disrupt the electrical charge that makes hair stand on end," says Dr. Cohen, "and it will minimize breakage."

POUR ON SOME HORSETAIL. The very name of this herb conjures the image of a shiny, swishy ponytail—and that's exactly the promise of using horsetail. It contains a large amount of the trace mineral silica, says Dr. Flewelling, and can restore strength and shine to burned-out tresses. Check your health food store for horsetail tincture and massage 50 to 60 drops into wet hair. Leave it on for 15 minutes, then shampoo.

BEAT DANDRUFF WITH BIOTIN. One of the B-complex

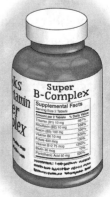

vitamins, biotin is essential for healthy hair and can help discourage those ugly flakes. All you need is a handful of soy nuts a day, says Jeanette Jacknin, M.D., a dermatologist in Scottsdale, Arizona. You can also take supplements, available at health food stores.

OIL YOUR FLAKES. Tea tree oil contains an essential oil called terpinen-4-ol that penetrates and disinfects the top layers of the scalp. You can either use a shampoo that contains tea tree oil or apply the oil directly to your scalp. At the health food store, look for tea tree oil that contains a hefty percentage of terpinen-4-ol (more than 30 percent), then massage a few drops into your wet, washed hair, suggests Kristi Fuhrmann, a TV studio stylist in New York City. Wrap your head in a towel for a half-hour, then rinse.

ZAP IT WITH ZINC. For really stubborn dandruff, look for anti-dandruff shampoos containing zinc pyrithione and selenium sulfide—and purchase both. These two minerals scruff up the scalp, initiate cell turnover, and can break cornflake-size flakes into less noticeable ones. Just be prepared to alternate brands each week, since these products tend to lose effectiveness with continued use, says Samuel Selden, M.D., assistant professor of clinical medicine at Eastern Virginia Medical School in Chesapeake.

OIL AWAY THE ITCHIES. In a small pan, warm a few drops of almond, sesame, olive, or vitamin E oil, then gently comb it through your dry hair. Wrap a towel around your head and leave it on for at least 15 minutes, then shampoo. "The oil will help loosen dry scales and make your hair shiny, not greasy," says Dr. Jacknin.

BELLY FAT

Melt It Away

───────◆◆◆───────

I have a friend whom I consider a real peach, but when it comes to body shape, she's strictly an "apple." That's because, unlike my pear-shaped friends (who have cinched waists and ample hips), her weight tends to settle in a pudgy roll around her waistline. And that puts her at greater risk for serious conditions such as heart disease, stroke, diabetes, and breast and colon cancer— even though her overall weight is within the normal range.

In fact, studies indicate that women who have spare-tire fat (whether they're over-weight or not) have higher blood sugar levels, higher total cholesterol counts, and lower

WHAT WORKS

One recent study of women who lost 30 pounds and kept it off revealed a couple of surprisingly basic secrets behind their success: They simply ate less and exercised more. In fact, the women ate about 1,400 calories a day (less fat and sugar and more fruits and veggies than they were previously accustomed to eating). They burned an average of about 400 calories a day (the equivalent of about an hour of brisk walking). No tricks, no gizmos—just a good, solid strategy. And it worked!

levels of high-density lipoprotein (HDL—the good cholesterol) than women who don't, making them worse off than overweight women without excess tummy fat.

What makes this intra-abdominal visceral fat, as the scientists call it, such a threat? The answers aren't entirely clear.

"One reason may be that deep, central fat literally surrounds and squeezes the heart and other internal organs so that they are unable to function properly," explains Leslie Bonci, director of sports nutrition at the University of Pittsburgh and a spokesperson for the American Dietetic Association.

A second possibility is that abdominal fat may find its way into the bloodstream more readily than other types of fat, precipitating a buildup of fatty acids that results in high cholesterol and high blood pressure—two prime factors in heart disease. Excess fatty acids can also lead to higher resistance to insulin (the hormone that snatches excess blood sugar from the bloodstream), which can set the stage for diabetes.

There's also evidence that carrying fat around your middle may increase estrogen activity in the body, which may explain why the incidence of breast cancer—considered an "estrogen-fueled" disease—is higher among women with belly fat than

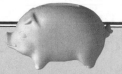

THE ONLY BELLY-BUSTING AID YOU'LL EVER NEED

Sure, you can buy the latest ab-burning aid for just four easy payments of, say, $29.95. But why would you? All you really need to keep your crunches honest is a stability ball (really a giant beach ball), which isolates your abdominal muscles so you work them hard without straining your back, says Peter Francis, Ph.D., professor of biomechanics at San Diego State University. If you're under 5 feet tall, choose a 45-centimeter ball; if you're taller, choose a 55-centimeter ball. The harder the ball, the more difficult the exercise, Dr. Francis adds.

Here's how to use it: Sit on the ball with your feet flat on the floor about shoulder-width apart. Let the ball roll backward slowly so it lies beneath your lower back and hips, while your thighs and lower torso are parallel to the floor. Position your feet farther apart for greater balance. Place your hands behind your head or cross your arms over your chest, then tuck your chin in slightly toward your chest. Next, raise your upper torso (no more than 45 degrees) by contracting your abs. Repeat as many times as you can.

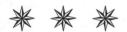

among those with overall fat, according to findings from the long-term Framingham Heart Study.

WHY ME?

"The apple literally does not fall far from the tree," Bonci says with a chuckle. In other words, weight distribution is inherited. In fact, it's likely that your genes are largely to blame for your apple-esque profile—even more so, many researchers venture, than the food you eat. While gorging on buttery sauces, rich desserts, and other high-fat foods will certainly make you gain weight, it won't make you gain it in your belly, the experts say, unless you were genetically programmed to do so.

Also, recent studies have shown that high levels of cortisol—a hormone triggered by stress—can expand your waistline. When your body is under stress, your adrenal glands pump out excess cortisol, which in turn releases the glucose your body needs for energy as it prepares to fight or flee your stressor. Normally, cortisol levels ebb as stress subsides. But if you are chronically stressed—as most of us are anymore—your cortisol levels remain high, prompting your body to keep releasing glucose it never uses up (because you don't fight or flee). The glucose is then stored as fat around your organs. If you often drink a glass of wine to unwind, you only make matters worse, since the presence of alcohol increases cortisol production.

10 WAYS TO DEFLATE THE SPARE

Yes, being apple-shaped can be rotten for your health. And yes, you probably inherited a tendency toward it—but that doesn't mean you can't do something about it. In fact, you should, if your waist-to-hip ratio is more than 0.8 (calculated by dividing your waist measurement by your hip measurement).

What exactly might that something be? "Your goal should be to shrink your bulk from the inside so your lungs and heart work better than they did before," says Bonci, "not from the outside." In other words, no expensive ab flex gizmos or toning tablets—they won't work anyway. You simply need to whittle your waist the old-fashioned way (with the help of a few new-fangled tips)—by eating less and exercising more.

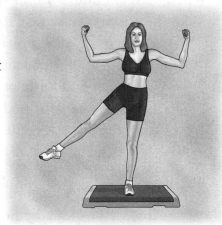

MOVE, BABY, MOVE. Any exercise that raises your heart rate is excellent for losing overall body fat because it builds muscle, which naturally burns more calories than fat, and boosts your metabolism—not only while you're working out but also long after you've stopped. In fact, researchers found that when women ages 50 to 75 (when middle fat tends to accumulate) walked for 45 minutes three times a week, they lost 16 percent of their abdominal fat. "In the past, many postmenopausal women turned to hormone replacement therapy [HRT] to control estrogen levels and keep their middles slim," says Bonci. "But the newly discovered risks of HRT make this no longer an option." Besides, exercise won't simply cut inches—it'll also cut your risk of heart disease, breast cancer, and diabetes.

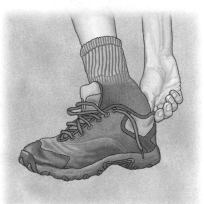

EXERCISE IN SMALL SPURTS. "Abdominal fat responds to 30 to 60 min-utes of accumulated continuous movement through-out the day," says Bonci. That means you don't have to carve an hour out of your day to spend at the gym or train for a marathon to slim your middle. What you do have to do is move for a *total* of 30 to 60 minutes—perhaps by walking briskly for 15 minutes after lunch and 20 minutes after dinner. Bonci suggests slipping in 5 minutes of activity before and after breakfast, 5 minutes before and after lunch, and 10 minutes after dinner. As your fitness level goes up and your waistline goes down, your motivation will soar—and you may find you're able to carve larger chunks out of your day for continuous exercise.

SWALLOW SOME PSYLLIUM.
Taking a fiber supplement such as psyllium before meals could help reduce the number of calories absorbed by your body. Plus, psyllium helps you feel full and stabilizes blood sugar levels, which may help control food cravings, notes Glen Rothfeld, M.D., clinical assistant professor of medicine at Tufts University School of Medicine in

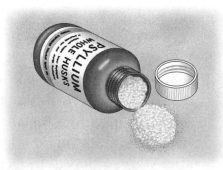

Boston. Check your supermarket, drugstore, or health food store for psyllium powder and take 1 to 3 tablespoons dissolved in water or juice three times a day before eating, he suggests. Just be sure you swallow a full glass of water with your psyllium and drink 8 to 10 glasses of water throughout the day, since the extra bulk will pull water from your body. (Water intake alone can dull your appetite somewhat, anyway.)

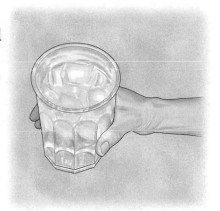

DRINK YOUR MILK. And make it from grass-fed cows, if you can. Aside from calcium (which some researchers think may help regulate weight), milk contains an abundance of conjugated linoleic acid (CLA)—a fatty acid that may promote weight loss. Cows fed on grass produce milk with 500 percent more CLA than milk from grain-fed cows.

In one recent study, researchers gave CLA to overweight people with diabetes every day for eight weeks. As a result, their blood sugar levels decreased fivefold; they had less leptin hormone, which can promote weight gain in already overweight people; and they each lost an average of 3.5 pounds. "Although we're not sure how it works, CLA seems to trick the body into not storing fat," says Martha Belury, Ph.D., associate professor of human nutrition at the Carol S. Kennedy Research Center at Ohio State University in Columbus. Other studies have shown that supplementing your diet with CLA reduces abdominal fat in particular.

The CLA supplement dosage in the studies ranged from 3 to 4 grams (3,000 to 4,000 milligrams) a day, taken with meals. You'd need to drink about three glasses of milk to get one-fifth that amount, but even that may be beneficial, since milk is loaded with calcium. To get about 1,000 milligrams of calcium a day (plus a healthy dose of CLA), drink a cup of fat-free milk

(300 milligrams) and eat an ounce of Cheddar cheese (204 milligrams), a cup of yogurt (400 milligrams), and a cup of broccoli (140 milligrams) every day.

COOK WITH FAT-BURNING SPICES. Certain common kitchen spices, such as ginger, red pepper, mustard, and cinnamon, may help raise both your body temperature and your metabolism, so you burn calories for fuel rather than store them as fat. Plus, they may speed your digestion. Red pepper, for instance, contains the compound capsaicin, which stimulates saliva, and that in turn can help the digestive process. People with sluggish digestion tend to gain weight, says Dana Myatt, N.D., a naturopathic physician in Phoenix. In fact, in one small study, dieters who added 1 teaspoon of red-pepper sauce and 1 teaspoon of mustard to every meal raised their metabolic rates by 25 percent.

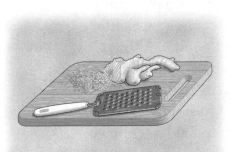

Perhaps what these tasty spices do best, though, is make food savory, so you need less fat (such as oil) to make it palatable, and you can feel satisfied with smaller portions. To start, sprinkle some red pepper on your baked potato or some grated ginger on your veggies instead of butter. Like the results? Break open an ethnic cookbook, then let 'er rip.

PRACTICE PORTION CONTROL. Studies show that larger portions do indeed mean larger bodies. "Biggie eyes translate to biggie thighs—or in this case, biggie bellies," quips Bonci. But you can use the following tricks to rein in both your portions and your pants size. When you go out, order an appetizer for the main meal or split an entrée with a friend, and get used to asking for doggie bags. At home, dole out pretzels or other snacks on a plate or in a bowl—never put out the whole package (it's simply too easy to mindlessly dip your hand into a bag, and before you know it, the bag is empty). Serve meals on individual plates—don't put out bowls family-style. And along those lines, avoid giant platters—the temptation to fill them is too great. Finally, read the serving sizes on packages. "We have been so fixated on looking at fat content, we have overlooked the serving size," says Bonci. "If the cereal box says a cup, get out a measuring cup, pour some in, and learn just what a cup of cereal really looks like."

WORK YOUR JAWS. Chewy, high-fiber foods not only slow down your intake, they enter your bloodstream in turtle-like fashion, preventing your blood sugar from spiking and then dropping—along with your energy and your resistance to Milky Way bars. Choose hearty, whole grain bread instead of soft white bread. A mound of crisp greens sprinkled with crunchy carrots, broccoli florets, and sesame seeds instead of a squishy burger. A bowl of steel-cut oat bran instead of sugary, melt-in-your mouth cereal. You get the picture. Just make sure you include a fiber source at every meal.

BLADDER LEAKS

Tighten Up

❦

If you travel even short distances with women, you know that the first order of business upon arriving at a destination is often to scan for the nearest ladies room. Experts call it toilet mapping—locating bathrooms in case you get the unbearable and sometimes almost uncontrollable urge to go.

Some women wear dark, baggy clothes in case of accidents. For others, traveling long distances or sitting for hours on end is out of the question. As my friend Gina put it, "I sometimes wonder—am I headed for adult diapers?"

The quick answer is no. While thousands of people—most of them women, by the way—have bladder leakage known as urinary incontinence, it is possible to make your bladder behave. "Just because bladder leakage is common doesn't mean it's normal or that it can't be curbed—no matter what your age or gender," says Lonny Green, M.D., associate clinical professor of urology at the Medical College of Virginia and director of the Virginia Continence Center in Richmond.

WHY ME?

If you dribble when you laugh, sneeze, lift, or otherwise jostle your abdomen, you have what's called stress incontinence. It occurs because the muscles supporting the bladder have become saggy, possibly due to pregnancy, childbirth, excess belly weight, or even estrogen loss at menopause.

If you feel an overwhelming need to go and can barely make it to the bathroom, your problem is urge incontinence, or overactive bladder. For reasons scientists haven't yet been able to pinpoint, the muscle that controls urination goes into spasm even when your bladder isn't completely full. Eating foods that irritate your bladder, such as chili and chocolate, can set it off, as can antihistamines, heart medicine, and other drugs. Other possible causes include a urinary tract infection and any condition that affects the bladder nerves.

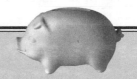

SAVE YOUR MONEY!

Don't Sit on It

Imagine lounging, fully clothed, in a recliner chair for 20 minutes several times a month—then walking away cured of bladder accidents. It could happen, but it could also cost you a bundle. The NeoControl chair, now available at some bladder-control centers, emits a pulsing magnetic field that stimulates the pelvic floor muscles to contract and relax. Sitting sessions could cost $20 or more, which may not sound so bad, but the therapy may require 10 sessions—and Kegel exercises do the same thing for free.

By menopause, most women have both forms of leaky bladder to some degree. The estrogen loss associated with menopause makes the urethra more sensitive to the "gotta go" spasms, while pelvic muscles that have grown lax fail to slow the flow.

NO-GO THERAPIES

Your doctor may suggest devices to prop up your sagging pelvic muscles (such as a vaginal ring that presses the neck of your bladder closed) or potent drugs to decrease bladder spasms, among other therapies. But odds are, you can nip your dribble in the bud on your own. The key is to start now. If you usually urinate more often than eight times a day or more than twice during the night, try one—or a combination—of these no-go therapies.

Do pelvic pushups. Exercises known as Kegels, which involve lifting and squeezing the muscles of the pelvic floor, can help stop leaks. "Strengthening these muscles can help even severe leakers stay drier," says Dr. Green. Use the same muscles you would if you were trying to hold back gas. Squeeze them and hold the contraction for 5 seconds before releasing. Repeat the sequence for a total of 5 minutes at least three times a day, gradually working up to holding each contraction for 10 seconds. Within two months, you should notice a tighter grip and more bladder control.

ON-THE-SPOT RELIEF

Ready, Set, Squeeze!

Whether you're about to sneeze, guffaw, or lift your sofa, slip in a quick pelvic squeeze beforehand. It lets your bladder know what's coming. Whenever possible, cross your legs, too. You'll avoid an accident and be able to stroll, not sprint, to the bathroom.

Delay the urge. "Going to the bathroom every time you feel the need trains your bladder to empty more frequently than it has to," says Dr. Green. To retrain it, delay the urge to go. Do a Kegel contraction and distract yourself by taking slow, deep breaths and focusing on relaxing the muscles outside your pelvis, such as your belly. Try not to panic. When you think you're ready to burst, make your way to the bathroom. Even if you can delay for only 3 counts, consider it a victory. Eventually, you'll be able to hold it for 5 counts, then 15, and then 50. Gradually lengthen the intervals between bathroom visits until you've reached 3 to 4 hours, which is normal.

DITCH THE IRRITANTS. "I've seen overactive bladders disappear when people revamp their diets to exclude substances that irritate the bladder lining," notes Milton Krisoloff, M.D., a urologist in Santa Monica, California. Cut back on caffeine, chocolate, spicy sauces, hot mustard, citrus fruits, and artificial sweeteners, all of which can irritate the bladder. And talk to your doctor if you're taking medicines such as antihistamines, tricyclic antidepressants, diuretics, and heart medications, which may also be irritating.

MAKE SURE YOU CAN GO. Counterintuitive though it may be, chronic constipation can contribute to stress or urge incontinence by placing pressure on the bladder or pelvic floor muscles. "If you clear up constipation," says Dr. Green, "you may clear up bladder leaking." To that end, eat more whole grain cereals and breads and at least two servings of juicy fruit, such as prunes, daily. Include one cooked fruit, since it passes through your system more easily. Then help your digestive tract get things moving by heading out for a brisk walk every day.

BIOFEEDBACK FOR BETTER KEGELS

It's a lot easier to beef up your pelvic floor muscles if you have a home biofeedback kit to help you figure out where the darn things are. All you have to do is place a painless, pressure-sensitive probe in your vagina. The probe is hooked to a monitoring device, so when you give your muscles a squeeze, the device "feeds back," or tells you when you've hit your mark—which, by the way, many more women do after using these kits. In fact, biofeedback can improve the success rate of Kegels by a whopping 70 percent! Look for the kits for sale on the Internet (they can run up to $60), or ask your doctor where you can buy one.

Biofeedback
MIND MACHINE
POWER

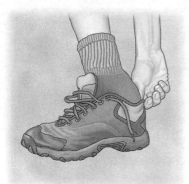

WHITTLE YOUR WAISTLINE. Studies show that women who lose 5 percent of their body weight—especially if it's bunched around their middles—have less than half as many leaking episodes. Kick-start your metabolism and shore up your bladder by doing at least 20 minutes of continuous aerobic exercise, such as walking, three times a week.

CONSIDER SUPPLEMENTS. Scan your health food store for bladder-control formulas that contain the amino acid arginine. "Naturally found in meat and other high-protein foods, arginine is converted to nitric oxide in the body, which helps prevent the bladder from going into spasm," says Dr. Green. Doctors who recommend arginine for bladder control usually suggest starting with 100 milligrams a day.

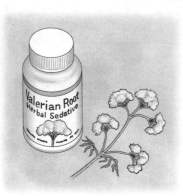

RELAX WITH VALERIAN. This Native American plant has a soothing effect on the smooth muscles of the body. "The bladder is really just one big smooth muscle," points out Dr. Green. "I recommend that patients take valerian capsules before bedtime so they don't have to hop out of bed for bathroom trips every few hours." You can find valerian at a health food store, then follow the label directions. Don't use this herb if you're taking any other medications.

BLEEDING GUMS

Protect Your Teeth and Heart

———⟩⟨⟨⟨———

Ever since I was a child, I've had a recurring dream of losing my teeth. My teeth are actually rock solid, and all of the elders in my family have similarly strong teeth, so my dream isn't necessarily rooted in reality. Nevertheless, it nags at me, and when I spied a pale pink tinge on my toothbrush, I didn't exactly panic, but I did consider it a giant red flag, a wakeup call, if you will, to pay more attention to my gums.

Gum disease, or gingivitis, develops when sticky, bacteria-laden plaque hardens into yellowish, rock-hard tartar. The bacteria release toxins that attack the gums and slowly

> ## SOMETHING TO CHEW ON
>
> Double your pleasure, double your fun—with chewing gum that contains pine bark extract, or Pycnogenol. Studies show that chewing Pycnogenol-packed gum (available at health food stores) after each meal reduces inflammation and helps slash gum bleeding by half.

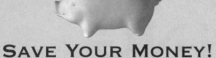
wrench them away from the teeth. Over time, the bacteria can seep below the gum line, spread to the roots of the teeth, and begin to gnaw at the ligaments and bones surrounding them. What's worse, gum disease can even predispose you to heart attacks, since inflamed gums may provide a portal through which bacteria can slip into your bloodstream and wend their way to your heart.

WHY ME?

How come your gums bleed—and your infrequently flossing friend's don't? The answer may be rooted in your genes, habits, diet, or even the time of the month.

You may come from a long line of excess plaque producers. You may be inviting swollen, bleeding gums by gorging on cookies and pastries and skimping on the milk, broccoli, and other calcium-rich foods that strengthen bones. You may be experiencing a hormonal surge—during pregnancy, before menopause, or in the midst of the menstrual cycle—that tends to pump fluid into tissues and make them more vulnerable to plaque. You may be torturing your gums with your brushing technique. Or you may be unable to wash away sticky plaque because you're short of saliva from "dry mouth," and bleeding gums could be the result.

The good news is, just as there are myriad ways to develop gum disease, there are many ways to combat it—starting with a bevy of rinses and rubs that are far more gentle than hydrogen peroxide (a standard antiseptic for diseased gums)—and a lot more tasty. Just don't delay. Even a little bleeding means that there's an infection brewing that you should take care of, pronto.

ROOT OUT BLEEDING

If your gums are bleeding and/or sore, make an appointment to have your teeth checked and cleaned by your dentist. In the meantime, try one of these do-it-yourself ways to stomp out that first invasion of bacteria before the troops really get riled up.

SWAB WITH ALOE. The gel of that kitchen-windowsill staple, the aloe vera plant, heals all tissues—including inflamed gums, notes Flora Parsa Stay, D.D.S., a dentist in Oxnard, California. Simply slice open an aloe leaf, dip a cotton swab into the gel, and apply it to your gums. Don't eat or drink for a half-hour afterward—and don't use aloe if you're pregnant.

EXPERIMENT WITH CoQ$_{10}$. "Coenzyme Q$_{10}$ is a potent antioxidant that helps tighten gum tissue so plaque can't become trapped in it," says Darin Ingels, N.D., director of New England Family Health in Southport, Connecticut. Plus, studies show it speeds the healing process and repairs tissue. While you can find CoQ$_{10}$ in some toothpastes, your best bet is to take a 30-milligram capsule (available at health food stores) with food twice daily. Or break open a capsule and dip your toothbrush in it, then press it lightly to tender gums.

GET PLENTY OF C AND E. Oranges, broccoli, and tomatoes practically drip with vitamin C, an antioxidant that toughens gums, reduces swelling, and squelches infection. Its partner

HOMEGROWN SOLUTION

◆ ◆ ◆

Gargle with Garden Flowers

The volatile oil from the daisy-like chamomile flower acts as an anti-inflammatory and can heal mucous membranes in the mouth, says Flora Parsa Stay, D.D.S. Unless you're allergic to ragweed, steep 2 tablespoons of chamomile flowers (either right out of your yard or from a health food store) in 2 cups of boiling water for 10 minutes, then strain and sip.

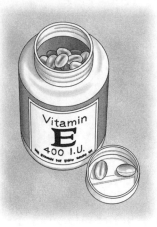

antioxidant, vitamin E, which is found in nuts and seeds, fights cell damage caused by renegade oxygen molecules called free radicals. The less you get of this potent pair, the more serious your gum disease. If you don't have kidney or stomach trouble, Dr. Stay suggests downing 1,000 milligrams of vitamin C and 400 IU of vitamin E daily. For extra protection, break open a vitamin E capsule and rub the contents on tender gums twice daily after brushing.

SPLASH WITH FOLIC ACID. Rinsing once or twice daily with a mouthwash that contains folic acid (check labels to find one that does) can help stop gum bleeding. Or you can pick up some liquid folic acid from a health food store and dab it directly onto your gums to hasten healing.

GO FOR THE GOLD. "Goldenseal should be in everyone's medicine cabinet," recommends Dr. Stay, "because it not only reduces inflammation and fights bacteria, it also contains a host of minerals, including calcium, phosphorus, potassium, and vitamins that keep gums healthy." You can mix 1 tablespoon of goldenseal powder (available at health food stores) with enough water to make a paste and apply it directly to

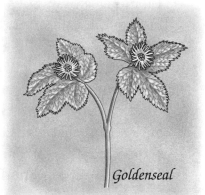

Goldenseal

tender gums. Or add 1 tablespoon of goldenseal powder and 1 teaspoon of baking soda to 1 cup of warm water, then swish and spit. Look for toothpastes that contain goldenseal, too.

TREAT IT WITH TEA TREE. The extract from the Australian malaluca tree has made its way into everything from mouthwash to dental picks to lip balm. And for good reason: It's highly antiseptic but less harsh than hydrogen peroxide. Mix the extract, which you can find at health food stores, with a little water, then rub the combo directly onto inflamed gums to fight infection.

GO GREEN. The extract from the wintergreen mint is milder than tea tree oil, but it's an excellent antiseptic that has long been used to treat wounds and stop hemorrhages, says Dr. Stay. Soak a cotton ball in wintergreen oil and dab it onto fiery gums.

SWISH WITH A SPOT OF TEA. To stop your gums from bleeding, rinse your mouth with black tea for 1 minute. Studies show that if you do this 10 times a day, you may decrease plaque buildup, which could be at the root of the bleeding. Certain chemicals in black tea, called polyphenols, suppress the growth of cavity-causing bacteria in plaque and inhibit acid production.

BRUSH WITH BAKING SODA. Baking soda provides an abundance of oxygen, and bacteria hate oxygen, says Sara Grossi, D.D.S., director of periodontal disease research at the University of Buffalo in New York. You can dip your toothbrush in a paste made with baking soda and water, or buy commercial toothpaste that lists baking soda as an ingredient. If you opt for the latter, avoid brands that contain sodium lauryl sulfate, a harsh foaming

WHEN TO DIAL THE DOC

• • • • • • • • • •

If your gums continue to bleed and feel tender despite your best self-care efforts, see your dentist. In all likelihood, he'll use a metered probe to measure the grooves, or pockets, between your gums and teeth. The deeper the probe goes, the more serious your gum disease. If you need more than a routine cleaning, a gum specialist called a periodontist can scale off the plaque and tartar from your teeth all the way down to the roots.

PURE BAKING SODA
FOR BAKING & DEODORIZING

ingredient that can irritate gum tissue.

BRUSH BELOW. Experts recommend starting your daily brushing with the insides of your lower teeth. That's the most likely site for plaque buildup because it's often the most neglected.

SPLURGE ON A SONIC. Available at most drugstores, sonic toothbrushes are three times faster than ordinary electric toothbrushes and have been shown to reverse gingivitis and help shrink gum pockets. They're pricey—costing anywhere from $75 to $100—but if you have the beginnings of gum disease, they may be well worth the investment.

MAKE YOUR MOUTH WATER. A dehydrated mouth is an ideal spawning ground for bacteria. Toss the drying, alcohol-

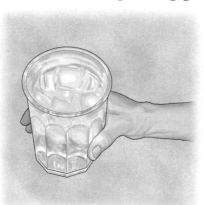

based mouthwash, cut back on those mocha cappuccinos (caffeine is dehydrating), and drink at least eight glasses of water a day. And as long as you're not pregnant, you might even consider rubbing aloe gel onto your gums in the evening to keep them moist. (Just don't eat or drink anything afterward.) If you have serious dry mouth from medica-

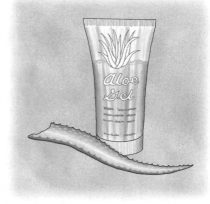

tions, look for an artificial saliva product such as Xero-Lube or Salivart at the drugstore, where you'll also find Biotene toothpaste and mouthwash. Both contain natural salivary enzymes that can be helpful.

A chronically dry mouth can be a sign of systemic conditions. Be sure to tell your doctor if this one of your symptoms.

BLOATING

Lower Your Water Level

———⧓⧓⧓———

It's never really comfortable to have a bloated belly, ankles so swollen your socks leave dents in your shins, or fingers so puffy you need a crowbar to pry off your rings. It should come as welcome news to hear that you can deflate "water weight" fairly easily—and wear whatever you want any day of the year.

WHY ME?

If you're a woman, it's probably the increase in estrogen right before menstruation that causes your bloating. Fluid that normally flows effortlessly through your bloodstream and lymph ducts accumulates in the spaces between the cells, making tissues swell and your skin plump up. In fact, some women gain a whopping 10 pounds of water weight in the week prior to their periods, when higher estrogen levels spur the body to retain sodium—which in turn makes tissues hold onto more water. Estrogen replacement drugs used to treat menopausal symptoms such as hot flashes can also make you retain water.

There are other reasons as well: Gorging on salty pretzels or tortilla chips, for instance, can leave you looking like a cream puff the next day. "Proper fluid regulation requires a balance of

A REASON NOT TO WEED

Avid weed whackers may consider it a nuisance, but bloaters should think of it as a plus—the lowly dandelion, that is. The fresh, young leaves of the dandelion plant (which the French call *pissenlit*, or "urinate in bed") act as a natural diuretic. In fact, in head-to-head tests, dandelion leaf tea was shown to be as effective as the prescription diuretic furosemide (Lasix). Drink two to four cups of tea (which you can buy prepackaged at health food stores) a day to deflate swollen tissues, suggests Michael DiPalma, N.D. Or take up to two standard capsules of dried dandelion leaf daily. You can even toss fresh leaves into your summer salads to benefit from their cleansing effect.

If you have fluid retention due to heart problems, talk to your doctor about slowly adding dandelion and decreasing your dosage of pharmaceutical diuretics and potassium supplements. Do not, under any circumstances, do it on your own.

salt and of potassium gleaned from fruits and vegetables," explains Michael DiPalma, N.D., a naturopathic physician in Newtown, Pennsylvania. "Most of us gorge on the former and skimp on the latter." As a result, our kidneys retain too much sodium and water, bulking up body tissues.

Other puffiness promoters include corticosteroid medications, blood pressure–lowering drugs, and inflammatory reactions to everything from insect bites to sunburn to bread. Belly bloating in particular can be an allergic reaction to foods (especially the gluten in wheat) or a result of lactose intolerance—a lack of the lactase enzyme that breaks down the milk sugar (lactose) in dairy foods. The lactose ferments and forms a gas, which puffs the belly.

BLOATING BE GONE!

The conventional treatment for bloating related to simple water retention is water pills, or diuretics. These drugs help the kidneys excrete excess sodium and water in the tissues, but they can also flush out important minerals such as potassium, which actually battles fluid retention. For occasional bloating—such as when you've overdone the tortilla chips or are about to menstruate—try these more natural ways to siphon off the fluid without draining your body.

SIP MINERAL-RICH TEAS. Beat bloating (and retain ample potassium) by sipping potassium-rich teas. Parsley is a good choice, as is cleavers, a nineteenth-century herb once known as bedstraw because it was used to stuff beds. "It's a common weed that acts as a diuretic and clears waste and excess fluid," explains Judith Boice, N.D., a naturopathic physician in Portland, Oregon. Just be sure to have only one cup of one of these teas a day—too much can drain minerals from your body.

CHUG ASPARAGUS JUICE. When you steam asparagus, save the water, let it cool—then gulp it down (it'll taste vaguely of asparagus, but mostly like water). "Asparagus drippings make a great diuretic," says Dr. DiPalma. Other excellent diuretic foods include artichokes, watercress, and watermelon.

ON-THE-SPOT RELIEF

Make a Silky Tea

The next time you're shucking corn, don't chuck the silk—instead, dry it and save it to make cornsilk tea, a time-honored folk remedy that will help your kidneys flush out fluids. Because cornsilk is rich in potassium, it will help balance the sodium in your system that may be making you hold water. Steep 1 tablespoon of dried silk in 1 cup of boiling water for 5 minutes. You should see an effect within an hour or two, and you can continue to drink up to three cups a day for no more than four days.

DRINK UP. That's right: Although it may seem counterintuitive, drinking ample water—at least eight glasses daily—is crucial for combating fluid retention, especially fluid that pools in your belly after eating. "Food allergies can irritate the digestive tract and cause the body to retain more fluid to try and dilute the irritating substances," says Dr. Boice. "Drinking water helps the kidneys flush it all out."

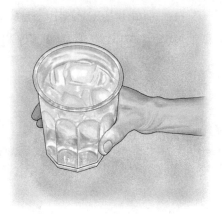

LINGER LONGER IN PRODUCE. That's where you'll find literally piles of potassium-rich foods that send puffiness packing. Among the best are sunflower seeds, dates, figs, oranges, peaches, bananas, tomatoes, and all the leafy greens—even the tops of celery stalks are rich in this precious mineral! When you finally roll into the prepared and processed food aisles, read the product labels with an eagle eye. Sodium, or salt, which promotes fluid retention, hides in everything from cereal to cheese to colas. Your goal is to keep sodium intake between 1,000 and 2,000 milligrams a day. And that can be tough: Just 2 ounces of American cheese packs 800 milligrams, and 3 cups of microwave popcorn contains 500 milligrams.

TRY TANGY SPICES. You can

WHEN TO DIAL THE DOC

• • • • • • • • • •

If you have an underlying liver, heart, or kidney condition, you need to consult your doctor if you begin to retain fluid. Likewise, talk to your physician if simply pressing on your skin leaves a dent (you may have edema, or very serious fluid retention, which can block blood flow), if you're pregnant and have sudden swelling in your face and hands (which could signal the beginning of preeclampsia—life-threatening, pregnancy-induced high blood pressure), or if you suspect that a food allergy may be behind your bloating.

use them as salt substitutes. A single teaspoon of table salt contains 2,000 milligrams of sodium, so try paprika on your popcorn or flakes of basil on your green beans instead. These and other salt substitutes can keep your sodium intake low—and the buttons on your slacks intact.

CONSIDER B$_6$. "Bloating can occur if you're deficient in vitamin B$_6$, which helps your body metabolize hormones—including the hormones that cause premenstrual bloat," says Dr. Boice. "That's why I recommend that women regularly take a B-complex supplement," she says—but you should avoid individual B vitamin supplements.

GET PUMPED. Look for a massage therapist near you who specializes in what's called lymphatic massage, a rhythmic pumping and kneading of the lymph nodes on the sides of the neck, under the arms, and in the groin to boost circulation and flush away fluid buildup. The technique works especially well for hormonal bloat, notes Dr. DiPalma.

BODY ODOR

Lose the Stink

———◦◦◦◦◦———

A woman I know carries a supply of baby wipes with her everywhere—and her son hasn't worn diapers in 15 years. "I use them to wipe my armpits so odor doesn't seep into my clothes," she reveals. "I'm sick of throwing away silk blouses."

Odds are, you know the feeling. We've all had occasions when no matter how frequently or ferociously we've scrubbed, we smell more foul than fresh, and the lingering odor has made our favorite sweater sets into instant castoffs. The culprits are bacteria that thrive on skin. When they devour the fatty sweat produced by the apocrine glands in the underarms, scalp, and genitals, the result is a very pungent smell.

WHY ME?

Aside from general odor that makes you feel the need to rub Ban all over your body, you could have genital odor from a vaginal infection, bad breath from gum disease, or fetid feet from a foot infection. You could also have an underlying condition, such as liver disease, diabetes, or a zinc deficiency, that causes unfamiliar and even unsavory smells. The most likely reason, however, that your natural scent has turned somewhat sour is that you have a digestive problem of some sort.

"Just as old garbage can stink up your whole house, the odor from decaying matter in your intestines can radiate throughout your body," says Daniel DeLapp, N.D., instructor of dermatology at the National College of Naturopathic Medicine in Portland, Oregon. For instance, some people can't metabolize foods that contain large amounts of the nutrient choline, which is found primarily in eggs, organ meats (liver and kidneys in particular), nuts, milk, and legumes. Eating these foods can cause a fishy body odor. Red meat can also create a stink. "Protein is harder to break down in the gut," says Dr. DeLapp, "and the more food that's left hanging around, the more chance for smelly bacterial by-products to hang around, too."

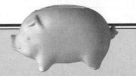

SAVE YOUR MONEY!

Go for the Stone

If you're going through deodorants and antiperspirants like there's no tomorrow, consider trading your stick for a stone—a crystal deodorant stone, that is. Not only will one stone last much longer than a standard stick, it may be much kinder to your system. Standard antiperspirants contain aluminum chloride, which completely plugs up the sweat glands; crystal stones contain alunogenite, a natural astringent that may only partially block the glands.

STANCH THE STENCH

Regardless of the source of your odor, Dr. DeLapp suggests skipping the conventional treatments, which range from injecting botulinum toxin to paralyze the sweat glands to loading up on antibiotics to even having surgery to snip the sweat glands. "These approaches don't really get at the heart of your odor problem," he says. "My view is that if you change your internal environment by watching what you eat, you discourage the proliferation of bacteria, and the smell will disappear."

Of course, if you want to keep your season stadium seats, you may need to try some gentle stopgap measures to squelch odor while you're improving your waste disposal system. Here are some ways to do both.

GET THE GOOD BUGS. The best way to control odor-causing "bad" bacteria in your gut is to fill it with "good" bacteria. You can do this by eating yogurt that contains live, active cultures of *Lactobacillus acidophilus* (check the label; frozen yogurt and yogurt-covered snacks don't have live cultures) or down-

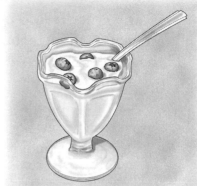

ing acidophilus capsules, which you can find at any health food store.

CRUNCH ON CRUDITÉS. Uncooked veggies and fruits provide roughage that helps escort smelly waste through—and out of—your intestinal tract. Cooked foods, on the other hand, are slower to move through your intestines. Plus, says Dr. DeLapp, "when you cook foods, you change the oxidation, which can prompt more odor during digestion."

SLURP YOUR SALAD. "Using a juicer is a great way to get a range of chlorophyll-rich foods such as kale, chard, and other dark green vegetables all in one shot," explains Jennifer Reid, N.D., a naturopathic physician at the Columbia River

LEMON AID

Giving your body a steady stream of water—no fewer than eight glasses a day—is one of the best ways to flush out toxins and eliminate the stink. But Jeanette Jacknin, M.D., a dermatologist in Scottsdale, Arizona, offers a twist on this advice: Every evening, add a squeeze of fresh lemon juice and 1 teaspoon of chlorophyll—available at health food stores—to your glass. Both will help restore the pH balance of your blood and give any "bad" bacteria in your gut the boot.

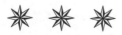

Natural Medicine Clinic in Troutdale, Oregon.

Chlorophyll can restore the pH balance of blood that's too acidic—and therefore too friendly to bad bacteria—due to a diet heavy in meat and other proteins. Not ready to invest in yet another kitchen appliance? Look for a commercial wheatgrass beverage at your health food store and drink it with yogurt at lunch.

SNACK ON PUMPKIN SEEDS. They provide a good, concentrated supply of the mineral zinc, a deficiency of which can prompt odor. If you're not keen on the seeds, you can take 30 to 50 milligrams of zinc in tablet form daily to help reduce body and foot odor—but not without your doctor's guidance. If taken continuously, zinc can deplete copper and other minerals, and it could be toxic. "In fact, I wouldn't exceed 15 milligrams a day without guidance from a health-care practitioner," warns Dr. Reid.

SLAP ON SODA. That lowly box of baking soda you use to keep your fridge moisture-free and smelling sweet can do the same for your feet and underarms, says Nelson Lee Novick,

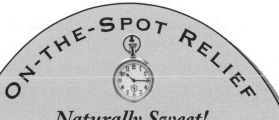

ON-THE-SPOT RELIEF

Naturally Sweet!

Fennel tea is a sweet postmeal drink—especially if you've had garlic, onions, or other smelly foods that not only cause bad breath but may also make odor pour from your pores. In fact, fennel is such an excellent natural deodorizer that Indian restaurants often offer fennel seeds instead of after-dinner mints. Another on-the-spot secret: Parsley is a great source of odor-eating chlorophyll, so if you mistakenly ordered a garlic-heavy dish, simply gobble up your garnish.

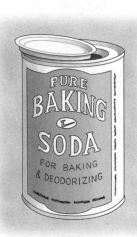

PURE
BAKING
&
SODA
FOR BAKING
& DEODORIZING

M.D., associate clinical professor of dermatology at Mount Sinai School of Medicine in New York City. Pat the nonirritating, hypoallergenic powder under your arms and on the soles of your feet. Repeat at least twice daily, if you can.

ADD ANTI-ODOR HERBS. That tangy-smelling sage you use to season poultry stuffing contains compounds that can tame wetness, plus oils that fight bacteria. Piney-scented rosemary is another natural antibacterial herb. Mix 1 tablespoon of each ground herb with 1 cup of baking soda and sprinkle on any odor-causing body part.

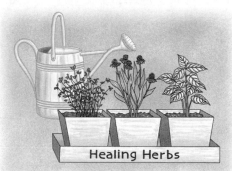

Healing Herbs

SIP YOUR SAGE. Sage tea can help curb sweat gland activity and may be especially helpful when your perspiration is stress induced. Simply steep 2 teaspoons of dried sage in 1 cup of boiling water for 10 minutes, then strain and savor in small doses—but only during tense situations. Ingesting sage on a regular basis may cause dizziness, hot flashes, and other problems. Don't drink sage tea if you're pregnant or nursing.

GET SWEATY. Encouraging sweating—say, by sitting in a sauna—can help detoxify your system, keep your liver and gastrointestinal tract functioning at optimal levels, and diminish body odor, says Dr. DeLapp.

SOAK YOUR STINKY TOES. Immerse your smelly feet in a solution of 1 part warm water and 1 part vinegar for 10 minutes twice a day for three weeks. Vinegar baths can often eradicate an offensive smell for good, says Dr. DeLapp.

RUN OFF ATHLETE'S FOOT. Stamp out smelly athlete's foot fungus by steeping your feet in a basin of warm water spiked with 2 to 3 teaspoons of tea tree oil. Soak them for 15 minutes twice daily, and during treatment, go barefoot or wear open-toed shoes as often as possible. Also change into clean socks several times a day.

CAN THE CAFFEINE. You probably already know that odorous oils in garlic, onions, fish, and exotic spices can linger in your body. But coffee and tea are also bad news because they increase the activity of the apocrine sweat glands. Try eliminating these offenders and see if that foul odor fades. Also, keep in mind that a high-fat, high-sugar, low-fiber diet can upset the balance of bacteria in your intestines, throw a monkey wrench into your digestion, and provoke odor.

QUESTION YOUR MEDS. Like fatty, sugary, low-fiber foods, antibiotics can upset the pH balance in your intestines, inhibit your digestion, and increase body odor. But they aren't the only pharmaceutical offenders: betaine (Cystadane), which removes excess homocysteine from the blood; bupropion (Wellbutrin) and venlafaxine (Effexor), which are prescribed for depression; and pilocarpine (Salagen), which is used to treat dry mouth, can all raise a stink, says W. Steven Pray, Ph.D., professor of non-prescription drug products at Southwestern Oklahoma State University in Weatherford. If you suspect medications may be at the root of your trouble, talk to your doctor.

BRITTLE NAILS

Sheath Them in Velvet

———◦◦◦———

Iwield my fingernails like tiny, built-in Swiss Army knives. I use them to slice open packages wrapped with yards upon yards of tape, tighten the minuscule screws in my eyeglasses, and clean unidentifiable, crusty gunk from between my keyboard buttons. They're fabulously functional, those fingernails—but stubby, brittle, peeling, and unbeautiful. Over the years, though, I've learned that they don't have to be.

WHY ME?

According to the experts, while you can inherit fingernails that tend to be brittle, the most common reason for frail nails is that we abuse them by dunking them in and out of water and exposing them to a waste dump's worth of caustic chemicals—often without even knowing it. Nail polish remover, which contains the harsh drying agent acetone, is among the worst. Frequent applications of the smelly stuff can make nails peel and the tips snap like potato chips.

TOUGH AS NAILS

Strengthening fingernails is considered a cosmetic, do-it-yourself job, so your doctor isn't likely to offer much help. The good news is, you don't need him: There are many ways you can make weak nails strong all on your own. Here's a handful of tricks to try.

QUAFF CARROTS. Carrot juice contains loads of calcium and phosphorus and is great for strengthening nails, says Jeanette Jacknin, M.D., a dermatologist in Scottsdale, Arizona. Try replacing your O.J. with the other orange-colored juice several times a week.

CRACK AN EGG FOR CRACKED NAILS. Eggs are packed with protein and sulfur, both of which speed nail growth. Plus, they're rich in biotin, the B vitamin that helps your body make and use amino acids, the building blocks of protein. Long ago, biotin was found to strengthen horses' hooves, and more recent studies have shown it works similarly for us two-legged types. Does the thought of eating eggs regularly have your stomach feeling, well, scrambled? Soybean flour, brewer's yeast, cauliflower, and peanut butter are also rich in biotin.

TAKE A MULTI. Bendable, easily breakable nails could indicate a deficiency of zinc, iron, essential fatty acids, or silica and

ON-THE-SPOT RELIEF

Butter Up Your Nails

I recently hit upon a method to keep my nails strong and pliable when the mercury dips: Before bed, I coat each nail with shea butter, a super-thick, velvety-smooth cream made from the African mangifolia tree. It naturally contains iron, vitamin B, and calcium—all nutrients said to be necessary for harder nails—but it's also laced with lavender to heal cracked cuticles. Once my nails are slathered, I cover my hands with cotton gloves and hit the pillow. After just three nights of this routine, my nails were noticeably stronger.

other trace minerals. Try popping a multivitamin/mineral supplement and see if your nails improve. Dr. Jacknin suggests looking for a formula that contains 1,200 milligrams of calcium and about 15 milligrams of zinc, both of which contribute to nail strength.

AID ABSORPTION. Brittle nails can be a sign of poor digestion and protein absorption. To improve both, you can supplement with hydrochloric acid to boost the normal production of this acid in your stomach. First you have to determine if you're indeed acid deficient, though. Unless you have been diagnosed with ulcers, break a tablet of a digestive-enzyme formula that contains betaine hydrochloride (available at drugstores) and take half of it before the last bite of a meal. If you notice a burning sensation or feel as if you have indigestion, skip the supplements—you probably have plenty of stomach acid. If there's no burning, however, Dr. Jacknin suggests taking one or two tablets after each meal for at least three months. In that time, your digestion and protein absorption should improve—as should the strength of your nails.

DUNK IN DILL. Dill contains nail-strengthening calcium and other minerals, while horsetail is a solid source of silica, a mineral that gives hair, skin, and nails flexibility and strength, says Kathlyn Quatrochi, N.D., a naturopathic physician in Oak Glen, California. Steep $1/2$ teaspoon of extract from each herb (available in health food stores) in 1 cup of hot water, wait until the "tea" cools, then soak your nails in it three times a week.

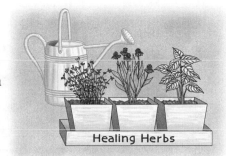

Healing Herbs

WEAR RUBBERS. Too much moisture makes nails brittle. In fact, "under a microscope, the cell arrangement in waterlogged nails looks like Swiss cheese—they lack solid bonding," says Jere D. Guin, M.D., professor of dermatology at the University of Arkansas for Medical Sciences in Little Rock. To keep your nails from absorbing too much water, have a pair of rubber or latex gloves handy when you're dunking your digits in dishwater.

MOISTURIZE YOUR MITTS. Check lotion labels and find a brand with alpha hydroxy acids (AHAs), then apply it to your nails whenever you've had your hands in water. AHAs can reverse brittleness by increasing the bonding of cells.

GO BARE. The problem isn't so much applying and reapplying nail polish as it is removing it. Most polish removers contain the harsh chemical acetone, which zaps the moisture—and the strength—right out of nails. Look for products that contain acetane, a gentler alternative. And skip the artificial nails entirely. "Nail glues wreck the nail bed," warns Dr. Guin.

BRONCHITIS

Quiet the Barking

———————◦⊶◦⊷◦———————

There are times when I call my mother that it almost sounds as if I've reached Vito Corleone of *The Godfather*. Her voice is raspy and cracked, and she's wracked with the dry, tickling cough of acute bronchitis—a temporary inflammation of the mucous membranes of the bronchi, the main, branching airways of the lungs.

These irritated passages swell and produce excess mucus, which your body attempts to clear by coughing. When your cough is dry and "unproductive," you don't bring up any phlegm. When you have a deep, window-rattling, "productive" cough that sounds like a seal barking, you bring up gobs of sometimes clear, sometimes white, sometimes yellowish-gray mucus. Both coughs are hallmarks of bronchitis, as are achy muscles from nonstop hacking, a runny nose, a slight fever—and a voice as hoarse as Brando's.

WHY ME?

The bug that's responsible for most cases of bronchitis is a virus—not bacteria, as was once thought. "You catch acute bronchitis in the same way you catch a cold—from touching someone with it, then touching your own nose or mouth," says David Zeiger, D.O., a family physician in Chicago. In fact, acute bronchitis typically follows a cold, when the virus travels from your nose to your air passages. For some people, however, the problem recurs at regular intervals—say, once in the spring and again in the fall—and is linked to airborne allergens or pollutants that inflame or irritate the bronchi.

Whatever their source, the symptoms of acute bronchitis usually last about a week. If you've been coughing—especially in the morning when you get up—for more than three months, you don't have acute bronchitis. You'll need to consult your physician for a definitive diagnosis (and to rule out asthma), but you probably have what's called chronic bronchitis, a separate and serious disease.

As its name suggests, chronic bronchitis is not temporary. The lining of the bronchial tubes becomes permanently inflamed and thickened, leaving you more prone to pneumonia and possibly serious lung disease. Cigarette smoking, toxic gases, and air pollution in the environment or workplace are often to blame.

HALT THE HACKING

Most cases of acute bronchitis, like most colds, disappear on their own after several miserable days. If you seek help to nudge it along, your doctor may prescribe an inhaler (the kind you

WHEN TO DIAL THE DOC

· · · · · · · · · · ·

Contact your doctor immediately if your coughing keeps you awake at night, interferes with your daily activities, or lasts longer than six weeks; if the mucus you're coughing up becomes thicker, darker green, yellow, or bloody; or if you become breathless or have a fever. You could have pneumonia or asthma, both of which require immediate treatment.

would use if you had asthma) to help open your bronchial tubes and clear out mucus. But there are literally dozens of gentle, do-it-yourself ways to accomplish the same thing. In fact, many of these strategies have the same effect as asthma drugs, but with fewer pesky side effects. Here's a rundown of the best remedies to check with your doctor.

SKIP THE SUNDAE. When you were a kid, you may have been given ice cream to soothe that tickle in your throat, but when it comes to bronchitis, it's a no-no. "You want to lay off foods that produce phlegm and those that cause inflammation," says Dr. Zeiger. This means skipping not only dairy foods but also wheat, soy, sugar, margarine, peanut butter, preserved meats, and processed foods. What's left? Namely fish, legumes, and green vegetables—all of which are rich in magnesium, which helps relax the smooth muscles of your bronchial tubes so you can breathe easier.

EAT GOBS OF GARLIC. One of garlic's key components—the volatile oil allicin—helps relax the bronchi and allows more air to pass through them. Garlic also stimulates the immune system and reduces phlegm. One suggestion: Try lacing your chicken soup—a tried-and-true respiratory infection fighter—with lots of garlic.

CONSIDER QUERCETIN. For a healthy, tasty twist, add curry to your recipes, especially if your bronchitis is allergy related. This Indian spice contains turmeric, which is a great source of quercetin, a bioflavonoid-antihistamine combo that can calm reactivity in the airways. Or simply supplement with three 200- to 300-milligram capsules of quercetin (available at health food stores) a day—one before breakfast, lunch, and dinner—for as long as your symptoms last, suggests Michael DiPalma, N.D., a naturopathic physician in Newtown, Pennsylvania.

TRY THE REISHI RX.
Studies indicate that the reishi mushroom—a reddish-orange fungus that grows on the bark of withered Japanese plum trees—may be highly effective for treating bronchitis. In fact, in one study, people with bronchitis who took reishi extracts had a 60 to 90 percent improvement in their symptoms. The typical adult dosage for acute bronchitis is 30 drops of reishi extract (available at health food stores) added to a glass of water every 2 to 3 hours while symptoms last.

APPLY AN ONION POULTICE. Like garlic, onions contain the volatile oil allicin, which can open your airways by relaxing your bronchi. Coat a cast-iron skillet with olive oil and add a handful of chopped onions, a teaspoon of apple cider vinegar, and a pinch of cornstarch.

Cook over low heat to make a paste. Let the paste cool and place it on a cloth. Lay the cloth on your bare chest and cover it with plastic wrap, add another cloth, and top everything with a heating pad set on low.

WRAP IT UP!

You can short-circuit bronchitis by flushing out mucus with hot-and-cold wraps. Here's how: Immerse a towel in water and wring it out, then heat it in the microwave until hot, says Jennifer Reid, N.D., a naturopathic physician at the Columbia River Natural Medicine Clinic in Troutdale, Oregon. Next, lay a wool blanket over your chest and cover it with a sheet. Place the steamy towel on top of the sheet and cover it with another blanket. Let your chest soak in the moist heat for 5 minutes to bring the blood to the surface. Next, repeat the process with a very cold towel, which will shunt blood away from your chest. All the while, have someone massage your legs, rubbing vigorously toward your heart for 10 minutes. The heat and cold, combined with the rubbing, create a kind of pump to flush out phlegm and draw white blood cells into circulation to kill off the virus that's behind your bronchitis.

"The onion will be absorbed into your body," says Dr. DiPalma. "You'll know, because you'll have the onion breath to prove it."

REACH FOR ECHINACEA. In one study, people who took echinacea twice a day for eight weeks reduced the duration of respiratory tract infections by half—possibly because the herb boosts the body's infection-fighting cells so they attack the virus with a vengeance. You can find tinctures at a health food store. "Drink 1 teaspoon of echinacea tincture added to a shot glass of warm water two or three times daily for the duration of your symptoms," suggests Dr. Zeiger. Disregard the slight numbness you may feel in your mouth from the herb, he says; it will quickly pass. But don't use echinacea if you have an autoimmune disease such as lupus, rheumatoid arthritis, or multiple sclerosis or if you are pregnant or nursing.

GET LOADS OF C. As long as you don't have kidney or stomach problems, you can safely dilute 1 to 2 teaspoons of buffered, powdered vitamin C—a nutrient shown to cut coughing and wheezing

ON-THE-SPOT RELIEF

Broncho-Buster Spread

To get mucus flowing, try this broncho-buster cracker spread suggested by James A. Duke, Ph.D., president and CEO of Duke's Herbal Vineyard in Fulton, Maryland. Mix small amounts of garlic, ginger, mustard, turmeric, chopped chile peppers, and horseradish into a paste. Spread very small amounts on crackers and nibble gingerly, one tiny bite at a time. The ingredients will make everything run, promises Dr. Duke—your eyes, your nose, and even the thick mucus clogging your bronchial tubes.

time in half—in a glass of juice or water and sip it throughout the day, says Dr. Zeiger. Or you can take a 500-milligram tablet every 4 hours while your symptoms last or until your stools become loose. Having diarrhea means you've reached your body's limit for vitamin C.

TREAT IT WITH TEA. Search your local health food store for teas containing mullein, colt's-foot, marshmallow root, and aniseed—all excellent bronchodilators, suggests Jamison Starbuck, N.D., a naturopathic physician in Missoula, Montana. "They're especially helpful for making unproductive coughs productive," he says. Combine equal parts of each and add 2 teaspoons of the mixture to 1 cup of boiling water. Cover and steep for 10 minutes, then drink four times a day. Prefer a different blend? Try one that includes thyme, fennel seed, and English plantain, all of which will also open your bronchial passages.

TAKE A BATH. Climb into a steaming tub laced with 2 drops each of eucalyptus, thyme, and rosemary oil, plus a cup or

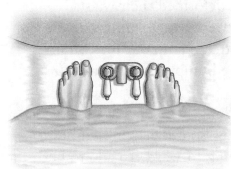

so of Epsom salts. "The steam will increase the flow of nasal mucus; the molecules from the oils will dilate your small airways, easing your breathing; and the Epsom salts contain bronchi-relaxing magnesium that's absorbed through the skin," says Dr. Starbuck.

BUNIONS AND HEEL SPURS

Keep Your Feet Happy

———◦◦◦———

We may think we've come a long way since women wore corsets that severely pinched and even deformed their waists, but sometimes I wonder. Here in the twenty-first century, after all, many of us willingly slip on shoes that cramp our toes, strain our arches—and, experts say, encourage bumpy growths and even painful deformities.

In fact, one woman I know with a longtime penchant for pointy-toed pumps has feet that are now so misshapen that her toes veer off to the sides instead of facing forward. To add to her discomfort, she also has a bunion—a protruding bump of tissue on the joint of her big toe. Wearing shoes with insufficient toe room forced her big toe to angle toward her other toes, and that unsightly bunion was the result.

My friend Ellen's feet look lovely, but they're actually just as problematic—and painful. Years of wearing comfy, skimpy-soled shoes strained her arch to the point where she developed a bony calcium deposit, or spur, within her heel. A spur is visible only on an x-ray, and by itself, it often doesn't hurt, but the pain from the overstretched arch that "spurred" its formation can be excruciating. "It felt like I had a knife stabbing my heel every time I chased after my toddler," the busy working mom says.

GIVE PAIN THE BOOT

Now that you know your feet can't take the pressure, you have extra incentive to nip bunions and spurs in the bud. Here's how to keep foot pain from ruining your stride.

SMOOTH ON A SOOTHER. "One of the best painkillers for bunions I've found is called Fortex," says John Hahn, N.D., D.P.M., a naturopathic physician and podiatrist in Bend, Oregon. "It packs aspirin-like salicylate in a peanut-oil base, and it can penetrate the skin and quell inflammation rather quickly." Check for Fortex at a health food store and smooth the cream on your bunion several times daily, if you can.

EASE THE PRESSURE. Surround your burgeoning bunion with over-the-counter, doughnut-shaped moleskin or a gel-filled pad to reduce pressure and friction from shoes. Check your drugstore or supermarket for protective pads impregnated with anti-inflammatory medicines. They'll deliver first aid to your

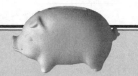

SAVE YOUR MONEY!

Forgo Fancy Foot Aids

It's not that orthotics—custom-made shoe inserts that subtly change the way your feet move when you walk—don't relieve heel pain. It's just that studies show that over-the-counter insoles, combined with exercises that stretch the arch, Achilles tendon, and calf, may offer the same relief at a fraction of the cost. Another tip: You're better off cutting a hole in a cushioned insole under the painful part of your heel rather than purchasing a heel cup.

bunion as they cushion it.

KEEP 'EM IN LINE. If your big toe is starting to drift and a bunion is sprouting, a sponge-rubber toe spacer, which you can find at any drugstore, can keep it from angling outward and relieve the pressure while you're wearing shoes. Start with a small spacer and gradually use wider ones until your toe feels comfortable.

STRETCH BEFORE RISING. "Stretching out heel pain is the very best way not only to get rid of it but also to prevent it from recurring," explains Ronald Jensen, D.P.M., a podiatrist with the Sutter Gould Medical Group in Modesto, California. Instead of just hopping out of bed in the morning, grab a towel, scarf, or belt and loop it around the ball of your foot. Pull the towel so that the front of your foot and your toes are pointing toward your face. Stretch your arch to the point of discomfort and hold for 30 seconds. Repeat three times, then rotate your ankles three or four times in each direction. Then you'll be ready to get out of bed!

SLEEP FLEXED. When your foot is relaxed, such as when you're sleeping, the muscles in the arch tend to shorten and contract. Then, as you step out of bed in the morning, those muscles are instantly yanked—and often overstretched—when your foot is forced into a flexed position. A removable, bracelike night splint can keep your foot flexed and passively stretch your arch and Achilles tendon so they don't seize up and cause stabbing pain in the morning. If you'd like to try it, talk to your doctor. Studies indicate you should see relief within three months—and not only if you buy the most expensive brand (some splints can set you back $100). All night splints, even the cheaper ones, are effective.

LOOSEN UP. Tight calf muscles can overstretch your heel and arch, so one of the best ways to keep your arches limber is to loosen up your calves with wall pushups. Stand facing a wall with your arms straight in front of you and your palms flat against the wall. Keeping your heels on the floor and your body straight, bend your elbows and lean forward until your nose touches the wall. If you don't feel the stretch in your calves and Achilles tendons, move farther from the wall and start over.

TOE A 2 X 4. Keep a short board on the floor near the

BRING ON THE HEAT

On your tongue, the fiery capsaicin in red pepper makes you want to guzzle a gallon of water. But when you apply capsaicin cream (available in drugstores) to a painful heel, you'll feel sweet relief. Capsaicin relieves pain by gradually decreasing the concentration of something called substance P, which transmits pain signals to the brain. Plus, it helps warm the muscles surrounding the heel that go into spasm due to an overstretched arch, says John Hahn, N.D., D.P.M. When these muscles bunch up, they can irritate the nerves in the heel. Applying capsaicin (following the package directions) can help short-circuit the pain-spasm-pain cycle. The cream stings, so be careful not to get it in your eyes or on any area of broken skin, and wash your hands well after using it.

kitchen sink. When you're doing dishes or washing vegetables, place the ball of your foot on the board and keep your heel on the floor. This will stretch out your arch.

WORK YOUR TOOTSIES. To flex your arches and Achilles tendons—and minimize heel pain—plop a towel on the floor in front of your TV chair and use your bare toes to grab it and pull it toward you. Or place a few marbles on the floor near a cup. Keeping your heel on the floor, use your toes to pick up the marbles and drop them into the cup.

SHELVE THOSE SLIPPERS. To reduce heel pain, you really need to wear thick-soled shoes with rubber heels and arch support whenever possible—and that means during your downtime, too. Slippers and flat sandals just don't offer enough support.

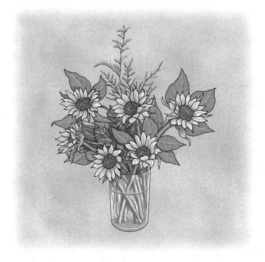

BURNS

Beat the Heat

———◦◦◦———

We have a lot of heat in our lives—and I don't mean the steamy stuff on premium cable. I'm thinking of dry heat from barbecues and ovens; moist heat from boiling pots of pasta and whistling teakettles; and electrical heat from space heaters and hair dryers. It's no wonder, then, that we get singed.

Recently, I seared my fingers on a spoon marooned in sputtering oil while I was stir-frying. In a flash, the burn stung and turned redder than a chile pepper. Experts classify burns like mine—the type that affect only the top layer of skin, or epidermis—as first-degree burns. A second-degree, or "blistering," burn penetrates to the second layer of skin, the dermis. A third-degree burn penetrates all the layers of skin, destroying the nerves and blood vessels there and leaving the skin looking charred or possibly white, yellow, or bright red. Finally, a fourth-degree burn—the worst type—damages the muscles, bones, and internal tissue. There's massive loss of body fluids, and the damage is always extensive and life-threatening.

DOUSE THE BURN

As you might guess, third- and fourth-degree burns aren't something the average person can treat—the risk of infection

MOTHER NATURE'S BEST BURN REMEDY

To hasten healing and guard against infection, you can't do much better than the thick juice inside the leaves of the aloe plant—even if you head to the hospital. "Aloe's so effective that it's included in a product developed for burn victims to reduce the need for skin grafting," says Jennifer Reid. N.D. Simply cut a notch in a leaf, squeeze until the juice appears, and apply it directly to the burn. The cooling liquid will ease pain, keep skin from blistering, stave off infection, and speed wound healing by helping fresh skin cells grow.

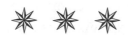

and scarring is simply too great. Burns that severe require hospital care, including surgical removal of burned tissue, grafts to replace damaged skin, antibiotics to manage any infection, and constant monitoring to guard against fluid loss.

For first- and second-degree burns, however, you don't need a medical degree to put out the fire, prevent infection, and reduce the chance of an ugly scar. All you need is a cool head—and the following tips.

COOL IT. "Put out the flames, wash off the chemicals, or break contact with whatever is causing the burn," says Jeanette Jacknin, M.D., a dermatologist in Scottsdale, Arizona. Then immerse the burn in cool water. If you can't hold the burned area under a running faucet, cover it very lightly with a cloth soaked with cool water. By immediately cooling a heat or chemical burn and continuing to immerse it in cool water for at least 30 minutes, you can reduce its size and depth. Just one caveat: Be sure the water is cool, not icy. Ice shunts blood away from the area, and as it returns, it creates throbbing pain.

HOLD THE OIL. "Putting butter or any oily substance on a burn is the worst thing you can do, because it will seal in the heat," says Jennifer Reid, N.D., a naturopathic physician at the

Columbia River Natural Medicine Clinic in Troutdale, Oregon. "After heat singes your skin, it continues to cook the tissues, so you want to try to cool the burn immediately. For that to happen, the heat has to be able to escape."

CLEAN IT WITH CALENDULA. This herb is an anti-inflammatory, astringent (cleanser), and antiseptic (germ killer), all rolled into one. Plus, it helps repair tissues and prevent scarring. "Some physicians advise applying calendula cream directly to a burn," notes Dr. Reid, "but I prefer to add several drops of calendula tincture to a cup of water, dip a cloth in the mixture, and dab the cloth onto the wound a day or two after the burn occurred so it won't sting the tissues." You can find both calendula cream and tincture at health food stores.

APPLY A POULTICE. The leaves and roots of the comfrey plant contain the healing agent allantoin, which stimulates healthy tissue growth. To make a cooling, cell-growth-encouraging poultice, simply mash 1 cup of fresh leaves or soak 1 cup of dried leaves in enough water to cover them (you can find both at health food stores). Then wrap the mash in a thin cloth and apply it to the burn as needed.

ON-THE-SPOT RELIEF

Season Your Singe

Did you ever accidentally brush against your piping hot grill and singe your finger? Instead of yelping all the way to the kitchen, where you keep your aloe, just mash up some of the raw garlic or onion you may have next to the grill, then apply it directly to the burn. This simple makeshift poultice will cool the area, act as an antiseptic, and help ease the pain.

PAINT ON PLANTAIN. If the blisters on your wound burst, dab the burn with water and apply plantain. This antibacterial Native American plant contains the healing agent allantoin and is sometimes called nature's Bactine because it's good for healing all kinds of wounds, says Michael DiPalma, N.D, a naturopathic physician in Newtown, Pennsylvania. Brew a tea (you can find packaged plantain tea at a health food store), let it cool, and apply the liquid to your burn.

SWAB WITH SWEET OIL. Ever since French perfume chemist René-Maurice Gattefossé healed his burned hand by plunging it in a vat of lavender oil, this scented herb has been used to guard against infection and prevent

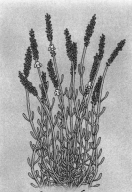

Lavender

scarring. Apply several drops of oil (available at health food stores) directly to your burn throughout the day, suggests Dr. DiPalma.

SLICK ON ST. JOHN'S WORT. You may know this herb for its reputation as a treatment for minor depression, but it also helps heal minor burns quickly and with minimal scarring, says Dr. Jacknin. Apply the extract (available at health food stores) directly to the burn several times a day.

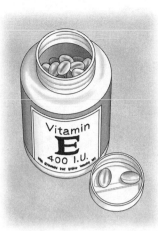

NOURISH YOUR SKIN. If your burn is serious, your body's supply of vitamin E may be diminished. To replenish your stores, take 400 IU daily until the burn heals, says Dr. Jacknin. When it's starting to heal, you can also break open a vitamin E capsule and apply the contents directly to the burn twice daily to help fight cell damage.

FEED IT WITH C. As long as you don't have kidney or stomach problems, you can take 1,000 milligrams of vitamin C a day to reduce cell damage as you heal. You can also use it topically to speed healing. Just stir 2 tablespoons of powdered vitamin C into 1/2 cup of aloe juice, then apply the mixture directly to the burn.

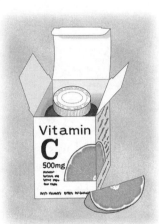

SNACK ON PUMPKIN SEEDS. They pack a lot of crunch and even more zinc, which helps wound healing, says Dr. Jacknin. So munch a bunch!

CANCER

Manage the Cure

———◆◆◆———

If getting cancer is one of the greater, more terrifying blows in life, being treated for it is like getting hit when you're down. "The diagnosis was scary enough," says Laura, my husband's colleague, who recently endured radiation therapy for cancer of the adrenal glands. "But when I was getting radiation, I had this equally strong fear that I was poisoning my body."

If you're among the more than one million Americans diagnosed with cancer each year, using a variety of resources to get you through the one-two punch of the disease and its treatment is vital. "First, you're zapped by the systemic effects of the cancer itself," explains Karen Lawson, M.D., director of integrative and clinical services at the Center for Spirituality and Healing at the University of Minnesota in Minneapolis. Then, whether or not you have surgery, your illness is likely to be compounded by the chemotherapy and radiation used to treat the cancer.

HANDLING SIDE EFFECTS

The drugs used in chemotherapy—the process of infusing the body with a toxin that destroys rapidly reproducing cells—

affect healthy cells as well as cancer cells. As a result, if you're undergoing chemotherapy, you may experience extreme fatigue, nausea, hair loss, and concentration problems as side effects. You may also develop mouth sores, which can discourage you from eating—and getting the wealth of healing nutrients your embattled body so desperately needs.

Radiation therapy—which focuses a beam of radiation on the cancer site—is also used to kill cancer cells, and like chemo, it destroys some healthy ones as well. Nausea and extreme fatigue are often the result.

The good news is, most of the side effects of cancer therapy fade after the treatment ends, when your healthy cells have a chance to grow again. The bad news is, the side effects can be pretty awful while they last.

BOOST YOUR IMMUNE SYSTEM

In a research study, more than half of a group of people with cancer who received regular massages experienced an increase in immune function. Both their white blood cell counts and their natural killer cell activity went up! Plus, massage after surgery can help drain off fluids that build up in the lymphatic system. Ask your cancer specialist for the name of a massage therapist near you who specializes in lymphatic drain massage, or contact the American Massage Therapy Association at (888) 843-2682 for a referral.

If your side effects are debilitating, your doctor may prescribe a prescription anti-nausea drug such as ondansetron (Zofran), which can settle your stomach—but can also cost up to $16 for a single pill. The doctor might also prescribe megestrol (Megace), which mimics the hormone progesterone, to jump-start your appetite. The trouble is, Megace can also jump-start hot flashes and other annoying symptoms. And when you're already grappling with serious side effects, you don't need any more.

IMAGINE NO PAIN

Picture this: A noninvasive way to reduce not only your nausea and anxiety but also the amount of pain medication you need—by half! That's exactly the promise of guided imagery, "a profound form of stress relief that can help lessen pain from cancer treatment," says Karen Lawson, M.D.

Here's what's involved: With either a tape or a practitioner to guide you, you learn breathing exercises and how to develop mental images that suggest relaxation or safety and evoke all five senses, which help you gradually gain control of your mood and decrease your feelings of anxiety. Studies prove that in the process, you'll reduce your pain and boost your immune function. To find out more, talk to your doctor.

HEAL YOUR BODY, MIND, AND SPIRIT

Complementary therapies, while not cure-alls, can often help ease queasiness, fatigue, and other debilitating side effects of chemo and radiation. Plus, nondrug therapies such as meditation have another edge: In addition to boosting your immune system, they may promote healing of the emotions and spirit that can be damaged by the stress and anxiety that accompany the disease and its treatments. "Stress relief is a major consideration in your ability to heal," says Dr. Lawson. "The less stressed you are, the better you heal in the aftermath of cancer, and the better your quality of life will be."

Here's a rundown of the methods that will help you get the nutrition, serenity, and rest your body needs to rebuild and continue the healing process.

EAT BY THE RAINBOW. The more nutrients you receive during treatment, the stronger and less prone to infections you'll be. "Relying strictly on supplements can place too much stress on the immune system," says Cynthia Thompson, R.D., Ph.D., assistant professor of nutritional sciences at the Arizona Cancer Center in Tucson. She suggests loading your lunch plate with a spectrum of red, yellow, and green foods to get the most cancer-

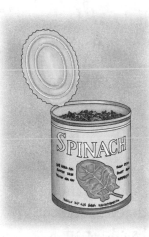

fighting nutrients possible. For instance, on a bed of dark leafy greens (such as spinach or kale), toss some red peppers (for vitamin C), carrots (for beta-carotene), and several cruciferous veggies, such as broccoli or cauliflower (for isothiocynates, which are potent, cancer-fighting compounds).

MAKE IT WITH MUSTARD. The brown variety that contains horseradish is a great way to get isothiocynates, says Dr. Thompson, especially when you don't feel up to eating broccoli.

MIX THINGS UP. "When even the sight of a fruit or vegetable makes you gag," says Dr. Thompson, "juicing these nutrient powerhouses into a drinkable pulp is a great way to get a high concentration of antioxidants and chlorophyll, both of which may help neutralize toxins from chemotherapy or radiation." Toss some sweet strawberries in with a few beta-carotene–rich carrots for a nutrient-dense alternative to O.J. Or opt for tomato juice, which is a super source of the antioxidant lycopene.

ON-THE-SPOT RELIEF

Fisherman's Helper

Research from the University of Rochester Cancer Center in New York indicates that those acupressure wristbands sold to fishermen to stave off seasickness may also ease any chemotherapy-related queasiness. The bands (also called acustimulation wristbands) have a button that pushes on an acupressure point called P6, which lies on the inside of the wrist along what acupuncturists refer to as the body's anti-nausea meridian. The wristbands are available in many drugstores.

SLURP CLEAR SOUPS. If keeping solid foods down is a problem, sip clear, salty vegetable broths or miso soup, made with a salty soybean paste. Soups high in sodium, as most canned soups are, can help replenish the electrolytes (minerals necessary for normal heart rhythm, muscle contraction, and a whole host of other regular body functions) you lose when you vomit.

SAVOR GREEN TEA. Green tea leaves are rich in polyphenols, special cancer-battling compounds that help cancer drugs attack bad cells and spare healthy ones, says Paul Riley, N.D., a naturopathic physician with the Seattle Cancer Treatment and Wellness Center. Plus, green tea protects the liver so it's able to function optimally as your body's detox center. Try to drink three to five cups daily, he suggests.

SNEAK IN SOME PROTEIN. If meat's on the list of foods you can't stomach, boost your protein intake by supplementing soups and sauces with a shot of milk. Simply add 1/4 cup of powdered milk to 1 cup of whole milk, then blend it into whatever you're cooking.

SETTLE YOUR STOMACH. Both peppermint and ginger teas, which you can find prepackaged at a health food store, have been shown to decrease nausea. Just avoid sweetening them with sugar, which can dampen your immune system and increase your risk of infection. Instead, try a grain-derived sweetener like rice syrup or barley malt or an herbal sweetener such as stevia.

IMBIBE BEFORE DINNER. Not only can wine help stimulate the appetite, but anthocyanins (the pigments that give red wine its color) are cancer-fighting antioxidants and may help correct an imbalance of B vitamins, which can be a result of cancer treatments and may cause mouth soreness, anemia, and nerve problems, says Dr. Thompson. Red wine also contains an antifungal compound that's converted in the body into a powerful cancer-fighting agent. If you have breast cancer, however, you should avoid alcohol altogether because it may boost estrogen levels and fuel cancer. Eating red grapes, though, is a good choice for anyone.

TRY CURRIED RICE. The sunshine-yellow color in curry comes from curcumin, a component of the spice turmeric. Studies indicate that curcumin can both strangle tumors by cutting off the blood vessels that feed them and protect against burns and blisters that can often occur during radiation treatments. Turmeric (which is also available as a tea; check your health food store) has also been shown to relieve nausea.

SNACK ON CITRUS. The pulpy white membrane on orange and tangerine wedges provides pectin, which may help reduce the spread of cancer, says Dr. Riley. If mouth sores make eating citrus impossible, you can buy pectin in powdered form at a health food store. Swirl a teaspoon or two into applesauce and eat it once a day until your mouth is better and you can savor citrus again.

SUCK ON PEPPER LOZENGES. Early studies indicate that lozenges made with capsaicin—the ingredient in red pepper that provides its bite—may help soothe chemotherapy-related mouth sores. It seems that capsaicin not only numbs inflamed sores in the same way that benzocaine or other topical anesthetics might, but it may also draw white blood cells to the site to heal them. Another plus: Capsaicin has antioxidant properties that may help fight nitrosamine, a cancer-causing agent. Look for the lozenges in any drugstore.

SNEAK IN SOME FLAXSEED. Flaxseed turns into a soothing, protective gel in your digestive tract, which helps promote intestinal functioning with none of the harshness of bran or other insoluble fiber—making it a great pre- or post-chemo addition to your diet. Plus, flax provides omega-3 essential fatty acids to help squelch the inflammation that results from chemotherapy. Stir a few teaspoons of ground flaxseed (available at health food stores) into your morning smoothie or yogurt, and your taste buds won't have a clue that you're getting your daily quota of roughage.

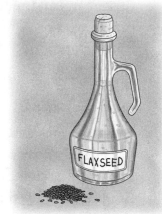

DRINK YOUR MILK...THISTLE. This spiny, purple-flowered herb protects the liver from damage, including damage from toxins infused during chemotherapy. As a result, it may minimize chemotherapy-related nausea, fatigue, and flu-like aches. The recommended dosage is 250 milligrams of standardized extract (which you can get at a health food store) three times a day. Check with your doctor before taking it.

BREATHE DEEP. Cancer is nothing if not scary. But in one of life's crueler catch-22s, when you're

THE GIFT OF THE MAGI

The mucous membrane of the gastrointestinal tract, which starts in the mouth, is very vulnerable to chemotherapy drugs, which can cause acutely painful canker sores. But there is an ancient solution: myrrh, the herb carried to Bethlehem by one of the biblical Wise Men. Long prized for its astringent properties, myrrh soothes sore mouth tissues and works as a fluoride alternative. Look for it in mouthwashes and toothpastes at a health food store, or buy an extract and make your own rinse by mixing 20 drops in 1/4 cup of water.

✳ ✳ ✳

frightened, your body releases stress hormones that can depress your immune system. To relieve your anxiety, lower levels of stress hormones, and bring yourself to a healing state, breathe slowly and fully from your lower abdomen. Keep your shoulders still and expand your lungs fully so your belly bulges out as far as it can, then exhale slowly. Your heart rate will slow, your anxiety will fade, and you may increase your feelings of control. "When I was facing surgery and later radiation, I inhaled the word *let* and exhaled the word *go*," Laura told me. "This really helped my state of mind."

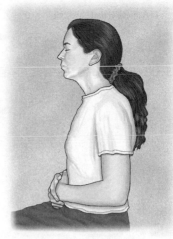

CANKER AND COLD SORES

Soothing Solutions

Several years back, I went through the torturous experience of wearing adult braces for a brief period. The worst part wasn't losing my smile behind stainless steel; it was trying to eat and speak with a mouthful of sores caused by all the wires! Needless to say, I was glad to get rid of all that metal, and my mouth healed quickly.

If you've ever had a mouth sore, you know exactly what I mean. Pain isn't always proportionate to size, especially when you're talking about minuscule, whitish-gray canker sores, or aphthous ulcers—which crop up inside the mouth along the gum line, tongue, or inner cheek—and cold sores, or fever blisters—those highly contagious, highly unsightly little blebs that occur on the outer lips.

WHY ME?

Canker sores can arise from injury to the mouth tissues—the kind you might get from wearing braces, as I did; being poked by the dentist; or even scrubbing with toothpastes that contain the harsh detergent sodium lauryl sulfate.

But there is a host of other causes as well. Pineapples, tomatoes, oranges, and other acidic foods, for instance, can irritate the tender tissues in your mouth and create the perfect environment for canker sores to develop. A deficiency of B vitamins or iron can do the same, as can an allergy to food preservatives, such as benzoic acid, or a sensitivity to gluten, the protein that's found in wheat and other grains.

Canker sores can also be triggered by stress, menstrual periods, and hormonal changes, and they commonly occur in conjunction with viral infections. Sometimes there may be no identifiable cause, just a tingling or burning sensation—then a fiery bump.

The pain usually goes away on its own in within 7 to 10 days, and the ulcer typically heals completely within two weeks after that. Once you've had them, though, canker sores can recur at the drop of a hat.

ON-THE-SPOT RELIEF

Lick It with Licorice

Licorice candy won't do the trick, but licorice gel will—thanks to the herb's chief constituent, which thickens the mucosal lining of the mouth (where canker sores form) and provides speedy relief. "When my patients use licorice gel, their canker sore pain disappears in 30 seconds," says Jennifer Reid, N.D., a naturopathic physician at the Columbia River Natural Medicine Clinic in Troutdale, Oregon. Check your health food store for licorice gel and apply it directly to sores several times a day.

COLD SORE WOES

Unlike canker sores, cold sores have a definite cause—the herpes simplex virus (HSV), which most of us probably caught as kids from kissing our moms and dads. Once it makes the person-to-person jump, HSV usually remains dormant, tucked into the nerves near our cheeks. But in a third of us, it awakens periodically when our resistance is low—usually due to fever, stress, overexposure to sunlight or wind, or the onset of menstruation.

As the bug begins reproducing, you may feel a slight tingling, itching, or burning near your lip. That's your signal that the virus is about to erupt on the skin as an ugly red blister. Within 10 days, the blister will burst, dry out, and go away on its own, but in the meantime, it can itch and sting like crazy.

SORE NO MORE

While antiviral cold sore remedies can keep HSV from reproducing, you have to use them the moment you feel the first tingle, before your blister blooms. Even then, points out Cynthia Thompson, M.D., a dermatologist with the Hennepin County Medical Center in North Carolina, "they really only hasten healing by a day."

As for cankers, there are drugs that can chemically close the pain-causing nerve endings on the surface of these vexing sores. Yet that solution may be even more painful than the sore! Before you resort to powerful drugs,

---

BAG YOUR BLISTER

Every type of tea imaginable—from good old Earl Grey to orange pekoe—contains tannic acid, an astringent that helps numb pain. Brew a cup of your favorite, let the tea bag cool, squeeze it to reduce its size as much as you can, and tuck it into your mouth to cover your canker sore. "The tea will help cauterize, or close, the nerve endings near the sore and ease your pain," says Cynthia Thompson, M.D.

---

try one of these kinder, gentler ways to soothe your sores.

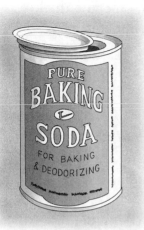

SWISH WITH SODA. That same box of baking soda you use to cut odors in your fridge can also be used to reduce the acidity in your mouth, which some people believe can not only set you up for canker sores but also aggravate existing ones. Just add 1 to 2 teaspoons of baking soda to a quart of warm water, swish it around in your mouth, and spit it out.

TURN TO MYRRH. You may know myrrh as the herb taken to biblical Bethlehem by one of the Magi, but herbalists know it as a highly effective treatment for mouth inflammations because of its astringent properties. You can mix a few drops of extract in a cup of warm water and swish daily. Or open a myrrh capsule and dab the powder directly onto your canker, suggests Jeanette Jacknin, M.D., a dermatologist in Scottsdale, Arizona. Both extract and capsules are available at health food stores.

GET MILK. Grab that dusty bottle of Maalox or milk of magnesia from the far reaches of your medicine chest—but instead of swigging

WHEN LIFE GIVES YOU LEMONS...

Use lemon balm! Studies show that *Melissa officinalis*, commonly known as lemon balm, helps cold sores heal faster with less crusting. "Lemon balm contains at least four antiviral compounds," explains Jeanette Jacknin, M.D., "so it's considered by some to be a first-choice herbal treatment." The key is to apply it at the first inkling of an outbreak. Make a tea by steeping 2 to 4 teaspoons of dried lemon balm leaves in a cup of hot water for 10 minutes or so, then apply the cooled solution directly to the sore. Or look for a commercial lip balm that contains lemon balm (also called melissa) and slather it on your sore.

it, swish with it. "The magnesium in liquid antacids will neutralize the acidity in the mouth," says Dr. Thompson, "and the thick film will coat your sore, making it easier to eat, drink, and talk." If you have a single canker, you can let the coating agent form in a spoon, then paint it on your boo-boo with a cotton swab. After a few minutes, rinse your mouth with water.

RINSE WITH FOLIC ACID. Since a deficiency of folate (the natural form of folic acid) may give rise to canker sores, rinsing with a folic acid mouthwash may send them packing. Find the mouthwash at a health food store, then follow the package directions.

SOOTHE WITH ALOE. Rinse your mouth with 1 to 3 tablespoons of aloe juice (which you can buy by the gallon at most health food stores) three times a day to dull canker pain and reduce the bacteria in your mouth. Be sure to get aloe juice, not gel.

EXTRACT IT. At the first indication of a blister outbreak, scan the shelves of your local health food store for extracts of calendula, tea tree oil, slippery elm, and myrrh—all off which are either excellent astringents or inflammation and infection fighters. Add several drops of each to a cup of hot water, let it cool, and dab the solution directly onto your cold sore for instant pain relief.

TAKE ECHINACEA. Echinacea isn't just a plain old cold fighter; it battles cold sores, too, perhaps by boosting the antiviral immune fighters in mucous membranes. Mix 1/4 teaspoon of extract (available at health food stores) in water or juice, then drink it three times a day for as long as your symptoms last, suggests Dr. Jacknin.

Don't use echinacea if you have an autoimmune disease such as lupus, rheumatoid arthritis, or multiple sclerosis, or if you're pregnant or nursing.

GO FOR THE GOLD. Goldenseal is another antiviral herb that can treat cold sores. Add ¼ teaspoon of extract (available at health food stores) to your echinacea drink three times a day. To relieve the pain of canker sores, make an antiseptic mouth rinse by dissolving ½ teaspoon of goldenseal powder and ¼ teaspoon of salt in 1 cup of warm water. Swish and spit four times a day.

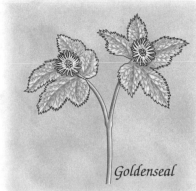

Goldenseal

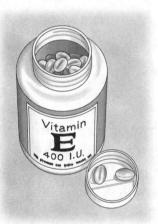

SQUEEZE ON SOME E. Studies show that if you apply vitamin E oil (from either a bottle or a capsule) directly to a cold sore, says Dr. Jacknin, you may speed your recovery and relieve the pain—possibly within a single day.

ZINC IT. The same white ointment that lifeguards use on their noses to protect against sunburn may heal cold sores in 5 days instead of the usual 10. The catch, according to research, is that you have to apply zinc oxide four times a day—and perhaps every hour—and start it within 24 hours of the first hint of an outbreak. You can find the ointment at drugstores.

CARPAL TUNNEL SYNDROME

Relieve the Squeeze

———◆◦◦◦◆———

Every night, thousands of people brush their teeth, put on their PJs—and slip into contraptions that keep their hands as stiff as a mannequin's. I know, because I've been one of them.

During my pregnancy and then during marathon stints at the keyboard, my wrists developed the telltale signs of carpal tunnel syndrome (CTS). I had a pins-and-needles sensation in my hands, and my fingers were so numb I couldn't feel them turn the pages of a book. My grip weakened to the point where I couldn't open a jar of spaghetti sauce, and the pain radiating up my arm made it tough to drag a brush through my hair.

WHY ME?

Any activity that calls for frequently bending your wrists—from typing to dicing onions to dealing cards—can make you prone to CTS. It arises when your wrist is flexed unnaturally for long periods of time, putting pressure on the median nerve that runs through the narrow passageway (the carpal tunnel) on the inside of your wrist. This nerve controls the feeling in your thumb, index finger, middle finger, and part of your ring finger. When you repeatedly bend your wrist, the tendons inside the tunnel swell and compress the nerve, and your fingers begin to feel numb.

GET A GRIP

Sure, a firm handshake can get you places, but a powerful grip on everyday objects can only get you CTS (and studies show that most people grip things like doorknobs a whopping five times harder than they have to). One suggestion: Loosen your grip and move your hands lower on the steering wheel when you're sitting in traffic to minimize stress on the nerves in your arms.

Women are three times more likely than men to develop the syndrome, partly because their wrists are smaller and the carpal tunnels are naturally narrower, says Robert Markison, M.D., a hand surgeon at the University of California, San Francisco. The median nerve can also be compressed by simple fluid retention—the kind that occurs naturally as a result of the hormonal surges women experience during menstruation, pregnancy, and menopause.

MAKE YOUR HANDS HAPPY

While untreated CTS rarely results in long-term nerve damage, you simply don't have to live with the pain—or, for that matter, the specter of impending surgery. "Because the carpal ligament doesn't automatically stretch to accommodate swelling, one option is to have the ligament snipped," says Scott M. Fried, M.D., a nerve and hand specialist at the Upper Extremity Institute in Blue Bell, Pennsylvania. "This provides more room for the soft tissues, reducing pressure. But the surgery is no cure, and it only works in half the patients."

Fortunately, you can stretch the ligament externally and soothe any CTS symptoms without the expense, pain, or extensive recovery time associated with the scalpel. In fact, with early, do-it-yourself treatment, "many nerve problems will calm down enough for the damage to be totally reversed," says Dr. Fried. Here's what to do when you start to feel those odd sensations creeping into your wrist and fingers.

SPLINT AT NIGHT. Wearing a rigid splint overnight will keep your wrist from overflexing while you sleep and relieve pressure on your nerve. As a result, the swelling within your carpal tunnel will go down, and your CTS will probably fade within two to three weeks, says Dr. Fried. Look for over-the-counter brands made with stretchy fabric and a rigid splint. Avoid neoprene splints, which don't provide adequate support. If you don't notice relief after wearing the splint for two weeks, talk to your doctor about having a custom splint made.

GO BARE DURING THE DAY. "I really don't recommend wearing splints while you're on the job," warns Arlette Loesser, an occupational therapist who specializes in body-friendly workplace design at the Ultimate Workplace in New

SAVE YOUR MONEY!

Resist the Rests

Whether they're filled with gel, foam, or buckwheat, the wrist rests you use with your keyboard to reduce pressure on your wrists may actually double the pressure inside your carpal tunnel—and increase the likelihood of developing CTS. Instead, position your keyboard on an adjustable platform so the space bar is higher than the function keys. When you're not typing, rest your hands on the arms of your chair or in your lap—anywhere but on your keyboard or mouse pad, which will cause your wrist to bend upward and increase the pressure inside that trouble-prone tunnel.

York City. "Splints can decrease circulation to your wrist and force you to overcompensate with other parts of your arm. You could transfer pain to your shoulder."

STRETCH YOUR WRIST. If you perform this simple exercise at the first hint of discomfort, you may head off a full-blown case of CTS. With your wrist straight and your palm facing downward, hold your fingers and thumb in a relaxed fist. Next, slowly straighten your fingers and thumb and extend your wrist backward, turning your forearm so your palm faces upward. Then, with your other hand, press lightly on your fingers to give them a gentle downward stretch. Repeat 5 to 10 times, then switch hands for one set. Perform three sets each day, gradually adding more sessions throughout the day or increasing the length of each session.

PRESS HERE. Gentle self-manipulation of the bones and soft tissues of the wrist can shift the fluids responsible for swelling, releasing the entrapped nerve. As an added benefit, it can keep your forearm agile. Here's what to do: Gently press your thumb into the soft bottom side of your wrist, 1 to 2 inches back from the crease, then slide it back and forth over one tendon at a time as well as up and down your wrist. Repeat several times throughout the day or as often as you feel you need to.

TRY A SOOTHING SALAD. Top it with hard-boiled eggs for vitamin A, red peppers for vitamin C, and sliced almonds for

> ## WORK THE DIRT, NOT YOUR WRISTS
>
> Fat-handled gardening tools may be the height of dirt chic, but all those big handles do (besides look cool) is add weight. If you're prone to CTS or are an avid gardener who's trying to avoid it, you're better off using "leverage-enhanced" tools. These gardening implements, from trowels to shrub rakes, have handles that allow you to garden with the strength of your upper arm and shoulders rather than with the weaker muscles of your hand or wrist.
>
>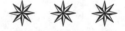

vitamin E. All these nutrients are excellent anti-inflammatories and may help reduce the swelling in your tendons that's causing your pain, says Andrew Lucking, N.D., a naturopathic physician in Minneapolis.

OIL IT WITH EFAS. Flaxseed is a rich source of omega-3 essential fatty acids, which are also anti-inflammatory. Drizzle 1 tablespoon of flaxseed oil (available in health food stores) on your salad daily, and your wrist woes may be over within two weeks.

WRAP YOUR WRIST. "A compress made from castor bean oil is a great way to get an anti-inflammatory to the source of the pain," says Dr. Lucking. Soak a cloth with castor oil (available in health food stores), heat it in the microwave until it's warm but not hot, and place it on your wrist. Cover your wrist with plastic wrap and leave the compress in place for several hours.

RUB IT WITH RED PEPPER. Capsaicin—the compound that makes red pepper so fiery—also reduces inflammation by blocking the release of pain-causing substances. You can pick up a commercial pain-relief salve that contains capsaicin at any drugstore, or simply make your own by mixing 1 teaspoon of red-pepper powder into 1/4 cup of skin lotion. Rub no more than 1 teaspoon of the mixture on the sore area, being careful not to get it on any area of broken skin or near your eyes. Wash your hands thoroughly afterward.

DRINK UP. Taking frequent breaks from the computer is one of the surest ways to keep CTS at bay, says Loesser—and one of the surest ways to force yourself to get up is to drink lots of water so you have to take frequent bathroom breaks.

CHRONIC FATIGUE SYNDROME

Coax Your Body Back to Health

———◆◇◆◇◆———

My neighbor Julie didn't care if her couch was littered with folded laundry or copies of *People* magazine; she'd plop down on it anyway. She was that tired. Every evening, after routine days of teaching dance, she'd sink with utter and achy exhaustion into that crowded couch and stay there, barely moving, for hours. "Yet the more I slept, the more tired I felt," she recalls. "And I couldn't think straight the next day. I'd forget dance steps I'd known since I was 10."

As it turned out, Julie had chronic fatigue syndrome (CFS), a condition that's characterized by disabling fatigue. In addition to exhaustion, its grab bag of symptoms includes muscle aches, low-grade fevers, sore throat, headaches, memory deficits, and sleep disturbances. Some people may have mild symptoms that

WAKE UP AND SMELL THE ROSEMARY

When your energy flags, don't go for a cup of joe—reach for rosemary instead. "Rosemary and other aromatic herbs trigger the trigeminal nerve, which induces beta brain waves normally produced when a person is alert and concentrating," explains Alan Hirsch, M.D., director of the Smell and Taste Treatment Foundation in Chicago. Simply place a rosemary plant on your desk and rub its leaves to help you focus, or dab rosemary oil (available in health food stores) on the pages of a lengthy report you need to absorb.

only slightly interfere with their daily activities, while others may be practically bedridden.

WHY ME?

According to the National Institute of Allergy and Infectious Diseases, CFS was once pegged as the "yuppie flu" because those who sought help for it in the early 1980s were mainly well-educated, well-off women in their thirties and forties. We now know, of course, that anyone can get it. What we still don't know is why they do.

One theory is that excess stress, hormonal changes, allergies, environmental toxins, and/or infections disrupt the function of the mitochondria in cells, which serve as the body's energy furnaces. This in turn throws off a part of the brain called the hypothalamus, which helps regulate the pituitary gland and its production of hormones that control metabolism, energy, and immune function.

There's also the possibility that an overactive response to stress, environmental toxins, digestive disorders, or other factors deplete magnesium and interfere with production of adenosine triphosphate (ATP), the body's energy storage molecules. "Think of ATP as the currency used by the mitochondria to generate energy," says Jacob Teitelbaum, M.D., director of the Annapolis Research Center for Effective FMS/CFS Therapies in Maryland. "If you don't have enough ATP, your body goes bankrupt energy-wise."

RENEW YOUR ENERGY

Some doctors prescribe antidepressants or sedatives to help those with CFS ease muscle pain so they can sleep. Others recommend taking glutathione, an antioxidant believed to stoke the body's furnace and detoxify the system. While these single-shot treatments may well ease some of your symptoms, they do have a few side effects. Glutathione, for instance, can rev you up, but you still may be too tired to go anywhere.

A better approach is to think of CFS as a circuit breaker, an internal switch that has suddenly clicked off to protect your body from further damage and from

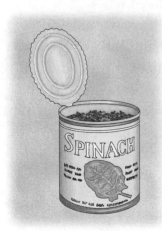

burning out, suggests Dr. Teitelbaum. Your goal shouldn't be to bypass the switch but to coax it back on—*gently*. Here are some ways to do it.

TOP A SPINACH SALAD WITH APPLES. Spinach (as well as other leafy greens, dried beans, lentils, and avocados) is loaded with magnesium—a mineral Dr. Teitelbaum calls "the most important nutrient for stoking energy and relieving muscle pain." Apples are packed with malic acid, which helps jump-start production of ATP. Together, they can help

---

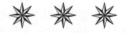

ROCK ON!

Rocking in a rocking chair may lull you to sleep, but it can have the opposite effect on long-dormant muscles. In fact, the rocking motion can actually move the fluid in the middle ear that helps stimulate the nerves in your muscles, remove the waste products that have accumulated there, and boost your energy, says John Reed, M.D. Think of rocking as a soothing springboard to walking, bicycling, and eventually to healing.

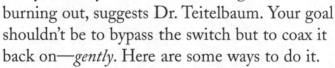

---

your body produce energy, ease achy muscles, and lift fatigue.

BOOST B₁₂. This nutrient, which is vital for maintaining energy, mental acuity, and immune function, is often absent in the brains of people with CFS. Help your brain and body along by "B-fing" up your diet with plenty of seafood, beef, lamb, and yogurt and by taking a vitamin B-complex supplement every day. You might also ask your physician about B_{12} shots, which Dr. Teitelbaum swears can make "all the difference" in just 10 weeks.

TAKE THIAMIN, TOO. All of the B vitamins can help improve energy, immune function, and mental sharpness, but one of the more important Bs is thiamin pyrophosphate—the activated form of vitamin B_1—which is necessary for the break-down and release of energy from carbohydrates. In addition to getting thiamin in a B-complex supplement, eat more of it by sprinkling wheat germ on your yogurt, choosing rice bran cereal for breakfast, and snacking on peanuts, pecans, and walnuts. Too much thiamin can cause nerve damage, though, so be sure to steer clear of high-dose supplements.

BET ON BROCCOLI. This vitamin C–rich veggie aids your body in making glutathione, the powerful antioxidant that helps your body rid itself of toxins. But many people with CFS are deficient in glutathione. Since it's questionable how well it works when taken on its own, John Reed, M.D., a physician in Arlington, Virginia, suggests that you load up on broccoli, red peppers, oranges, and other vitamin C–rich foods and take 750 milligrams of C in supplement form daily.

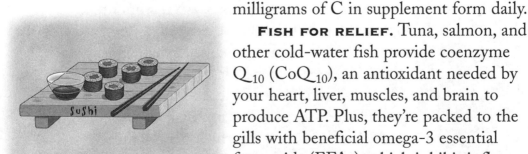

FISH FOR RELIEF. Tuna, salmon, and other cold-water fish provide coenzyme Q_{10} (CoQ_{10}), an antioxidant needed by your heart, liver, muscles, and brain to produce ATP. Plus, they're packed to the gills with beneficial omega-3 essential fatty acids (EFAs), which inhibit inflammation and can help minimize CFS pain, says Dr. Teitelbaum. Not fond of fish? Comb your local health food store for supplements of CoQ$_{10}$ and take 100 to 200 milligrams a day. As long as you're not taking aspirin or prescription blood thinners, you can also consider taking 1gram (1,000 milligrams) of fish oil twice a day.

SLEEP DEEP. Studies show that taking valerian and lemon balm—two well-known herbal relaxers—can improve deep-stage sleep. As long as you're not taking any other drugs, check your health food store for formulas that also include the mild sedatives passionflower, hops, and Jamaican dogwood. Follow the directions on the label.

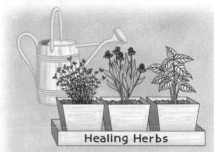

Healing Herbs

GET RID OF GLUTEN. In one study, people with CFS who eliminated wheat and other common food allergens from their diets showed a whopping 90 percent boost in energy. To gear up your get-up-and-go, scan food labels when you shop and avoid products with wheat or gluten in the ingredient list.

GET MILK. Many people with CFS are calcium deficient, which means they may be plagued by nighttime muscle cramps that prevent them from sleeping deeply. Dr. Teitelbaum suggests either guzzling a glass of the white stuff or taking 600 to 1,000 milligrams of calcium citrate and 75 to 150 milligrams of magnesium in powder or chewable form (available at health food stores) just before you hit the sack.

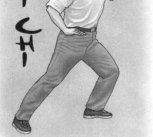

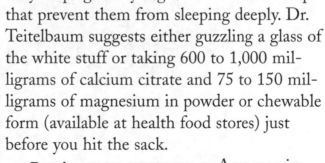

DON'T PUSH YOURSELF. Any exercise— from simply walking to the mailbox to regularly practicing tai chi—will force your body to use oxygen (which is energizing) and help decrease muscle weakness. In fact, one study showed that aerobic exercise relieved fatigue in 75 percent of the participants with CFS. But you have to address other aspects of your condition first. "Get your nutrition and sleep under control first, then aim for an exercise regimen that gives you a 'good tired,' not a 'wiped out' feeling," advises Dr. Teitelbaum. Begin with just 5 minutes of light activity a day, and then, as your strength improves, slowly increase the time you exercise.

TALK BACK. Studies show that talking yourself free of negative thoughts about your reduced activity level and capabilities may help you recover from CFS more quickly. For instance, each time your inner critic grouses that you "should be doing more" or calls you lazy for "just lying around," talk back. Remind yourself that you're rebuilding your energy renewal system through healthful eating and strategic bouts of activity—and you're following a proven plan for healing. If you stay positive, you'll also stay empowered, which can be a huge help to people with CFS.

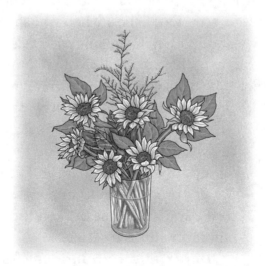

COLD HANDS AND FEET

No More Raynaud's

───────◆◇◆───────

Stuffing a clammy turkey on a crisp November morning can chill anyone's fingers to the bone. For one member of my family, though, simply grabbing the cranberries from the fridge is a numbing experience. The cold blast first turns her fingers waxy white, then, as the blood drains from her digits, they morph into a ghostly blue. After about 30 minutes, the blood returns, and her fingers turn red.

"Everyone gets cold hands and feet in lower temperatures," notes Frederick Wigley, M.D., director of rheumatology at Johns Hopkins University School of Medicine

MAKE YOUR OWN HEAT

To fashion a portable heat source, simply fill a cotton sock with white rice, tie the open end, and heat in the microwave for 2 minutes (don't let it get too hot to touch). Then tuck it in your glove or your pocket and take it with you wherever you go. It'll remain warm for hours and could help stave off a full-blown Raynaud's attack.

Don't Forget Your Rubbers!

Running icy-cold hands under warm water can quickly thaw them out, but if you have Raynaud's disease, your hands may be too numb to feel the water temperature—and scalding water can create a whole new problem. The solution? Slip on a pair of rubber dishwashing gloves before you stick your hands under the tap. Your hands will be safe—even under very hot water—and the warmth will feel sensational.

in Baltimore. "But for 10 percent of the population—most of them women between ages 15 and 40—it's an exaggerated and sometimes painful response."

It's called Raynaud's disease (or phenomenon). The condition occurs when blood vessels that channel blood to your hands and feet overreact to dipping temperatures, stress, and other factors. When the vessels spasm, your fingers or toes are starved of oxygen, so they become frigid and often turn ghostly white, then blue or purple. As the attack subsides and the blood vessels open up, your extremities flush a deep red and may throb.

WHY ME?

Scientists aren't sure why some people develop what's called primary Raynaud's (when the condition isn't caused by an underlying problem, such as disease) and others don't. The disease tends to run in families, and in some who have it, norepinephrine, a brain chemical that controls how blood vessels respond, is improperly regulated by the body for some reason.

But there are "mechanical" causes, too: Activities such as typing or playing the piano, which require you to bend your wrists repeatedly, may predispose you to intermittent episodes of Raynaud's. If they continue, you could experience tissue damage, and if circulation is obstructed for prolonged periods, small, painful skin ulcers can develop on the tips of the fingers. In the worst cases, gangrene can develop.

BEAT THE BRRR

Standard treatment for very serious Raynaud's is calcium channel blockers to pry open your blood vessels. These potent medications may have side effects, such as impotence in men, however, and most people can keep Raynaud's from progressing to that point, anyway. "The best nondrug approach is pretty simple," says Dr. Wigley. "Avoid the cold and protect your extremities from arctic blasts and shifting temperatures." Wear oven mitts to reach into the fridge, use insulated drinking cups, cover your steering wheel with lamb's-wool, and wear socks and even gloves to bed on chilly nights.

And if you do get chilled? Here are a few do-it-yourself ways to gently rewarm your fingers and toes, restore circulation, and minimize any chance of damage.

SWING LIKE A WINDMILL. You may be able to short-circuit a Raynaud's attack by briskly swinging your arms 360 degrees (as you would if you were releasing an underhand pitch in a softball game) for a full 1 to 2 minutes. The centrifugal force you create may shuttle the blood into your clamped vessels and relieve the spasm.

GET WIGGLY. Don't clap your hands or rub them vigorously, which could damage blood vessels. Instead, simply wiggle your frosty fingers and either run warm water over them or order a warm beverage and lace your fingers around the cup. Just steer clear of Irish coffee—both caffeine and alcohol are blood vessel constrictors. A better choice might be ginger tea, since it has a warming effect and boosts blood flow, says David Zeiger, D.O., a family physician in Chicago.

BRING THE HEAT. Capsaicin, the compound in red pepper that makes it hot, can give you some heat, too, by dilating your blood vessels. "If you don't love heavily peppered food, I recommend taking capsaicin capsules at every meal," says John Hahn, N.D., D.P.M., a naturopathic physician and podiatrist in Bend, Oregon. (The capsules are available at drugstores; follow the package directions.) You can even sprinkle a little red pepper straight from your spice rack into your shoes or gloves; you'll feel the heat instantly.

BOOST YOUR B. One way to increase blood flow to your extremities is with a form of the B vitamin niacin called inositol hexaniacinate. Dr. Hahn recommends taking 500 to 600 milligrams a day—but only after you check with your doctor. People with diabetes, low blood pressure, glaucoma, gout, liver disease, ulcers, or bleeding disorders should consult a physician before taking any form of niacin—as should anyone who's taking any medication.

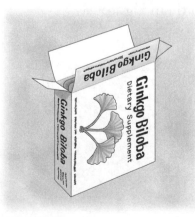

STOP THE SPASMS. Magnesium may relax tight blood vessels and return color and warmth to your skin, says Dr. Zeiger. Start with 200 milligrams twice a day and gradually increase to 400 milligrams twice a day, but talk to your doctor first if you have kidney or heart disease. If diarrhea develops, reduce the dosage.

GIVE GINKGO A GO. Ginkgo inhibits a substance called platelet activating factor, which tends to make blood stickier. As a result, it can improve blood flow in even the tiniest vessels. Check your health food store for standardized capsules that contain at least 24 percent flavone glycosides, take 60 milligrams three times a day—and be patient. You probably won't see a change for a month or so, warns Dr. Hahn. Don't take ginkgo with aspirin, ibuprofen, or prescription blood-thinning drugs.

TRY SOME GLA. Evening primrose oil and borage oil both contain gamma-linolenic acid (GLA), an essential fatty acid that can moderate pain. Studies of people with Raynaud's indicate that massaging some of either oil into your fingertips and toes can not only help them feel better, it can also help thaw them out. You can find the oils at health food stores.

Evening Primrose

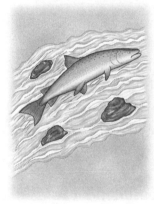

FISH FOR WARMTH. If your chilly fingers are caused by an underlying inflammation of the blood vessels that pinches off blood flow to your extremities, eating lots of fish, which contain omega-3 essential fatty acids, could increase your tolerance to cold by inhibiting inflammation. Savor cold-water fish such as salmon or tuna as many times a week as you can.

COLDS
AND FLU

Beat the Bugs

———◁◈▷———

My husband believes he's hit upon the way to beat the common cold and flu: Whenever he feels the slightest tickle in his throat, he slips into a pair of thick socks, drinks a gallon of orange juice, and then heads straight for bed. If his schedule permits and he can stay there for, oh, two or three days, he almost always wakes up symptom-free—no pricey commercial remedies required!

Of course, few folks with family or work responsibilities can take advantage of this particular "remedy." But the point is, commercial cold and flu medications aren't always needed to do the job. In fact, they don't always do the job at all, even when you want them to.

Antihistamines, for instance, will dry up a runny nose from allergies, but they won't affect the dripping and sneezing associated with the cold virus. Decongestants can leave you jittery. Aspirin and acetaminophen can dampen, rather than boost, your immune system. And those all-in-one nighttime cold remedies?

They come with a shot glass for good reason: The "knock-out" ingredient is alcohol. It may help your head hit the pillow, but it won't do a thing to fight infection.

SACK THOSE SYMPTOMS

Other than curling up in bed, what's the alternative? Enter all those "natural remedies" you may have noticed clustered around the drugstore checkout counter. A few of them—if taken at the first sneeze—can cut your sick time by more than half. They won't leave you groggy or jittery, and they're made to work with your immune system, not against it. Here's how to minimize your symptoms naturally.

DOWN BLACK ELDERBERRY. "Studies have shown that if you take the syrup at the first hint of flu, you may be able to cut your flu bout in half," says Isadore Rosenfeld, M.D., professor of clinical medicine at the Weill Medical College of Cornell University in New York City. Dr. Rosenfeld recommends downing 40 drops of black elderberry extract (available at health food stores) every 4 hours at the first sign of the flu.

ZAP IT WITH ZINC. Research indicates that zinc may cut the duration of colds by about two days by acting as a physical barrier to prevent viruses from entering the cells that line the nose and throat. All you have to

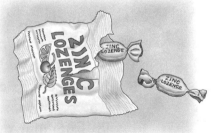

COLD REMEDIES AND DIABETES

Most commercial cough and cold medicines contain ingredients that are ineffective, make you groggy or jittery, and may even hamper your immune system. Even worse, however, many standard brands contain sugar in the form of dextrose. If you have diabetes and take these products as directed (typically every 4 to 6 hours), they could raise your blood sugar to unhealthy levels.

do is spritz an over-the-counter zinc nasal spray (which you can find in drugstores) in each nostril four times a day within 48 hours of the first inkling of a cold. Zinc lozenges require that you act even more quickly: within 24 hours of your first symptom. "Look for zinc gluconate tablets that aren't flavored with citric acid, tartaric acid, or sorbitol," advises David Zeiger, D.O., a family physician in Chicago. When these ingredients mix with saliva, they cancel out zinc's benefits.

SOUP UP YOUR SOUP. Smoky-tasting shiitake mushrooms amp up production of interferon, a protein that girds the body to defend against viral invaders, while reishi mushrooms may help ease respiratory tract inflammation. Either add these 'shrooms to your therapeutic chicken soup or look for them combined in extract form

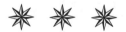

and follow the directions on the label, advises John Hahn, N.D., D.P.M., a naturopathic physician and podiatrist in Bend, Oregon.

TRY ECHINACEA. Studies have shown that the herb echinacea shortens the duration of colds from nine to six days and makes them less severe—possibly because the polysaccharides it contains boost the body's infection-fighting cells. The best way to take echinacea is as a tincture (an extract diluted in alcohol, which is available at health food stores) so it bypasses digestion and flows directly into your bloodstream.

At the first hint of a cold, Dr. Zeiger recommends taking 30 drops of tincture every 2 hours. After a week, go to 20 drops three times a day, for a total of 10 days. Use the herb only during your cold (with continued use, it loses its effectiveness), and never use it if you have an autoimmune disease such as lupus, rheumatoid arthritis, or multiple sclerosis, or if you are pregnant or nursing.

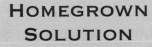
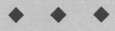
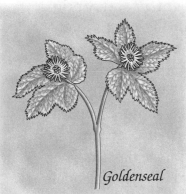

Goldenseal

ADD GOLDENSEAL. Goldenseal is an herb that has a drying effect on the mucous membranes. Jennifer Reid, N.D., a naturopathic physician at the Columbia River Natural Medicine Clinic in Troutdale, Oregon, suggests taking 500 to 1,000 milligrams of an echinacea-goldenseal combo, which you can find in health food stores. Try it in capsule form, or mix 30 drops of each tincture and take it every 2 to 3 hours.

OPT FOR OLIVE LEAF. Research shows that leuropein, the active ingredient in olive leaf extract, has powerful healing properties that may beat bacteria, viruses, fungi, and even parasites.

The recommended dose is a 300-milligram capsule three times a day for no more than two days. After that, gradually reduce your intake, suggests Dr. Reid. Check with your doctor first, and never take olive leaf in any dosage for more than seven days.

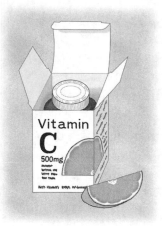

"C" IT THROUGH. Most people know that taking vitamin C on a regular basis can not only reduce the number of colds you catch but also minimize their symptoms and duration. My husband has his own special elixir: He drinks a gallon of orange juice, which he beefs up with 1 to 2 heaping tablespoons of powdered rosehips—a particularly rich source of vitamin C. He's definitely on to something there, says Dr. Hahn. Rosehips contain ascorbic acid (a form of vitamin C) and are a bioflavonoid (plant pigment) that enhances the absorption of C.

SNIFF MEDICINAL HERBS. Peppermint is cooling and may give you the sensation that your stuffy nose is clear, eucalyptus is a lung tonic and expectorant (meaning it clears congestion), and thyme is an antimicrobial that helps open tight airways. Sprinkle three to five drops of each herbal oil (available in health food stores) into a bowl of steaming water. Drape a towel over your head to trap the steam, lean over the bowl with your face about 12 inches away, and breathe in the soothing vapors.

APPLY A POULTICE. To ease a stuffy chest, add a few drops of water to a small amount of dry mustard to create a thin paste. Apply the paste to your chest and cover it with a layer of flannel and a hot water bottle or a heating pad set on low. The oils in mustard can easily burn the skin, though, so lift a corner of the flannel every 5 minutes to check for redness, and don't leave the poultice on for more than a total of 15 minutes. After several minutes, the congestion should start to loosen, possibly because mustard helps bring blood to the skin's surface and get fluids moving, says Mary Hardy, M.D., director of the Integrative Medicine Medical Group at Cedars-Sinai Medical Center in Los Angeles.

TRY HORSERADISH. This powerful herb contains allyl isothiocyanate, which stimulates the nerve endings in your nose and makes it flow like a faucet. Plus, horseradish has antiviral properties. "I suggest patients take a teaspoon of the freshly grated root or a half-teaspoon of horseradish extract three times a day," says Michael DiPalma, N.D., a naturopathic physician in Newtown, Pennsylvania. The extract is available in health food stores.

SIP LICORICE TEA. The steam from the tea will speed the flow of mucus from your nose, and the licorice will stimulate production of interferon, which helps the body defend against viral invaders, brings mucus up from the lungs, and soothes a scratchy throat. People with high blood pressure should not drink licorice tea.

SLIP IN SOME ELM. If you're coughing so much that your chest and back ache, try slippery elm tea. This time-honored expectorant will help break up the sticky mucus that may be clogging your bronchial tubes, says Dr. Reid. Look for it at health food stores and follow the directions on the label.

GIRD YOURSELF WITH ASTRAGALUS. This Chinese herb stimulates the release of interferon in the body and thereby boosts your immune system. Unlike echinacea, you can take astragalus, which is available at health food stores, every day during cold and flu season to bolster your resistance. Just follow the package directions.

CONSTIPATION

Get Things Moving Again

———◆———

I have a friend who makes herself a morning cup of coffee so strong that it doesn't so much "curl her toes" as keep her intestine on its toes. That's the whole point of the ritual, she says—to stay "regular." And sure enough, halfway through that high-test cup, she never fails to bolt to the bathroom to do her business.

WHY ME?

Not all of us are so fortunate. "Show me someone who is constipated, and I'll show you someone who regularly gorges on sugar, meat, bread, chocolate, alcohol, and dairy products, all of which plug up their digestion," says Christine Boorean, N.D., a naturopathic

---

HOT, COLD, AND GO!

Get things moving from the outside in by alternating hot and cold packs on your lower abdomen. First, heat a damp cloth in the microwave, remove it with tongs, and wrap it in a towel. Place the towel over your lower abdomen. After 3 minutes, replace it with an ice pack wrapped in a towel. Leave the cold pack on for 30 seconds, then repeat the sequence three times. "Your blood vessels will expand and contract, initiating a natural pumping action that will spur elimination," explains Christine Boorean, N.D.

---

physician in Portland, Oregon. "They probably skimp on fiber, which bulks up the stools so they press against the colon walls and stimulate peristalsis, the wave-like contractions that signal the urge to go. And they probably don't get enough liquids, which keep fiber soft," she adds.

Medications for high blood pressure or pain, excess stress, gulping your food, and severely limiting activity can also bring things to a standstill—as can being "toilet shy" and postponing the urge to go if you have to use a public restroom. The longer a stool stays in the bowel, the more water is reabsorbed by the intestine, the harder the stool gets, and the more you have to strain to eliminate it. As a result, you go less—and the cycle feeds on itself. Eventually, you could wind up with hemorrhoids or more serious intestinal problems.

MOVE IT IN MINUTES

Perform this yoga exercise, and you'll have a bowel movement within 10 minutes, promises Jeff Migdow, M.D., a holistic medical practitioner at the Kripalu Center for Yoga and Health in Lenox, Massachusetts. First, stand with your hands at your sides, inhale deeply through your nose, exhale through your mouth, and lift your arms over your head while inhaling deeply again through your nose. Next, exhale while lowering yourself into a squat, with your hands on your knees and your head lowered. As you finish the exhalation, still squatting, pump your abdomen in and out 20 times. Stand up and repeat the sequence three times.

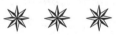

GET GOING—GENTLY

If you routinely use laxatives—the standard treatment for constipation—your colon will begin to rely on them to do its job. It will become lazy and weak and unable to function properly, says Gary Gitnick, M.D., chief of the division of digestive diseases at the University of California,

Los Angeles, School of Medicine. Once you have a "lazy colon," he warns, it will take bigger and bigger doses of laxatives to get things going. Eeventually, you may not be able to go at all.

Fortunately, there's a wealth of healthful, do-it-yourself measures to keep your stools loose—no laxative required. Get going with these.

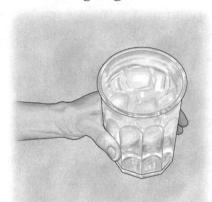

FILL 'ER UP. All experts agree that the simplest way to wake up your colon is to drink water—lots and lots of it. "Try to down 10 glasses [a total of 80 ounces] within 24 hours," recommends Dr. Gitnick. Need to get things moving now? Drink a large glass of water every 10 minutes for 1 hour to soften your stools and force elimination.

EAT YOUR OATMEAL. A certain type of gummy fiber called mucilage soaks up water, softening stools and making them easier to pass. Oatmeal is one food with lots of mucilage, which is why it's often recommended as an excellent breakfast choice to jump-start your system. Just don't top your bowl with bananas, which can be binding.

TRY PSYLLIUM. Not an oatmeal lover? Check your health food store for cereals or powdered laxatives that contain psyllium seeds, which are also mucilaginous. Once a day, add 2 tablespoons to a large glass of water or juice and drink it immediately, before it thickens. To avoid intestin-

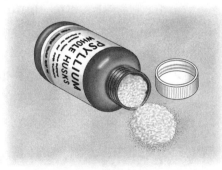

al blockage, be sure to drink lots of water throughout the day—at least six extra glasses—while you're taking psyllium. And don't use psyllium within 2 hours of taking any other supplements or medications, since it could delay their absorption into the bloodstream.

PIG OUT ON PRUNES. Ounce for ounce, prunes are packed with more fiber than almost any other fruit or vegetable—including dried beans. What's more, they contain dihydroxyphenyl isatin, a natural laxative. Down a glass of prune juice before bed to encourage a morning movement. Nibble on dried prunes (or figs and raisins, which also contain isatin) during the day. And for a tasty, high-fiber dessert, try baked apples stuffed with prunes, figs, or raisins.

SLURP POTATO JUICE. This old-time remedy really seems to loosen things up—even though scientists aren't able to ascertain why, says Dr. Boorean. Any time you boil potatoes, save the cooking water. The next morning, mix 2 tablespoons of potato water and 2 tablespoons of honey into a mug of hot water and drink it before breakfast.

ROOT FOR REGULARITY. Fresh dandelion roots (not leaves or stems) can have a mild laxative effect. Three times a day, either toss some rinsed roots into a salad or steep them in a cup of boiling water for 10 to 15 minutes, then strain and drink. Or look for prepackaged dandelion tea at your health food store. If you're taking diuretics or potassium supplements, check with your doctor before using dandelion.

SUPPLEMENT WITH C.

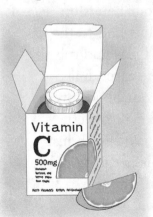

Diarrhea just happens to be one of the side effects of heavy vitamin C supplementation. As long as you don't have kidney disease or stomach problems, start by taking 1,000 milligrams of buffered vitamin C every couple of hours, suggests Dr. Boorean. "As soon as your stools loosen, back off to 500 milligrams a day."

GET MORE MAGNESIUM. There's a reason one of the best-known laxatives is called milk of magnesia: A magnesium deficiency can cause constipation. Make it a point to eat magnesium-rich spinach regularly, and check with your doctor about magnesium supplements.

TAKE TRIPHALA. This blend of Indian gooseberry (emla), beahera fruit, and tropical almond fruit is favored by practitioners of Ayurvedic medicine (the main system of healing in India) because it stimulates digestion as well as elimination. Check your health food store for triphala powder, then mix 1/2 teaspoon with 1 cup of warm water and drink it a half-hour before bedtime, suggests Vasant Lad, MA.Sc., director of the Ayurvedic Institute in Albuquerque.

RUB YOUR BELLY. "You can encourage a bowel movement with gentle abdominal self-massage," says Dr. Boorean—especially if your constipation is stress related. Here's how. Place your hands on your lower belly, below and to the right of your navel. Press and rub up the right side (the ascending colon), then move your hands over and press and rub down the left (the descending colon). Finish just above the groin. This is the path that waste takes as it passes through your system.

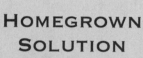

HOMEGROWN SOLUTION

◆ ◆ ◆

Have Another Slice of Pie...

Just make sure it's rhubarb—one of the yummiest natural laxatives around. Rhubarb stimulates mucus production in the large intestine to ease elimination, which typically occurs within 6 to 10 hours. You can also eat it stewed, or try this lip-smacking smoothie: Juice 3 cups of raw rhubarb stalks and 1 cup of fresh or frozen strawberries. Add 1/4 cup of water and 1/4 cup of honey, then sip and go!

CORNS AND CALLUSES

Rub 'em a New Way

———◆◯◯◯◆———

My sister's feet are incredibly smooth—so much so that I used to call her "marble feet." My feet are another matter: My heels are swathed in thick, dry calluses, and on occasion, my little toe sprouts a hard, painful corn that makes me prefer to go barefoot even in subzero weather. Don't feel too sorry for me, though: According to the experts, my mean little bumps and pads are actually gifts—from my feet.

WHY ME?

"Your feet produce extra skin cells to form padding that protects your bones from harm," explains John Hahn, N.D., D.P.M., a naturopathic physician and podiatrist in Bend, Oregon. This padding—a.k.a. corns, which tend to pop up on the tops of the toes or the sides of the small toes—usually develops in response to shoes with tight, narrow toeboxes that rub the feet. The corn starts out as a callus, then often thickens and develops a hard core, which can press against nerve endings and cause sharp pain. Soft corns can sometimes develop between toes when they rub together—but again, they're a result of wearing tight, narrow shoes and sometimes tight-toed pantyhose, too.

Most calluses that form on the bottoms of your feet cushion your bones as well. They arise because fat pads on the sole of the foot tend to thin with age, and the body produces calluses to make up for the suddenly skimpier soles.

STEPS TO SMOOTHER FEET

You can rid your dogs of any unsightly corns and calluses without going near the drugstore, with its pads, plasters, disks, and salves containing harsh salicylic acid. "These products are unwise to use, since their function is to burn skin, and they can't tell the difference between dead, bumpy skin and normal skin," says Ronald Jensen, D.P.M., a podiatrist with the Sutter Gould Medical Group in Modesto, California. Spare your skin and sock it to corns and calluses with these measures.

TREAT THEM RIGHT. Using a pumice stone or emery board is a great way to pare away dead skin cells, but you have to do some prep work first. After your daily shower or bath, pat your feet dry, then gently rub your corn or callus. "Don't rub like you're sanding down a cabinet, or you could abrade your skin and worsen your problem," warns Dr. Jensen. "The idea is to take off a little at a time, and do it often." After 10 to 15 sessions, the pads should disappear.

SQUEEZE. Bathe as usual, then squeeze the juice of an aloe plant onto your corn and massage away, says Dr. Hahn. Aloe moisturizes and helps remove dry, dead skin so fresh skin cells can rise to the surface.

ADD CHAMOMILE. If you have very thick calluses and want to soak them, try this remedy suggested by Suzanne M. Levine, D.P.M., clinical assistant podiatrist at Mount Sinai Hospital in New York City. Brew some chamomile tea and add it to your soaking water. Your skin will soften, but it may also turn slightly yellow. Don't worry, though: The tint is easily removed with soap and water. You can buy chamomile teas at health food stores and some supermarkets.

TURN TO GENTLE ACIDS. Lactic acid, a naturally occurring substance in milk, can get rid of dead skin cells without destroying your skin, says Dr. Hahn. To halt newly formed corns, massage a cream that contains 12 percent lactic acid into your skin at the first hint of pressure or pain. Look for the creams at drugstores and check the labels for lactic acid content.

RESIST THE RAZOR. Don't set foot near razor-bladed instruments to shave off corns or calluses, especially if you have diabetes, says Dr. Hahn. Blood supply to the feet is diminished in people with diabetes, so the skin heals more slowly. Besides, such "bathroom surgery" could lead to serious cuts and long-lasting infection. If you have a painful corn, see a podiatrist for treatment.

CUTS AND SCRAPES

Heal Minor Battle Wounds

————◦⟨◦◦◦⟩◦————

When spring finally arrives and I'm lured outside by the scent of moist, fertile soil, I sometimes rush to tackle gardening chores without protective clothing. For a while, I thrill at the feel of the warm sun on my bare arms and winter-white legs. By the time I've cleared prickly tree limbs, divided stubborn peony roots, and transplanted thorny rose bushes, though, my arms and legs are usually so covered with cuts and scrapes that I look as if I've been wrestling with a Bengal tiger.

Unfortunately, the standard disinfectants used to flush out wounds—alcohol, iodine, and hydrogen peroxide—can irritate tissues and

MAKE A HEALING POWDER

Raid your spice rack for whole cloves, which contain the chemical eugenol—an excellent antiseptic and painkiller. Crush the cloves into a powder, then sprinkle it directly onto your wound to speed healing.

actually slow healing, says Alison Clough, M.D., a physician in Tucson. Plus, they can sting like the dickens—and who needs that on top of the pain of the cut?

COMMONSENSE FIRST AID

If your wound is gaping, gushing blood, or the result of a puncture, head straight to the hospital. Other than tightly binding the entire wound to try to stem the flow of blood, don't attempt to doctor it on your own. For less serious, more manageable injuries, however, here's what to do.

CLEAN AND PRESS. Hold your cut or scrape under running water or pour cool water from a cup over the wound. Using a mild soap—the brand you normally use when you bathe should be just fine—and a soft washcloth, thoroughly clean the edges of the wound and the surrounding skin, being careful not to let any soap stray into the open skin. If dirt is embedded in the wound, use tweezers (cleaned by dipping them into rubbing alcohol) to pick out the particles. Better yet, use a very soft, clean nailbrush to remove any tiny, deeply embedded bits of debris.

Once the cut or scrape is clean, press a clean cloth or tissue on the wound for 15 minutes—about how long it takes to

WHEN TO DIAL THE DOC

• • • • • • • • • • • •

Head to the hospital or call your doctor immediately if:
• Blood gushes from the wound in spurts, which may mean you've nicked an artery.
• You're unable to stem the flow of blood after 10 minutes.
• The wound is on your face or lips, where scarring is most likely.
• The wound resulted from a puncture. You may need a tetanus shot if you've been punctured by a rusty object and it's been more than 10 years since your last booster.
• You can't get the edges of the wound to stay together (no matter how small it is). You may need stitches.
• You see red streaks around the wound or develop a fever, both of which may indicate infection.

stanch the flow of blood—especially if the cut is on your scalp, hand, or foot, where blood vessels are close to the surface of your skin. If blood seeps through the cloth, add another layer and reapply the pressure gently but firmly. If the cut is on your arm or leg, you can raise it above the level of your heart to help slow the bleeding. *Note:* If your cut bleeds in spurts, or blood drenches the bandage after 10 minutes of firm, direct pressure, go to the emergency room immediately.

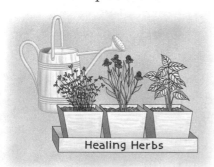

FIGHT THE BUGS. Calendula fights a broad range of bugs, including bacteria and fungi. "I like to use it as a poultice to clean out debris," notes Sharol Tilgner, N.D., a naturopathic physician and director of the Wise Acres Herbal Education Center in Eugene, Oregon. To prepare a poultice, saturate a piece of sterile gauze or cloth with calendula extract (available at health food stores), place the soaked material on your scrape, and leave it there for about an hour to help soften the skin and make any debris easier to remove. Afterward, pour a drop or two of extract directly onto the wound to keep it germ-free and reduce the chance of scarring.

WASH WITH ROSEMARY. To cut your risk of infection, wash your wound with rosemary extract, available at health food stores. This aromatic herb is a mild antiseptic that appears to penetrate the skin and may allow the wound to dry out better than antibiotic creams and ointments, which can smother the skin and may seal in germs.

COMFORT WITH COMFREY. The leaves and roots of the comfrey plant contain the healing agent allantoin, which stimulates healthy tissue growth, speeding healing and reducing scar formation. You can find comfrey cream at your health food store, or you can

Healing Herbs

crush fresh, clean leaves to apply to your wound as needed. Since comfrey encourages scab formation, however, use it only on shallow cuts that you've cleaned thoroughly, warns Dr. Tilgner. Otherwise, you may inadvertently seal in some germs.

USE A SWEET SALVE. When crude, undiluted honey was applied to infected wounds in a recent study, they healed twice as fast as wounds treated with antiseptics. "The thick honey covers the wound and may serve as an antibacterial to keep infection at bay," explains Manfred Kroger, Ph.D., professor emeritus of food science at Pennsylvania State University in University Park. Plus, honey appears to reduce swelling and pain. Just be sure to thoroughly wash your cut, use pasteurized honey (which won't harbor bacteria of its own), and watch for signs of infection, such as red streaks around the wound, a fever, or increased tenderness, cautions Dr. Kroger.

GIVE ECHINACEA A TRY. If you have a severe laceration or puncture wound, this natural immune booster will help bring white blood cells to the area to fight infection, says Dr. Tilgner. "I usually suggest taking two capsules three times a day for one week." Don't use echinacea if you have an autoimmune disease such as lupus, rheumatoid arthritis, or multiple sclerosis, or if you're pregnant or nursing.

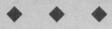

HOMEGROWN SOLUTION

◆   ◆   ◆

Use Yarrow

"Yarrow is my favorite herb for healing minor wounds," says Sharol Tilgner, N.D. "It's easily found, and it acts as both an astringent to stem the flow of blood and an anti-inflammatory to calm the pain." Simply rinse some fresh yarrow leaves, chew them into a paste, and spit out the mashed poultice directly onto your wound. The fresher the leaves, the more quickly the bleeding will stop.

DEPRESSION

It's Not Just Feeling Sad

———✦———

We all have times when we pull into ourselves like little box turtles, preferring to be alone with our thoughts or feelings. But if you've been inside your shell for longer than usual, or you're interacting with people with barely contained irritation, you could be depressed, like my friend Lee, and not even know it.

Normally very social, gracious, and energetic, Lee began getting really teed off with difficult customers at her gift store. She also started canceling dinner dates with friends and stopped browsing through flea markets—two activities she usually adored. "I just felt 'blah' about every-

---

GET TOGETHER WITH THE GIRLS

Studies at the University of California, Los Angeles, indicate that when one woman spends time with another woman, her body releases a brain chemical called oxytocin that counters the kind of stress that can contribute to depression. To take advantage of this phenomenon, one woman I know meets her girlfriends at a neighborhood restaurant once a week for a rip-roaringly funny girls' night out!

---

thing," she says.

Because Lee didn't really feel sad and was able to carry on with her life, she was surprised when she was diagnosed with depression, a condition that she, like most of us, associated with despair.

While depression can manifest itself as sadness and despair, it can also show up as irritability and a lack of pleasure in normally pleasurable activities. Even overfocusing at work can be a symptom of depression—a disease that springs from an imbalance in brain chemicals that powerfully affect moods, appetite, and sleeping habits, among other things.

WHY ME?

Genes, which help determine our levels of various brain chemicals that affect mood, may be partially to blame, but depression is usually a one-two punch. Genes set the stage, and then a stressful event tips your brain chemistry into the abyss. And chronic stress—the kind that arises from constantly trying to meet too many daily obligations—floods the body with the hormones cortisol and prolactin, which can lower levels of the mood-stabilizing brain chemical serotonin.

There are other causes of depression as well. The spikes and dips in hormones that normally occur during the menstrual cycle (giving rise to the irritability and general moodiness of premenstrual syndrome, or PMS), after giving birth (triggering postpartum depression), and before menopause can also affect brain chemistry and send you spinning. Abnormalities in the thyroid, pituitary, and adrenal glands can also precipitate a low mood.

Even the gloomy days of winter or simply being cooped up in a dark house or windowless office can add to your doldrums, since inadequate exposure to sunlight can inhibit the release of serotonin. This sleepy, moody type of low is called seasonal affective disorder (SAD) and usually lifts during the sunny spring and summer months. If you're underexposed to light in general, however, it can contribute to general depression year-round.

NATURAL MOOD BOOSTERS

Depression can be life-threatening, so if you think you may be depressed, consult your doctor immediately. Ask him for a referral to a mental health professional, such as a psychiatrist, psychologist, or licensed clinical social worker, who may recommend that you take an antidepressant medication, such as fluoxetine (Prozac) or sertraline (Zoloft). Both of these drugs block the reabsorption of serotonin into the brain, so people who take them always have a constant level of this mood-stabilizing hormone available. You should also be advised to have at least short-term cognitive therapy. Studies show that the two together are much more effective than any other treatment regimen.

For people with moderate or serious depression, the benefits of medication clearly outweigh the side effects (which often include lack of energy, weight gain, and zero libido or sexual function). If your depression is mild, however, you might talk to your doctor about starting with gentler, more natural alternatives such as those listed below. Just one caveat: If you're already taking prescription antidepressants or have bipolar disorder (also called manic depression), avoid the herbal antidepressants recommended here.

B GOOD. Nearly 80 percent of people with depression are deficient in vitamin B_6, says Hyla Cass, M.D., assistant clinical professor of psychiatry at the University of California, Los Angeles, School of Medicine. To get B_6 plus the rest of the Bs (all of which your body needs to deliver oxygen to the brain, turn blood sugar into energy, and keep feel-good brain chemicals in circulation), Dr. Cass suggests popping a B-complex supplement that supplies 20 milligrams of B_6, 500 micrograms of B_{12}, and 400 micrograms of folic acid. Take it with food.

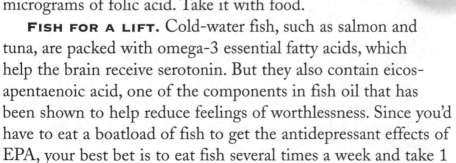

FISH FOR A LIFT. Cold-water fish, such as salmon and tuna, are packed with omega-3 essential fatty acids, which help the brain receive serotonin. But they also contain eicosapentaenoic acid, one of the components in fish oil that has been shown to help reduce feelings of worthlessness. Since you'd have to eat a boatload of fish to get the antidepressant effects of EPA, your best bet is to eat fish several times a week and take 1

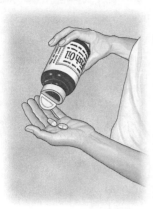

gram (1,000 milligrams) of fish-oil supplements (available at health food stores) twice a day. Just be sure your supplements contain at least half EPA and half docosahexaenoic acid (DHA). Since fish oil can thin your blood, avoid it if you take aspirin or prescription blood thinners.

TURN TO TURKEY. Don't wait until the holidays to get your dose of tryptophan, an amino acid that's ultimately converted into serotonin in the body. In one study, when women who were depressed feasted on tryptophan-rich foods, such as turkey, chicken, fish, dairy products, soybeans, nuts, and avocados, their depression eased without the help of medication, reports Dr. Cass. One idea: Buy bags of frozen soybeans at the supermarket, pop a bowlful in the microwave to cook, and snack on them (they're crunchy!). Or mash up some avocados to make some yummy, mood-lifting guacamole.

PAIR IT WITH POTATOES. When you're eating turkey or another tryptophan-rich food, pair it with a lower-fat carbohydrate, such as whole grain bread, brown rice, or mashed potatoes. Carbohydrates trigger the release of insulin, which allows tryptophan to freely enter your brain so that eventually, serotonin levels rise.

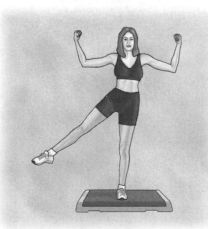

GET AEROBIC EXERCISE. A study at Duke University Medical Center revealed that people with major depression who exercised aerobically for 30 minutes three times a week experienced the same relief from depression as people who took antidepressants. There are several reasons for this effect. First, aerobic exercise forces oxygen into your cells, increasing energy production. Second, it signals the brain to release "feel-good" brain chemicals called endorphins, which boost mood. Finally, it enhances sleep and curbs weight gain, both of which can increase energy.

WORK OUT OUTSIDE. If you do your aerobic exercise outdoors, you may boost its antidepressant effect, says Marie-Annette Brown, R.N., Ph.D., professor of nursing at the University of Washington School of Nursing in Seattle. Exposure to sunlight— even on dim, overcast days—helps boost levels of vitamin D, which then helps the body maintain higher levels of serotonin. In fact, even in a downpour, there is 30 times more light outside than in, she says.

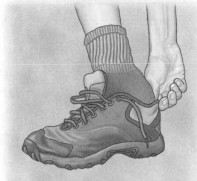

LIGHTEN UP. Try what's called a dawn simulator—essentially a bedside lamp whose glow increases gradually from dim to more intense light, mimicking a natural sunrise in mid-May—to self-treat SAD. All you do is program the "fake dawn" to start 1 to 3 hours before you awaken, and your body detects the changing light through your closed eyelids. Look for 250-lux models on the Internet and in catalogs and stores that sell personal health care products.

RUB THE BLUES AWAY. Preliminary studies indicate that massage may help reduce symptoms of depression, perhaps by combating a buildup of the stress hormone cortisol, says Valerie Raskin, M.D., clinical associate professor of psychiatry at the University of Chicago Pritzker School of Medicine. To enhance the effect, use some mood-boosting herbal oils, such as bergamot, geranium, jasmine, neroli, or ylang-ylang, all available at health food stores.

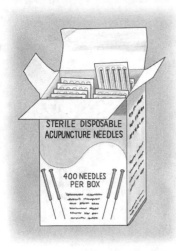

GET AN ACUPUNCTURE ATTITUDE ADJUSTMENT. A study from the University of Arizona found that three months of twice-weekly acupuncture treatments reduced depression in more than half of the women tested, although researchers aren't sure why. It's possible that insertion of the thread-thin needles stimulates the release of mood-lifting endorphins or corrects a chemical imbalance involved in depression. Ask your doctor to recommend a reputable practitioner in your area.

TRY ST. JOHN'S WORT. A slew of studies since the 1970s have shown that St. John's wort can ease mild (but not severe) depression, says Dr. Cass—perhaps by inhibiting the reabsorption of serotonin. Check with your doctor first, then check your health food store for a high-quality brand such as Kira or Nature's Made and take 300 milligrams three times a day. You may not feel its full effect for up to two months, and in some people, it can cause stomach upset, allergic reactions, and heightened sensitivity to the sun. Do not take St. John's wort with other medications.

SWALLOW SAM-E. SAM-e (short for S-adenosylmethionine)—a compound that helps regulate the breakdown of feel-good hormones—may be a more effective and faster mood booster for people with mild to moderate depression than St. John's wort. "You get results with SAM-e in less than a week with no major side effects," says Robert Brown, M.D., professor of psychiatry at Columbia University Medical School in New York City. Check with your doctor first, then look for quality brands such as Nature's Made coated tablets (to reduce the risk of stomach upset) at health food stores. Follow the package directions, and don't take SAM-e with any other medication.

DIABETES

Steady Your Bouncing Blood Sugar

———⊰⊱———

Some conditions announce themselves with obvious symptoms—a sharp pain in the chest, difficulty breathing, or stiffness in the joints. Not so with diabetes. It's stealthy, which is why many of us are walking around with the beginnings of the disease and don't even know it. For example, the only clue my friend Evie had that something might be out of whack was that she was always running to the store for creams to treat repeated yeast infections. Her doctor eventually tested her blood and found that her blood sugar (glucose) level was high—a hallmark of diabetes. When you think about it, the link makes sense, because yeast infections thrive in high-sugar environments, which is exactly what diabetes creates. When you eat, the food is converted to blood sugar. Your pancreas then secretes the hormone insulin, which whisks the glu-

> ## IT'S GOOD TO GO GREEN
>
> A banana that's a bit underripe—that is, still a little green at the tip—produces half the glycemic response of a ripe banana and is less likely to spike your blood sugar, says Thomas Wolever, Ph.D.

cose from your bloodstream and plunks it into your cells for energy. Any leftover glucose in the bloodstream is stored in your liver as glycogen. If your insulin level should drop too low, the liver releases glycogen into the bloodstream so you always have a ready supply for energy.

In diabetes, however, this tidy system for controlling blood sugar goes awry. In the rarer type 1 diabetes, the pancreas makes little or no insulin. People typically develop this type as kids or young adults and must take injections of insulin for the rest of their lives to keep their blood sugar stable.

In type 2 diabetes—which accounts for 90 percent of cases and can develop in people of any age—the body makes adequate or even high amounts of insulin, yet the cells are unable to use it because they've become insulin resistant. The result? Blood sugar isn't absorbed into the cells and is left to wander around the bloodstream, where it can wreak havoc. It not only feeds yeast infections but also damages major organs and sets the stage for a heart attack, stroke, or other serious diseases.

WHY ME?

Type 2 diabetes is about lifestyle. "We were not meant to gorge on huge quantities of simple

---

SUBDUE YOUR SWEET TOOTH

Ever feel helpless to resist the lure of a candy bar? Well, help is here, in the form of an Indian herb called gymnema, which means "sugar destroyer" in Sanskrit. When the leaf is chewed, it decreases the ability of the taste buds to detect sweetness. Gymnema capsules, which you can find at health food stores, also make sugar distasteful, says Diane Guthrie, Ph.D. "I suggest taking 200 milligrams twice a day, about a half-hour before breakfast and then again before supper." Just one caveat: Gymnema can lower blood sugar too much, so consult your doctor before you take it.

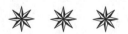

---

sugars like soft drinks or starches like potatoes and then just sit around," says Robert K. Bernstein, M.D., a physician specializing in diabetes and obesity in Mamaroneck, New York. Whole grains are digested slowly, but refined grains and sugar—"fast-acting carbs," as Dr. Bernstein calls them—literally flood the system with glucose. If you don't immediately burn off the glucose (and, honestly, how many of us go off for a sprint after wolfing down a Cinnabon?), the pancreas sends out a surge of insulin to get the sugar out of circulation. Over time, the pancreas poops out on producing insulin, the cells become insulin resistant, and blood sugar takes over.

> ## TUB THERAPY
>
> Who said controlling your blood sugar has to be hard? According to a small study at the University of Colorado Health Sciences Center in Loveland, taking a 30-minute soak in a hot tub six days a week for one month may inch down your glucose level enough for you to reduce your insulin dose. The hot water may simulate exercise by increasing the blood flow to muscles, thus reducing insulin resistance. Talk to your doctor before trying hot-tub therapy, though; if you have nerve damage or impaired circulation, it may not be right for you.

Beyond flooding your system with glucose, those fast-acting carbohydrates also just make you fat—often around the midsection, which is another contributing factor for diabetes. Carbs from your Cap'n Crunch breakfast quickly spike your blood sugar, a crash soon follows, and you become hungry again. So you eat more—and you gain weight. Today, a third more Americans have diabetes than eight years ago, and this expanded figure is directly related to our expanding waistlines.

THE WAY TO STABILIZE

If you are 20 pounds above your ideal weight, have a spare tire around your middle, or have other risk factors (such as a

Dunk Your Spuds—In Vinegar!

Gram for gram, potatoes are converted to blood sugar faster than any other food—including sugar sprinkled on cereal, says Richard K. Bernstein, M.D. If you're a spud lover, you could opt for potato salad made with unpeeled potatoes and vinaigrette dressing. The acid in the dressing will reduce the effect on your blood sugar. To do the same with French fries, simply eat them the British way—doused with vinegar.

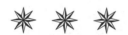

family history of diabetes; Hispanic, African-American, or Native American heritage; or high blood pressure), two tests—the fasting plasma glucose test and the glucose tolerance test—could help you head off diabetes. They can determine if you have prediabetes, meaning that your glucose levels are higher than is healthy but too low to be diagnosed as diabetes.

Whether the tests reveal diabetes or prediabetes—or neither—all of us would benefit from steadying our bouncing blood sugar levels, and there are myriad ways to do just that. Even the smallest changes in your diet and activity level can lower your glucose to healthier levels—and, if you're taking medication to control blood sugar, you may be able to cut back on or even eliminate your doses.

Here's where to start—with your doctor's approval, of course.

Go low. Those Cinnabons, along with ice cream, pasta, potatoes, and even corn and carrots, rank high on the GI, or glycemic index, which is basically a list of foods ranked by how much they boost your blood sugar after eating them. By eating foods lower on the GI scale at every meal for a month—for example, trading Cheerios for rice bran, having rye bread instead of a Kaiser roll, and eating more legumes and whole, unpeeled veggies—you may reduce your blood sugar and insulin by a third, according to research conducted by Thomas Wolever,

Ph.D., professor of nutritional science and medicine at the University of Toronto. Be sure to bypass packaged, processed foods as well, since they're all rated super-high on the GI.

BUMP UP YOUR FIBER. Getting 50 grams of fiber daily—double the amount normally recommended—may lower insulin resistance, studies show. Those fiber-rich psyllium powders sold in drugstores and grocery stores could help you meet that quota, but select brands without sugars or laxatives, follow the package directions, and consult your doctor before using them.

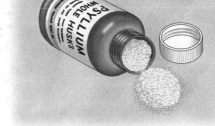

GULP MILK FROM GRASS EATERS. Compared with milk produced by grain-fed cows, milk from grass-fed cows contains twice as much conjugated linoleic acid (CLA), which, in supplement form, has been found to decrease blood sugar levels fivefold in people with diabetes. While CLA looks promising for reversing insulin resistance, says Diane Guthrie, Ph.D., a nurse practitioner with the Mid-American Diabetes Association in Wichita, it's not clear how much you need in order to benefit. "I suggest you make sure you get CLA from food sources," she says. Besides milk, these include beef, lamb, eggs, and turkey.

> ## DON'T OVERCOOK PASTA
>
> The starch isn't broken down as much in al dente (firm) noodles, so they're digested more slowly—and released more slowly as glucose into your bloodstream.

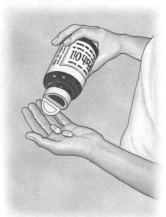

OPT FOR OMEGA-3'S. Cold-water fish such as tuna and salmon are the prime source of omega-3 essential fatty acids, which appear to help cells become less resistant to insulin. If you're not much of a fish eater, consider supplementing with 1 to 2 grams (1,000 to 2,000 milligrams) of fish oil in capsule form or 1 to 2 tablespoons of flaxseed oil a day for the same effect. Both are available in health food stores. *Note:* If you already have diabetes, fish oil may have no effect. Also, people taking aspirin or prescription blood thinners should not take fish oil or flaxseed oil.

MIND YOUR Bs. "I tell my patients to make sure that they take a B-complex vitamin that includes vitamin B_3 [niacin], the primary B that may help lower blood sugar and can often become depleted in people with diabetes," says Dr. Guthrie. It's not advisable to take niacin alone, but its chemical cousin niacinamide, a safe form, may be able to help keep prediabetes from turning into full-blown diabetes. Check with your doctor about taking niacinamide for this purpose.

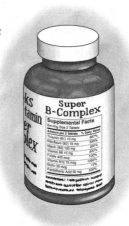

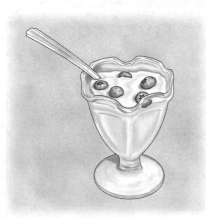

FIND FENUGREEK. Nutty, maple-flavored fenugreek seeds are used to flavor Indian curries, but the oil may provide more than taste: It may also lower blood sugar, says Kathi Head, N.D., a naturopathic physician in Sandpoint, Idaho. To get enough, she suggests adding about 2 tablespoons of defatted fenugreek powder (available in health food stores) to yogurt or a smoothie once a day. If you're taking diabetes medications, however, check with your doctor first.

GET BITTER. Whether it's called bitter melon or bitter gourd, the seeds of this Indian herb seem to work as a natural plant insulin, says Dr. Head. In one small study, people who took dried, powdered seeds for three weeks experienced a 25 percent drop in blood sugar. Those who received a liquid extract had a whopping 54 percent drop. The only problem is that the liquid extract lives up to the herb's name. If you can stand the tart taste, try the extract, or you can look for standardized extract in capsule form. Both are available in health food stores; follow the label directions.

FERRET OUT FRUCTOSE. A high intake of high-fructose corn syrup—now the leading sweetener in packaged foods—may put you on the road to insulin resistance. "Stay away from foods that have ingredients ending in '-ose' at the top of the list," advises Dr. Bernstein. And don't be conned into thinking that brown sugar, raw sugar, or any other sugar is "healthy." To your body, sugar is sugar.

GET MORE SHUTEYE. It'll not only enhance your beauty, it will also help your blood sugar. In fact, studies show that if you're shortchanging yourself by as little as 2½ hours of sleep a night, you may be 40 percent less sensitive to insulin than you would be if you got your full 8 hours.

DO YOU HAVE POS?

If you have polycystic ovary syndrome (POS), as 10 percent of American women of childbearing age do, you should be tested for diabetes. Having POS puts you at seven times the normal risk of getting diabetes, although it's unclear why. One theory is that because the ovaries are part of the endocrine system, which regulates not only when you get your period but also your insulin output, a glitch in one may cause a glitch in the other.

DIARRHEA

Stop the Trots

————⊶∞∞⊷————

I was having a heart-to-heart recently with a friend who is normally very attentive. On this occasion, though, she had to interrupt our conversation several times to dash to the bathroom. While I was left to stare at her empty chair, my poor pal was enduring something far worse: the agony of loose, watery stools.

We've all been there, of course—marooned miserably in the loo, wondering what in heaven's name could have given us the runs. There are no fewer than a dozen possibilities—everything from stomach flu to stress.

WHY ME?

If you tend to make beelines to the bathroom shortly after drinking espresso, there's no great mystery to your misery: Coffee is a natural colon stimulant. The culprit is also easy to pinpoint if you've been either gorging on fruit (say, snacking your way through a bag of cherries or a bunch of grapes in one sitting) or eating scoop after scoop of ice cream.

"I call this the 'eat-and-boom' form of diarrhea," says Christine Boorean, N.D., a naturopathic physician in Portland, Oregon. "For some people, sugar in any form—whether it's the fructose in fruit or the lactose in milk—is simply not well digested and can cause intestinal distress." Artificial sweeteners, alcohol, antacids, and megadoses of magnesium and vitamin C can also cause the runs, as can antibiotics—which is what had my friend running repeatedly to the ladies'.

Diarrhea can also signal more serious problems, such as food poisoning, a digestive disorder, or irritable bowel syndrome (which occurs when your colon goes into spasm, often in response to stress). It can even indicate that you're not absorbing nutrients due to anemia, diabetes, a thyroid disorder, or some other underlying condition. If the diarrhea is laced with blood, it can point to an infection or even a tumor. In other words, it's potentially quite serious.

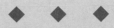

HOMEGROWN SOLUTION

◆ ◆ ◆

Please Eat the Daisies!

When Rover has an internal upset, he grazes on grass, but I suggest you bypass the lawn and head straight for your chamomile patch. A small handful of these daisylike flowers can provide a soothing and effective remedy for diarrhea. Simply wash them and leave them to dry out for a while, then steep 1 tablespoon of the dried flowers in a cup of hot water for 10 to 15 minutes. Strain out the herb and drink several cups of tea a day until your runs subside. Don't use chamomile if you're allergic to ragweed.

NO MORE RUNS

Fortunately, there are many nondrug remedies that will slow the passage of food and get to the root of the problem—all within 24 to 72 hours. Here's where to start.

BIND WITH BLACKBERRY. "The tannins in the blackberry root dry the mucous membranes in your intestine and bind up the bowel," says Michael DiPalma, N.D., a naturopathic physician in Newtown, Pennsylvania. Check

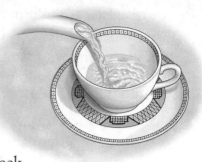

your health food store for blackberry tea (the real McCoy—not simply tea flavored with blackberry) and follow the package directions. Drink several cups a day.

EAT BARLEY. Bland though it may be, this grain can slow intestinal motion and curb diarrhea. To make it tasty, prepare pearl barley according to the package directions and add 1 cup to beef broth. The mixture will replace lost fluids and electrolytes in addition to calming your intestinal turmoil.

DRINK RICE WATER. The next time you prepare a batch of rice, add an extra 1½ cups of water to the pot. When the rice is cooked to the texture you want, drain off the extra water, chill it if you like, and drink it as a hydrating, bind-

---

NO MORE TRAVELER'S DIARRHEA

While everyone else on your tour was oohing and aahing at the Sun God's ruined temple, you were stuck on the throne in the hotel bathroom—but never again. Next time, you'll pack Culturelle, the only probiotic (good bacteria) formula made from a new strain of bacteria called lactobacillus GG (LGG), which has been shown to not only treat but also prevent traveler's diarrhea. In one study, yogurt laced with LGG limited diarrhea to two days instead of the normal eight. The usual dosage is one or two capsules daily with food. Ask your doctor about it if you're planning a trip. At this point, Culturelle is sold only through physicians and on the Internet.

ing tonic. If you need a sweetener, use a small amount of sugar or honey.

GET BUGGED. "Beneficial bacteria—so-called good bugs—are incredible healing agents that literally wipe out the bad bugs that may be causing your diarrhea, usually within a day or so," says Skye Weintraub, N.D., a naturopathic physician in Eugene, Oregon. While some brands of yogurt contain active cultures of beneficial *Lactobacillus acidophilus* bacteria, eating dairy products isn't the best way to treat diarrhea. Instead, get acidophilus in liquid or capsule form at a health food store and follow the package directions.

LULL YOUR INTESTINES. Valerian, an herbal sedative long recommended as a sleep tonic, can settle intestinal spasms and is especially helpful if you're doubled over with crampy diarrhea, says Dr. Boorean. She suggests you take one or two capsules, or 100 to 300 milligrams, a day for as long as you have symptoms. Since valerian is a sleep aid, it can cause drowsiness, so it's best to take it before bedtime. And don't take it if you're 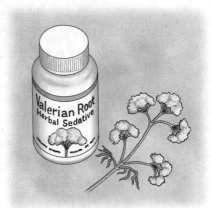 using any other kind of medication, particularly antidepressants or anti-anxiety drugs.

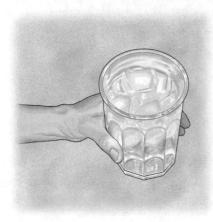

BET ON BARK. Slippery elm bark soothes the mucous membranes of the bowel with few or no side effects. Stir 1/4 teaspoon of slippery elm powder into a cup of applesauce and eat it three or four times a day. Or add 30 to 40 drops of tincture to a glass of water and drink it every 2 hours until your diarrhea stops. Both forms of the herb are available at health food stores.

COOL THE BURN. "If you have burning diarrhea, marshmallow tea can minimize your irritation by attracting moisture to the intestinal walls," says Dr. Boorean. Look for the tea in your local health food store. Make it according to package directions and drink a cup several times a day until the burning subsides.

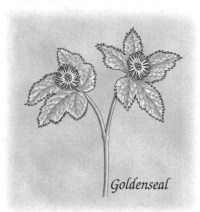

MAKE A STINK. "Garlic is one of the best ways to fight infection internally—whether your diarrhea is caused by a flu virus or bacteria that you picked up from food," says Dr. DiPalma. Pick up some garlic capsules at a health food store or drugstore and take 200 to 400 milligrams three times a day until your diarrhea subsides.

GRAB SOME GOLDENSEAL. If "something you ate" is at the root of your diarrhea, you've probably been hit by one of three nasty bacteria—*E. coli*, giardia, or salmonella. Dosing with goldenseal, an herb that can slightly dry up the mucous membranes in your intestine, can beat these bugs. The tea is bitter, so look for goldenseal capsules at a health food store and take 250 milligrams three times a day until your diarrhea subsides, suggests Dr. DiPalma—unless you're taking antibiotics or are pregnant or nursing.

Goldenseal

GIVE GRAPEFRUIT SEED A TRY. Made from the seeds and pulp of grapefruit, grapefruit seed extract (GSE) can knock out any bacterium, parasite, or virus that may be behind your diarrhea. "Add two drops to a glass of water and take it twice a day until you've killed whatever you picked up," suggests Dr. Weintraub. Never take GSE straight, or it may wipe out the beneficial bacteria along with the troublemakers. Also, if you're taking cholesteral-lowering medication, you should avoid GSE.

Dizziness

When the World Spins

As a kid, I used to love the head-spinning feeling of riding a roller-coaster. A few years back, though, I experienced a similar sensation while coasting in my own car, and it was scary in a whole different way. I made it home, my knuckles white from gripping the steering wheel. My husband rushed me to the doctor's office, where my stomach churned as the room spun faster than the fruits in a slot machine.

I was terrified; my doctor was mystified. In fact, he never did determine the cause of my dizzy spell, which thankfully vanished after a few miserable days.

WHY ME?

The most common cause of dizziness is a disturbance in a part

WHEN TO DIAL THE DOC

If a spinning sensation hits you suddenly or is accompanied by chest pain, a racing heartbeat, numbness, or blurred vision, you need to see a doctor immediately; you may be having a heart attack. Pressure or pain in the ears, deafness, or nausea after a dizzy spell also warrants a doctor's attention, since this could signal a nerve problem or other disorder.

of the inner ear that provides your sense of balance. If the room spins when you get up, flip over in bed, or tilt your head backward, your inner ear is probably full of rocks—bits of calcium carbonate that have broken off from a pouch called the utricle, also in your inner ear. Normally, these "ear rocks," or otoconia, simply dissolve and are reabsorbed by cells in your inner ear. As the utricle degenerates with normal aging, however, or is affected by an infection, a head injury, or even migraines, bits may break off and become lodged in the wrong part of the ear canal. Then, when you move your head or body, the misplaced bits stimulate nerve sensors there, and you experience that roller-coaster wooziness, minus the thrills.

These spells—formally called benign paroxysmal positional vertigo, or BPPV—can come and go and eventually fade away on their own after weeks or months. But while BPPV is harmless, the lightheadedness and unsteadiness that accompany it can leave you fatigued, nauseated, and unable to concentrate.

Other causes of dizziness include reduced blood flow to the inner ear due to hardening of the arteries, poor circulation from diabetes, or anything that constricts blood vessels, such as caffeine or anxiety. The spinning sensation, called vertigo—which isn't a fear of heights, as the classic Alfred Hitchcock film suggested—arises when your brain doesn't properly receive messages from your eyes, inner ears, or nerves in your skin, muscles, and joints. These three systems monitor where your body is in space. If one of them isn't working or your brain is getting conflicting messages, you feel dizzy, woozy, and nauseated.

STOP THE SPIN CYCLE

Because dizziness can result from a decidedly dizzying array of conditions, treating it appropriately can be difficult—but it isn't impossible. In fact, in most cases, you can stop the spinning with surprisingly basic, drug-free measures you can take on your own.

For instance, if you have occasional dizziness, the first thing you'll want to do, says Timothy C. Hain, M.D., professor of neurology, otolaryngology, and physical therapy/human movement science at Northwestern University Medical School in Chicago, is limit your intake of caffeine and salt, both of which can impede blood flow throughout your body—including to your inner ear. Here are more super-simple but super-effective spin stoppers to try.

PROCEED GINGERLY. Ginger in any form—including ginger tea,

GET RID OF THE ROCKS

For dizziness linked to benign paroxysmal positional vertigo—a disorder caused by bits of calcium carbonate, or "ear rocks," lodged in your inner ear—try this simple but effective head-positioning exercise, called the Brandt-Daroff maneuver. It will literally get the rocks out of your head.

Sit on the edge of a bed, then throw yourself onto the bed with one ear against a pillow. Don't move until your vertigo disappears. Next, return to an upright position and remain there until your dizziness fades, then repeat the rapid fall on the opposite side of your body. This is 1 repetition. Three times a week, do 10 to 20 repetitions twice daily. Your symptoms should start to fade within the first few days, although complete relief could take weeks, notes Timothy C. Hain, M.D.

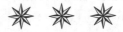

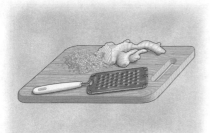

ginger candy, and fresh ginger—dampens the vestibular impulses in the brain that nauseate you, says William Warnock, N.D., a naturopathic physician in Shelbourne, Vermont. In fact, studies have shown that ginger is superior to dimenhydrinate (Dramamine) when it comes to curing nausea related to motion sickness. To brew a stomach-soothing tea, get some ginger tea at a health food store or supermarket and follow the package directions. Or grate 2 teaspoons of fresh ginger into a cup of boiling water, steep for 10 minutes, strain, and sip.

MAXIMIZE MAGNESIUM AND CALCIUM. Both minerals act as antispasmodics to ease open narrowed blood vessels that may be causing your dizziness by reducing blood flow to your inner ear, says Michael D. Seidman, M.D., director of neurotologic surgery at Henry Ford Hospital in Detroit. Check with your doctor first, but you can probably take a "cal-mag" supplement widely available in drugstores. Your goal should be to get 400 milligrams of magnesium and 1,000 milligrams of calcium a day.

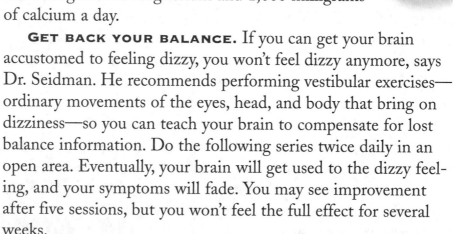

GET BACK YOUR BALANCE. If you can get your brain accustomed to feeling dizzy, you won't feel dizzy anymore, says Dr. Seidman. He recommends performing vestibular exercises—ordinary movements of the eyes, head, and body that bring on dizziness—so you can teach your brain to compensate for lost balance information. Do the following series twice daily in an open area. Eventually, your brain will get used to the dizzy feeling, and your symptoms will fade. You may see improvement after five sessions, but you won't feel the full effect for several weeks.

• Sit on the edge of your bed with your legs straight out in front of you, then quickly flop down on your back. Wait for the dizziness to fade, then quickly sit up again. Wait for the dizziness to subside, then repeat three times.

• Sit upright in a chair and turn your head rapidly left and right, five times in each direction. Wait for the dizziness to fade, then repeat three times. Next, move your head up and down, five times in each direction. Wait for the dizziness to fade, then repeat three times.

• While sitting in a chair, quickly bend forward, bringing your head halfway to your knees. Wait for the dizziness to subside, then quickly sit up again. Wait for your dizziness to fade, then repeat three times.

• Sit in a chair with one arm outstretched in front of you and your index finger pointing toward the ceiling. Staring at your finger, slowly turn your head to the left and then to the right. Begin slowly and increase the speed as you move your head back and forth 10 times. Stop, wait for the dizziness to subside, then repeat three times. Next, turn your finger sideways so it points either left or right. Repeat as above, only this time, move your head up and down.

TRY TAI CHI. The slow, graceful movements of this gentle martial art can help diminish dizziness associated with balance problems in about two months, says Dr. Hain. Tai chi helps you move your head and eyes in such a way that it recalibrates balancing systems that may be impaired, he says. The measured movements also force you into a variety of dizzying positions, so your brain learns what it's like to function with steadiness while you're dizzy.

DRY SKIN

A Reason to Pamper Yourself

———◈◇◇◇◈———

There comes a time in every woman's life when she makes the switch in her daily skin-care routine from sopping up excess oil in a battle against breakouts to slathering on moisturizers in a war against wrinkles. I won't tell you when I crossed this dermatological line, but suffice it to say, it's been a while since I arrived on what I think of as "the other side."

Doctors have another word for the dry skin that develops due to natural aging as well as exposure to harsh soaps, hot water, dry air, and improper nourishment: They call it xerosis. It occurs when so much water has evaporated from the top layer of the skin (or stratum corneum) that it can begin to look and feel like a shriveled autumn leaf.

BRUSH UP

Starting at the soles of your feet and moving up your legs toward your heart, gently rub your body in a circular motion with a super-soft, dry-bristle brush. Then do the same with your hands and arms. "Brushing will help stimulate your sebaceous glands to produce more sebum and will remove dead skin that makes your skin look dry, dull, and old," says Jeanette Jacknin, M.D.

WHY ME?

As we get older, the uppermost layer of our skin naturally loses some of its ability to hold water, explains Jeanette Jacknin, M.D., a dermatologist in Scottsdale, Arizona. In fact, by age 65, more than half of us have xerosis, she says. While natural aging isn't within our control, many other factors that contribute to dry skin are: Dry indoor heat; prolonged sun exposure; long, leisurely baths; frequent air travel (the air on planes is always very dry); frequent exposure to chlorinated water in swimming pools; the lack of fruit, seeds, and fish in our diets; and overuse of citrus-, alcohol-, or menthol-based skin-care products all do their share of damage.

MOISTURE MATTERS MOST

Almost always, you can treat dry skin on your own by following this simple equation: Add things that seal in moisture and take away things that encourage evaporation, says Leslie Baumann, M.D., associate professor of dermatology at the University of Miami School of Medicine in Tampa. This means, among other things, adding nutritionally rich foods and plenty of H_2O and subtracting frequent and/or lengthy showers. Of course, regularly using a moisturizer—any moisturizer—certainly can't hurt your skin. Choosing the best type from the three described below could actually help it.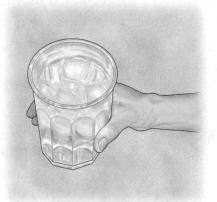

• Humectants attract water from both the atmosphere and the underlying layers of skin and bind it to the skin's surface. They include glycerin and alpha hydroxy acids.

• Emollients, including mineral oil, petroleum jelly, and lanolin, soften and smooth the skin.

• Occlusives coat the skin to lock in water and prevent evap-

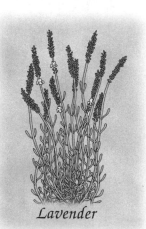
FINDING THE SOURCE OF DRY LIPS

If your lips always seem to be dry, check out the ingredients in your toothpaste. If it contains cinnamate—a flavoring agent that can be drying—you've nailed the culprit. Simply switch to a brand that's cinnamate-free and isn't labeled "tartar control." Like long-lasting lipsticks and mouthwashes that contain alcohol, tartar-control products can also dry out your lips.

oration. They tend to be quite greasy, oily, and/or waxy and include petroleum jelly, lanolin, and mineral oil (which are also emollients; the difference is in the concentration and how heavily they're applied), as well as grapeseed oil and beeswax.

If you have very dry skin or live in a very dry area, occlusive creams or oils may be the most effective moisturizers for you—at least until your skin responds to all your slathering. Then give these simple but effective solutions a try.

SELECT THE RIGHT SOAP. Check your health food store for oil-based bars that contain super-moisturizing olive oil or coconut oil, are not labeled as soap (which is drying), and are scented with palmarosa, rosewood, and/or sandalwood. All of these can help stimulate oil production.

OIL UP. After bathing, pat your skin to remove most of the water. Then, while it's still damp, slather on almond or sunflower oil (the same oil you use for cooking). Both are brimming with vitamin F, which provides unsaturated fatty acids that may help regulate the oil glands. If you'd rather not smell like a Caesar salad, simply add a few drops of lavender oil.

GET STEAMED. An herbal facial steam can deep-six dryness—especially if you use an oil that encourages oil production in your skin, says Kathi Keville, an herbalist in Boulder, Colorado. Simply bring 3 cups of water to a boil, then remove the pot from the stove. Add one drop each of rose, geranium, rosemary, fennel, and peppermint herbal oil. Drape a towel over your head and tuck the ends around the pot so the steam is captured inside a "mini-sauna." Be careful not to get close enough for the steam to burn your face. Limit your steam sessions to about 5 minutes once a week.

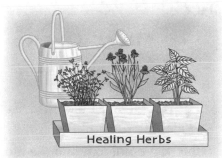

Healing Herbs

REFRESH WITH ROSEHIPS. Alcohol-based toners strip away much-needed oils, but rosehip oil has a high linoleic acid content, which studies show can both tone and moisturize skin. Look for the oil at your health food store, then douse a cotton ball with it and dab it all over your face, neck, and upper chest.

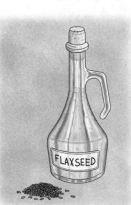

FLAXSEED

EAT FISH AND FLAX. Boost your intake of cold-water fish, such as tuna and salmon, and take 2 tablespoons of flaxseed oil (available at health food stores) daily, says Dr. Jacknin. Both provide omega-3 essential fatty acids (EFAs), which help your skin retain water to keep it plump, supple, and smooth. Don't take flaxseed oil if you take aspirin or prescription blood thinners.

USE EPO, ASAP! EPO, or evening primrose oil, contains the EFAs linoleic acid and gamma-linolenic acid, both of which may alleviate dryness and reduce the potential for future water loss. Check your health food store for EPO and take 1,000 milligrams (about a tablespoon) of oil three times a day, says Dr. Jacknin. Or get gel caps and follow the dosage instructions on the label.

Evening Primrose

GET AN A. Vital for proper skin growth and repair, vitamin A is one of a family of natural and synthetic derivatives known as

MOVE OVER, VASELINE

For years, dermatologists have lauded petroleum jelly as the thickest emollient and therefore the best treatment for very dry skin. Now there's evidence that moisturizers with large amounts of glycerin (which has a less greasy feel) may work just as well, if not better. "Glycerin appears to increase space between cells in the stratum corneum," explains Leslie Baumann, M.D., "creating a reservoir of moisture-holding ability that makes the skin more resistant to drying." Look for glycerin in commercial moisturizers or simply make your own. Purchase pure glycerin from a health food store and combine 1 part glycerin and 2 parts rosewater.

retinoids, which are the primary ingredients in many anti-aging prescription drugs, such as tretinoin (Retin-A). You can get pretty much the same protection (at a fraction of the cost) simply by filling your plate with foods rich in beta-carotene (which converts to vitamin A in the body), such as cantaloupe, carrots, and apricots.

DON'T FORGET E. As an ingredient in lotions or as oil, topical vitamin E—particularly the form known as alpha tocopherol—reduces skin roughness, the length of facial lines, and wrinkle depth. When it's combined with topical vitamin C in the form of ascorbic acid (which seems to help promote the growth of collagen, the skin's underlying support), the effects may be enhanced. Check your health food store for E and C combined in skin-care products.

OPEN SESAME. Indian women have long used sesame oil, which is rich in both vitamin E and linoleic acid, to moisten and soften dry, cracked hands and feet. Dr. Jacknin suggests pouring 1/2 cup of sesame seeds and 1/4 cup of warm water into a blender and processing for 3 minutes. Strain the lotion, apply it to your skin, and leave it on for as long as possible. Rinse with warm water, then cool water, and blot dry.

EARACHE

Soothe the Pain

———————◆◆◆◆———————

I wandered into the kitchen in the middle of the night recently to find my husband sitting at the table with a steaming mug of tea pressed to his ear, not his lips. As funny as this odd little scene appeared, my husband wasn't looking the least bit amused: He was using the warmth of the mug to ease an earache. Although it was working, he was still hurting.

The infection behind an earache, known as otitis media, obviously can cause excruciating pain. Interloping bacteria or viruses travel the length of the eustachian tube, which connects the throat to the ear, and take up residence in the middle ear—a pea-size, air-filled cavity separated from the outer ear by the paper-thin eardrum. Excess mucus then plugs the eustachian tube, barricading the bugs inside. Infected mucus builds up behind the eardrum, resulting in pain, swelling, and redness— usually for a week or longer.

WHY ME?

Middle-ear infections tend to occur with a cold, because of nasal congestion, or, as in my husband's case, in conjunction with a sinus infection. But you can also take home a souvenir

PREVENTION IS BEST

Here are three ways to stop earaches before they start.

DOUSE 'EM WITH VINEGAR. Anytime you're going to swim in an unchlorinated body of water, such as a lake, a river, or the ocean, take along a mixture of two drops of vinegar to two drops of rubbing alcohol (a drying agent), suggests William Warnock, N.D. Dry your ears well, then dribble the solution into them after each dip.

BET ON BORIC ACID. "If you're prone to ear infections, ask your pharmacist to mix up a 3 percent boric acid, 70 percent alcohol solution," says Michael D. Seidman, M.D. The boric acid will acidify the ear canal, discouraging any bacterial or fungal invaders from venturing down that path, while the alcohol will dry it up. Squeeze a few drops into your ears every day, he says, to keep yourself infection-free.

STOP THE POPS. Painful fullness in the ears during airplane travel is caused by a difference between the air pressure in the middle ear and the atmospheric pressure in the aircraft. If you pick up some pulsatilla extract from your health practitioner before your flight, however, you may be able to stop the pops—and the pain. This herb can help reduce inflammation in the eustachian tubes. "For flying-related pain, I recommend mixing 10 drops to one dropper of pulsatilla extract in a glass of water and drinking it 20 minutes before your descent and soon after landing," says Dr. Seidman.

earache from a weekend at the lake or beach. Lingering moisture in your ear may harbor bacteria that set up shop in the outer ear as well as in a portion of the ear canal leading to the eardrum. This can result in otitis externa, an itchy, achy infection commonly known as swimmer's ear.

You don't even have to do anything to get an earache: You can get one that's actually the result of pain elsewhere in your body, such as in your jaw, your teeth, or your throat. And you can get a whopper just sitting innocently on a plane. During the descent, the intense pressure in your ears can make you feel as if they're about to burst, and the fullness and ringing may not go away until hours after you've landed.

RELIEVE THE ACHE

Most earaches aren't serious and simply fade away on their own, but if you have ear pain for more than a day or two, you need to see a doctor. If fluid has accumulated, the doctor may use a small suction device to remove it. For bacterial infections, the standard treatment is an antibiotic, but natural infection fighters, such as the ones that follow, can often do the job just as effectively, says Michael D. Seidman, M.D., director of neurotologic surgery at Henry Ford Hospital in Detroit. Since these remedies are for adults only, you'll need to check with a pediatrician for specifics on how to treat earaches in infants and children.

HOLD A HOT ONION. Like my husband's steamy mug, this old-time remedy soothes an earache—and perhaps stimulates the flow of mucus—with warm, moist heat. Simply heat an onion or a potato in the microwave (boiling works, too), then cool it slightly, put the toasty sphere in a clean cotton sock, and rest your sore ear against it.

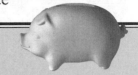

SAVE YOUR MONEY!

Keep the Candles for Romance

Have you ever been tempted to try ear candling, an alternative procedure touted to draw out excess earwax or ease earaches? It involves lying on your side with your affected ear facing up while the narrow end of a foot-long, hollow, candlelike cone soaked in beeswax is inserted into your ear. The top of the cone is lit like a candle and left to burn for several minutes. The thinking is that the vacuum created by the heat helps draw earwax into the cone and ease your pain, but studies indicate that the only thing that collects in the cone is melted beeswax—not earwax.

SOOTHE WITH SWEET OIL. Rubbing oil behind your ear (where your lymph glands are located) or placing a cotton ball saturated with oil inside your ear may soothe the ache and help stimulate the lymph glands to remove infectious agents. "Many of my patients find that something called sweet oil—which is really olive oil with other oils such as lavender, tea tree, chamomile, and hops mixed in—works really well," says Dr. Seidman. Check your health food store for

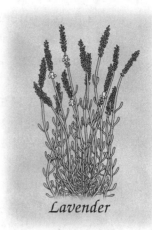

Lavender

sweet oil, or simply make your own. Just mix the oils together in equal amounts.

SNIFF SOME SALTWATER. Dissolve as much table salt as you can in a glass of warm water without the water becoming cloudy, then pour a little of the saltwater into the cup of your hand and sniff the mixture into one nostril, then the other. Repeat several times. "This nasal wash acts as a natural decongestant to shrink swollen tissues and unplug the eustachian tubes," says William Warnock, N.D., a naturopathic physician in Shelbourne, Vermont.

GET STEAMED. Eucalyptus is another herbal decongestant that may help ease the pressure in your eustachian tubes and nudge drainage of fluid that has been

WHEN TO DIAL THE DOC

· · · · · · · · · · ·

If your ear pain is severe, your hearing is diminished, you have blood or pus oozing from your ear, or you had severe pain that stopped abruptly and was followed by hearing loss, contact your doctor immediately. Your eardrum may have burst. While a ruptured eardrum usually heals on its own within two months (and hearing spontaneously returns to normal), your physician needs to watch it closely to ensure that it doesn't become infected and that any hearing loss doesn't become permanent.

dammed up in the middle ear—especially if you combine it with steam, which also encourages the flow of mucus. Fill a bowl with boiling water, add several (as many as 10) drops of eucalyptus oil (available in health food stores), and lean over the bowl (but not so close that you could burn your face). Drape a towel over your head and the bowl to capture the steam, then inhale the mist for at least 5 minutes. You can also place a few drops of eucalyptus oil in your bathwater, but don't put it directly into your ears.

REACH FOR A NATURAL ANTIBI-OTIC. Grab one like garlic, suggests Dr. Warnock. Simply mash a garlic clove with a fork and saturate it with several drops of olive oil. Let the mash absorb the oil overnight, strain out the garlic, and warm the oil so it's pleasantly tepid, not hot. Tilt your head with your sore ear facing up and plop two or three drops of the garlic oil into your ear. Lie down—again, with your sore ear up—and let the oil settle for 2 or 3 minutes before you raise your head. Do this a few times a day, and your discomfort should disappear within a day or two.

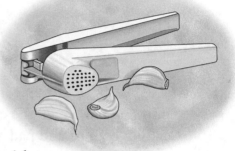

ENDOMETRIOSIS

Reduce Hormones, Inflammation, and Pain

————◦◦◦◦————

One of the women in my family still refers to her monthly period as "the curse"—and for good reason. The excruciating cramps and pad-soaking flows she endures due to endometriosis—a disease in which tissue resembling the endometrium, or lining of the uterus, grows outside the uterine cavity—make her feel as if she's living under a hex.

Just like the uterine lining, the misplaced tissue builds up, breaks down, and bleeds each month. Unlike normally positioned endometrial tissue, however, the stray tissue has no way of leaving the body, so it can result in inflammation, internal bleeding, the formation of scar tissue, and a host of other painful problems.

If the rogue endometrial

SWEET RELIEF

Sweet, unassuming cinnamon is a time-honored Asian remedy that may help ease cramps as well as curb yeast overgrowth that can disrupt the immune system, says Deborah Metzger, M.D. "I find that taking four cinnamon capsules a day—or swirling a heaping teaspoon into applesauce as needed—can help ease mild endometriosis flare-ups," she says. You can find cinnamon capsules at health food stores.

tissue has attached itself to the bladder or bowel, for instance, you may feel pain when you urinate or have a bowel movement. If the tissue is on the floor of the pelvis or attached to the ligaments that support the uterus, intercourse can be extremely painful.

EASING ITS GRIP

Unfortunately, no one has a clue as to why endometrial tissue migrates in the first place. That's why many women work with their doctors to develop a more natural approach that focuses primarily on lowering estrogen levels and inflammation and reducing symptoms. Here's just a sample of what they're coming up with.

ON-THE-SPOT RELIEF

Roll Away Pain

Many women who have taken mind-numbing narcotics for excruciating pelvic pain are finding that Menastil, an FDA-registered roll-on herbal pain reliever made from calendula (which is often used to reduce menstrual pain) brings swift relief for a few hours. And it has no side effects to speak of. For more information, call (800) 636-2784, or visit the Web site at www.menastil.com.

EASE KILLER CRAMPS. Studies show that more than half of women with endometriosis have less pain when supplementing with magnesium (a mineral that relaxes muscle spasms and can help quell severe cramps) and calcium (another cramp buster). Talk to your doctor about taking 400 milligrams of magnesium glyconate and 1,200 to 1,500 milligrams of calcium once daily with food (to increase absorption). And why not make those meals do double duty by including mineral-rich foods? Spinach is brimming with magnesium, and bok choy is an especially good source of calcium.

FISH FOR RELIEF. Meat, dairy products, and caffeine trigger the release of pain- and inflammation-causing prostaglandins, explains Eileen Kinder, R.N., a certified nurse consultant at the Helena Women's Health

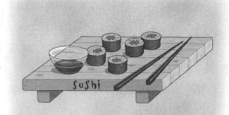

Center in Palo Alto, California. Fish will provide you with lots of omega-3 essential fatty acids (EFAs), which inhibit inflammation. So eat fish often, and for extra pain relief, talk to your doctor about taking 3 grams (3,000 milligrams) of fish oil in capsule form daily, along with 2 to 3 tablespoons of flaxseed oil (use it in place of salad dressing or spoon it into a smoothie). Both oils can thin your blood, so avoid them if you take aspirin or prescription blood thinners.

SAY SO LONG TO JOE. The caffeine in coffee (as well as tea and cola) can drive up your blood sugar and contribute to high estrogen and low progesterone levels in the body, notes Deborah Metzger, M.D., medical director at Helena Women's Health. All of that can aggravate endometriosis symptoms.

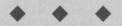

HOMEGROWN SOLUTION

◆ ◆ ◆

Flower Power

Yarrow's ability to balance hormones makes it especially helpful for women with endometriosis who need to flush out excess estrogen, says Jennifer Brett, N.D., a naturopathic physician at the Wilton Naturopathic Center in Stratford, Connecticut. Plus, yarrow's anti-inflammatory and antispasmodic effects may help ease menstrual cramps. To prepare a tea, steep 1 to 2 teaspoons of dried yarrow flowers (available at health food stores) in a cup of boiling water for 10 to 15 minutes, strain, and drink as needed. Check with your doctor before using yarrow, and don't take it at all if you are pregnant or breastfeeding or have pollen allergies.

Can't go cold turkey? Limit your intake to a cup a day or mix half decaf and half full-strength. This switch alone will go a long way toward easing cramps, promises Kinder.

BET ON BRUSSELS SPROUTS AND BROCCOLI. These veggies—along with cauliflower, cabbage, and kale—contain an abundance of phytoestrogens, compounds that are structurally similar to but weaker than the estrogen found in your body. When you eat these vegetables, the phytoestrogens you ingest compete with your body's own estrogen to bind to receptors in your body. When the phytoestrogens bind, they exert a weaker estrogenic effect, thereby reducing overall estrogen activity in your body and perhaps decreasing endometriosis symptoms.

EXAMINE EPO. Evening primrose oil (EPO), named for the late afternoon opening of its yellow flowers, is rich in EFAs that may help block the release of the inflammatory substances that put the pinch in menstrual cramps. Kinder suggests squashing cramp pain by taking 1,000 to 2,000 milligrams of evening primrose oil daily (divided, with meals) as needed. Look for it at health food stores.

Evening Primrose

BARK BACK AT CRAMPS. Before Midol hit the market, women used cramp bark to relax the uterus and ease the pain of menstrual cramps. Debi Smolinski, N.D., chair of the women's integrative medicine department at the Southwest College of Naturopathic Medicine in Tempe, Arizona, suggests mixing 30 drops of a standardized tincture of cramp bark (available in health food stores) in a glass of water and drinking it twice a day as needed. You can also dilute the tincture with water and swab it lightly on your abdomen to soothe your tense muscles.

GET MILK. Search your health food store for "lipotropic" supplements that contain milk thistle, choline, and dandelion, all of which help the liver metabolize estrogen, says Kinder. Follow the label directions.

ASK ABOUT ACUPUNCTURE. More than half of women with endometriosis report becoming pain-free after acupuncture

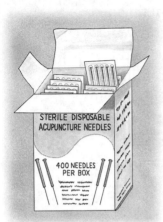

treatments, says Mary Lou Ballweg, director of the Endometriosis Association in Milwaukee. Perhaps it's because those hair-thin needles stimulate the release of "feel-good" endorphins. Willing to give it a try? Ask your doctor to recommend a reputable practitioner near you.

STAY ON TOP OF PAIN. Women with endometriosis who have a tipped uterus and a few inconveniently located tissue implants on pelvic organs can find the missionary, or man-on-top, position for intercourse intensely painful. If you're one of them, don't give up sex, urges Dr. Metzger; just find a way to have greater control over the depth of penetration. For many women, for instance, the woman-on-top position is more comfortable.

PACK IT ON. Some women swear by hot castor-oil packs to ease cramps. Supposedly, the packs increase circulation and decrease inflammation when placed on the lower abdomen. Just soak some folded flannel cloth in castor oil and place it over your abdomen, covering your liver and reaching from your breastbone to your pubic bone. Top it with some plastic wrap, a hot water bottle, and a towel, then relax for 30 to 60 minutes. You can use castor-oil packs three to seven days a week, but only when your cramping isn't accompanied by heavy bleeding. For best results, though, use this remedy between periods.

FIBROMYALGIA

Make the Ache Go Away

W hen the flu bug blows in for a visit, every muscle fiber in your body screams out in agony. Mercifully, after a few days of bed rest, the symptoms almost always hit the road. But when you have fibromyalgia (FM), a chronic pain condition affecting the soft, fibrous tissues of the muscles, tendons, and ligaments, your flu-like symptoms never leave. They linger and torture you like a houseguest from hell, as a friend of mine puts it.

If fibromyalgia has taken up residence in your body, you may feel deep muscle soreness or burning, throbbing, or shooting pains. You may ache all over and/or have extreme tenderness at specific spots—

THE HERBAL EQUIVALENT OF CAFFEINE—ONLY BETTER!

If you don't get ample or restful sleep, you can feel both drowsy and edgy at the same time. Siberian ginseng—a restorative and stimulating tonic—can help you fight fatigue without making you feel wired, says Victoria Franks, N.D. As long as you don't have high blood pressure, she recommends taking 30 to 60 drops of ginseng tincture (available in health food stores) daily.

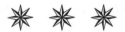
called myofascial trigger points—located in your neck, shoulders, lower back, elbows, and knees and beneath your buttocks. Pain and fatigue may be your constant companions or come and go, flaring during times of stress, before your period, or even when you're exposed to a draft. For my friend, even a slight chill on her shoulder prompts muscle tension that often leads to body-wide muscle pain. During these bouts, she's practically tethered to her chair.

That's the cruel irony of fibromyalgia: It makes you so tired and achy that you can barely move, but inactivity leads to poor sleep, which in turn makes your muscles ache more. You become so trapped in a pain-fatigue-pain loop that you may stop moving altogether.

WHY ME?

Although FM isn't uncommon, its cause remains a mystery. Scientists suspect that people who have it are born with a glitch in their brain's hormones, called neurotransmitters, which control everything from the adrenal glands that give you energy and respond to stress to the body mechanisms that control sleep, mitigate pain, and fight infection. The glitch may be awakened by emotional or physical stress—a strenuous workout, a bout with the flu, hormonal changes, exposure to environmental toxins, whiplash from a car accident, losing a loved one, or even just overstimulation from a hectic life.

People with FM have three times the level of substance P (a neurotransmitter involved in pain) than most folks, less of the growth hormone associated with muscle strength, and lower levels of serotonin—a "feel-good" brain chemical that controls sleep, pain management, and moods. They also lack adequate magnesium, a mineral needed to make adenosine triphosphate (ATP). Without ATP, your energy nosedives, your brain fogs, and your muscles are deprived of oxygen. They—and indeed your whole body—go into shutdown mode.

KNOCK OUT THE KNOTS

If you feel as though someone has yanked the plug on your energy, and you've had pain, stiffness, or aching in your upper and lower body for three months along with tenderness in specific trigger points, see a rheumatologist (a doctor specializing in musculoskeletal problems). The conventional treatments for FM all aim to reduce pain and increase sleep, but they can leave you with bothersome side effects. At best, the standard treatments work for only half of those with FM, anyway.

That isn't to say, though, that there's nothing you can do. A broad range of nondrug remedies can help release the knots, free you of pain and stiffness, and promote a good night's sleep—without grogginess or other, more troublesome side effects that you have to deal with the next day. Here's where to begin.

MOVE—BUT SLOWLY. When even a wave of your hand can be excruciating, exercise may be the last thing on your mind, yet it should be the first thing you do after you get

AN APPLE (OR MORE!) A DAY...

Just may keep FM pain away. Researchers have found that taking up to six tablets a day of Super Malic—which contains 200 milligrams of malic acid (found in apples) and 50 milligrams of magnesium—helped squelch pain in people with FM. As long as you don't have kidney problems, ask your doctor about Super Malic (available in health food stores), and give it about two months to work.

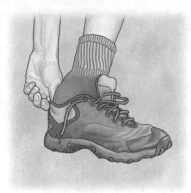

your diagnosis, says Robert Bennett, M.D., director of the Oregon Fibromyalgia Foundation in Portland. Studies show that nonimpact exercise can minimize pain and tenderness in just three months. Start by gently stretching your arms and legs to the point of resistance. Work up to holding each stretch for 1 minute. Then begin a walking or water exercise program. Start with three 5-minute sessions at a time, gradually upping the time you exercise and decreasing your rest time. Work up to 20 to 30 minutes without stopping, three times a week. Whatever you do, though, don't push through the pain, says Dr. Bennett. If you feel increased discomfort, stop, then resume your session the next day.

TRY TOUCH THERAPY. Common massage techniques (combining Swedish massage, which works the smooth muscles; Shiatsu, which uses thumb pressure at points along energy meridians in the body; and Trager therapy, which uses pressure on specific trigger points) can dampen pain, stiffness, and fatigue and help you snooze more deeply. In one study, FM patients who received twice-weekly massages using any one of these techniques reported more and better sleep, with less tossing and turning. They also had lower levels of substance P in their blood.

GO LIGHTLY. If even gentle massage is too much for your tender muscles, try craniosacral therapy, suggests Victoria Franks, N.D., a naturopathic physician in Cornwall, Ontario, Canada. To enhance mobility and release tension, a craniosacral therapist uses barely noticeable, rhythmic movements of the bones at the back of the head and bottom of the spine (sacrum) and of the connective tissue system. You can find a practitioner by calling the International Association of HealthCare Practitioners at (800) 233-5880 or visiting their Web site at www.iahp.com.

MAXIMIZE MAGNESIUM. A magnesium deficiency can literally leave you without the makings of ATP—the energy juice that powers your body—so eat plenty of leafy greens, dried beans, and lentils. You could also consider taking magnesium supplements in divided doses with meals, suggests Dr. Franks. Talk to your doctor before trying it, though, especially if you have heart or kidney problems, and ask how much magnesium is right for you.

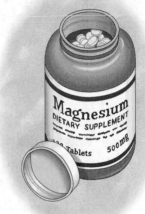

SPRING FOR SAM-E. Short for S-adenosylmethionine, SAM-e is a molecule in all living cells that helps regulate the breakdown of serotonin, the hormone that helps reduce trigger-point pain, prompt sleep, and even out moods. Some doctors who use it for FM suggest starting with 200 milligrams twice daily and working up to 400 milligrams two or three times a day, an hour before breakfast and lunch. At $2 a pill, relief could be costly, but the upside is that there seem to be no major side effects. If the potential to become pain-free is worth the price, talk to your doctor about taking SAM-e.

LOAD UP ON CoQ$_{10}$. Coenzyme Q$_{10}$ is a super antioxidant that also provides the spark that fires up ATP in your cells— which may mean less pain, more energy, and much better sleep. It's abundant in spinach, sardines, albacore tuna, and peanuts, but to ensure that you get enough, look for capsules or tablets (available at drugstores and health food stores) in an oil base. They are absorbed better than powder-based forms, says Jacob Teitelbaum, M.D., director of the Annapolis Research Center for Effective FMS/CFS Therapies in Maryland. He recommends taking 100 to 200 milligrams twice a day with food.

TURN ON THE HEAT. Applying an over-the-counter cream containing capsaicin—the ingredient that gives chile peppers their bite—to your most painful areas reduces soreness because capsaicin helps tamp down chemicals that transmit pain. Look for capsaicin creams in your drugstore or health food store and follow the directions on the label. Wash your hands thoroughly after applying the cream, and be careful not to get it in your eyes or on areas of broken skin. And just so you know, it may take several days to a week or two of daily applications to melt away pain.

GET NEEDLED. In one study, people with FM who tried acupuncture—the painless insertion of hair-thin needles to promote the flow of chi, or healing energy—reported less pain and depression after just one month of treatment. Acupuncture may also boost endorphins, the body's morphine-like painkillers. Ask your doctor for a referral to a reputable acupuncturist.

BE SURE TO GET B. Some doctors use high-dose B_{12} injections to chase away the fatigue and weakness of FM (B vitamins are crucial for energy production, immune enhancement, and fighting "fibrofog"). You can also battle those symptoms by eating foods rich in B vitamins (such as fortified cereals, eggs, meat, poultry, shellfish, and milk) and taking a B-complex supplement.

GARDEN BITES AND STINGS

Stop the Itch, Soothe the Pain

———◆◆◆◆———

I may have seen one too many "revenge of the giant ants"–type movies as a kid, but last summer, while I was puttering near my garden fence, I disturbed a hornet's nest and had the fleeting thought, "I hope they don't come back to get me." And wouldn't you know, a few days later, they did! I got a really nasty hornet sting on my upper arm, and it smarted for days.

Of course, insects aren't usually out for revenge—unless, of course, you get in their face (or their habitat) as I did. But even if you never go near a critter's nest, if you spend any time at all outdoors, it's nearly impossible to escape being stung or bitten by a bee, a tick, or a mosquito or two (or three).

WHY ME?

At family picnics when you were a child, your mom may have assured you that mosquitoes zeroed in on you because you

Mint of a Remedy

"I tell patients never to go camping or walking in the woods without a bottle of peppermint oil to carry along," says Sharol Tilgner, N.D. When you apply it to a bite, the cooling menthol will distract you from pain and encourage blood flow to the area to flush out the venom and disperse the inflammatory chemicals that have rushed to the site. The swelling and itch should fade pretty fast, she says. In a pinch, mint toothpaste will work, too.

were extra sweet. The truth is, in the case of mosquitoes and certain bees, at least, the allure was (and still is) more likely to be your fragrant shampoo or deodorant, the sugary soda you were sipping, or the doughnut you were munching. Mosquitoes also seem to be drawn by bright colors—particularly red—but your biggest attraction is carbon dioxide, which you exhale with every breath. To a mosquito, your breath is like a big dinner bell.

CLEVER WAYS TO BITE BACK

Ordinarily, when someone is stung by, say, a bee, her body reacts to the venom by producing antibodies that latch onto mast cells. These mast cells release inflammatory substances known as histamines, which spur the release of fluids to flush out the invading substance. The resulting swelling and itching usually recede within hours.

If you're allergic to insect venom, however, your antibodies remember the invader, and the next time you get stung, they react with a vengeance. Your system is overwhelmed with histamines, which trigger severe hives and rapid swelling that may block your breathing or shut down your heart, throwing you into anaphylactic shock. Head for the ER immediately if, in response to a sting or insect bite, you have rapid swelling of the eyes, lips, tongue, and throat; nausea; irregular heartbeat; and difficulty breathing.

Even if you're not allergic, however, insect bites and stings can smart. If you act really fast, you can take the sting out of your sting (naturally, no less) and return to your activity with a minimum of pain, swelling, or itching. Here's what to do.

STOP THE ITCH WITH VITAMIN C. To stop those reactionary histamines and ease that awful itching without the sleepiness associated with an over-the-counter antihistamine such as diphenhydramine (Benadryl), try vitamin C. This natural antihistamine works topically and internally to reduce the toxicity of the venom and the inflammation, says Jeanette Jacknin, M.D., a dermatologist in Scottsdale, Arizona. Mix vitamin C powder (available at drugstores or health food stores) with just enough water to make a paste, then apply it to your sting as often as needed.

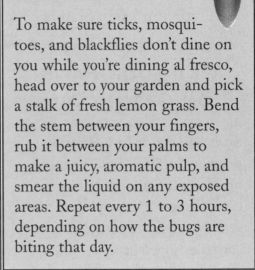

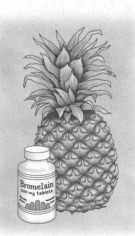

QUAFF QUERCETIN. This compound found in apples may help inhibit the release of histamines. It's often sold in formulations with bromelain, an enzyme found in pineapple that boosts quercetin's effect in the body and may reduce inflammation in its own right. If you take quercetin alone, the suggested dose is 250 to 500 milligrams three times a day on an empty stomach until symptoms subside. If you take a combination product, follow the directions on the label. Both are available at health food stores, but don't take bromelain if you take aspirin or prescription blood thinners.

SOOTHE IT WITH SODA. Bee stings release acidic venom, and baking soda is a well-known alkaline substance that can neutralize the reaction in a jiffy. Simply pour a little baking soda in your hand and add enough water to make a paste. Smear it on your sting and leave it there for at least 20 minutes to reduce pain, swelling, and redness.

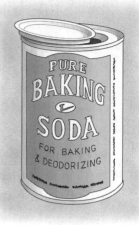

TRY LEMON AID. If a wasp got you, you're better off pouring an acid-based liquid such as vinegar or lemon juice on your sting to neutralize the alkaline effects of the wasp's venom.

APPLY ADOLPH'S. The same meat tenderizer that makes pork chops melt in your mouth can also melt bee sting discomfort. Meat tenderizers contain papain, an enzyme that breaks down the protein in venom to ease pain and itching, says Sharol Tilgner, N.D., a naturopathic physician and director of the Wise Acres Herbal Education Center in Eugene,

---

GET YOUR PAWS ON CATNIP OIL

Sure, you can treat bites and stings naturally—but you can prevent them naturally, too. In fact, catnip—the same stuff that sends your cat to kitty cloud 9—contains nepetalactone, which, according to studies at the University of Iowa, is 10 times more effective at deterring insects than DEET (short for diethyl-meta-toluamide, a powerful insecticide that does the job but can also cause skin rashes, lethargy, muscle spasms, nausea, and irritability). Check your health food store for products containing catnip oil.

Oregon. Mix 1 teaspoon of tenderizer with a few drops of water to make a paste, then apply it to your sting for no more than 30 minutes.

SWALLOW SOME ECHINACEA. This herb can relieve the pain and itching of bites and stings by battling the enzyme hualouronidase, which is injected by insects and breaks down tissue at the site of the bite. Immediately after a bite or sting, take 250 to 500 milligrams of echinacea in capsule form (available in health food stores), then take an additional dose every 2 to 3 hours for the rest of the day, suggests Dr. Jacknin. Don't use echinacea if you have an autoimmune disease such as lupus, rheumatoid arthritis, or multiple sclerosis, or if you are pregnant or nursing.

PLAY WITH CLAY. Check your health food store for a couple of powders: bentonite clay and goldenseal. Goldenseal is a well-known skin healer, and when the powder is mixed with a bit of the clay and enough water to make a paste, it makes a perfect poultice for easing the pain and inflammation of stings, says Dr. Tilgner.

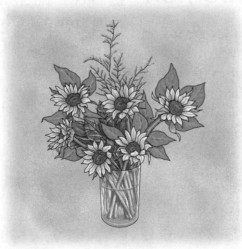

GAS

Clear the Air

⸻❖⸻

I was watching the cowboy spoof *Blazing Saddles* with a few 9-year-olds recently, and when it came to the part where the cowhands "pass wind" after eating beans around the campfire, the kids quite predictably howled with laughter.

Of course, real-life flatulence is rarely if ever funny for us grownups. In fact, it's downright mortifying if you release gas—an odoriferous mix of oxygen, nitrogen, hydrogen, carbon dioxide, and methane that forms from undigested food—in a meeting or crowded elevator! What's even less amusing, however, is excess gas that causes your belly to bloat up like a basketball or triggers sharp, abdominal cramps that

TRY AN ANTI-WHOOPEE CUSHION

If you have persistent, toe-curling gas that resists all your self-help measures, you may want to invest in a special seat cushion called the Flatulence Filter. Formerly known as the Toot Trapper, it's impregnated with charcoal and can instantly absorb the odor of intestinal gas. Each cushion costs approximately $40. To order—and de-odor—contact UltraTech Products at (800) 287-7573 or visit www.flatulence-filter.com.

make you feel as though you're being stabbed with a Ginsu knife.

WHY ME?

The laundry list of causes for excess gas is as long as the ladies' room line at the movies. Fortunately, it's matched by an equally long list of effective remedies. First, let's take a look at how you got so gassy in the first place.

You may have heard that if you gulp down your food, you also gulp down air that can cause you to burp and pass gas. While that's true, the problem has less to do with air than with digestion. Food that moves quickly through your mouth misses out on digestive enzymes that help break down food, so it must be broken down, or fermented, in your colon. It's that fermentation that causes gas. In fact, in most cases, gas arises from foods that aren't digested in the small intestine and must be broken down in the colon.

Beans, other legumes, onions, cabbage, broccoli, brussels sprouts, and cauliflower are among the worst offenders. These veggies contain cellulose, which, when eaten in its raw state, is indigestible in the small intestine, so the colon bacteria must take care of digestion. Fruits such as bananas, apricots, raisins,

THE PEPPERMINT TRICK

Ever wonder why waiters at most restaurants leave peppermints along with the check? It isn't, as you might suspect, a bribe for a fat tip but rather a nod to peppermint's ability to boost the flow of digestive juices and reduce gassiness and cramps. Too bad restaurants don't dispense them prior to meals! A recent study showed that nearly 80 percent of people who took peppermint capsules or tablets three or four times daily before meals had less flatulence. Check your local health food store for enteric-coated peppermint capsules (which are less likely to cause heartburn and just as effective for gas), then follow the dosage instructions on the label.

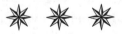

prunes, and figs can also cause flatulence since they contain fructose, which isn't well absorbed. Again, their digestion is left to the bacteria in the colon.

But fruits and veggies aren't the only culprits. Many adults—especially African-Americans—don't secrete enough lactase, the enzyme that breaks down lactose (milk sugar), so dairy products make them gassy. High-fiber foods and fiber supplements such as psyllium can also trigger flatulence, especially if you add them to your diet very quickly so they overload your digestive system. Fizzy, carbonated beverages such as beer, soda, and even sparkling water contain air, which (like gulping down air along with your food) can contribute to flatulence.

Finally, sugary foods and any foods (even chewing gum) that are artificially sweetened with mannitol, xylitol, or anything ending in "-tol" can cause gas because they're not easily digestible. In fact, fully half of all healthy people who eat these sweeteners develop gas and diarrhea.

Unfair though it may be, you can also get gassy without touching even a crumb of food. "Excess gas can result from an overproduction of acid in your stomach, such as what you might get from a bad case of nerves or an allergic reaction to pollen or other airborne inhalants," says Robert Pyke, M.D., Ph.D., a physician and pharmacologist who specializes in digestive diseases in Ridgefield, Connecticut. When your stomach overproduces acid, your body immediately produces bicarbonate to neutralize it, and it's the bicarbonate that liberates the gas. "There is actually a foaming-up in your stomach, just like when you put baking soda, which is sodium bicarbonate, in a glass of water," notes Dr. Pyke. Very high doses of vitamin C (which is, after all, an acid—ascorbic acid) can also prompt the body to produce bicarbonate—and excessive gas.

TURN OFF THE GAS

Are you constantly popping Tums, swigging Maalox, or taking some other antacid that contains calcium carbonate to reduce gas? You may well be making your problem worse, warns Dr. Pyke. The calcium contributes to more bicarbon-

MAKE A TOAST

Leave it to Europeans to come up with a very civilized—and tasty—way to sidestep gas. You know those patrons you see in sidewalk cafés along, say, the Champs Elysée, sipping liqueurs from tiny glasses? Many of those liqueurs help reduce gas.

One favorite is Pernod, which is made from anise, a Mediterranean herb that tastes like licorice and helps settle the stomach, reduce gas, and sweeten the breath. Another is "bitters," made from tart-tasting herbs such as gentian root, which stimulates the digestive tract and reduces gassiness.

Andrew Weil, M.D., director of the Program in Integrative Medicine and clinical professor of internal medicine at the University of Arizona in Tucson, suggests taking a teaspoon of Angostura Bitters (available in supermarkets and liquor stores) before or after meals. You can also add 10 to 20 drops of gentian root extract to a cup of water and drink it after meals.

ate, which fills you up with excess gas, resulting in "rebound acid"—and, yes, more gas! So save your money.

Fortunately, there is a slew of things that can help your digestive system do its job gas-free. The most obvious tactic is to limit—or avoid altogether—foods that promote excess gas and flatulence. Start by eliminating, say, all dairy products for a week, just to see if your problem fades. Or simply ask your doctor to help you pinpoint the culprit by doing a test called ELISA/ACT (enzyme-linked immunosorbent assay/activated cell test), which measures levels of IgG, the antibody involved in delayed food allergy reactions. In the meantime, however, here are additional gas cutters to try.

SLOW DOWN. As I mentioned earlier, when you wolf down your food without chewing it properly, you don't give salivary enzymes time to break down the food and ease digestion. "Type-A eating simply doesn't work," chides Dr. Pyke. "Try to really savor your food so it doesn't erupt in gassiness later."

GET STEAMED. Don't replace your raw veggies (which can give you gas) with, say, chips. Simply steam or stir-fry them until they're tender. The cooking process helps to break down the cellulose, which can be tough to digest.

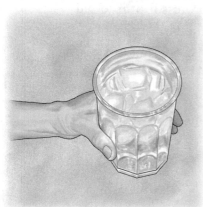

ADD FIBER...GRADUALLY. A high-fiber diet is a healthful diet—unless you add a bunch of gas-producing bulk all at once. To increase your health while babying your gut, add fiber gradually. For instance, if you're planning to start eating cereals that contain high-fiber psyllium seeds or bran, eat half the recommended amount along with plenty of water (8 to 10 glasses throughout the day) for several days before you begin eating the full amount.

BENEFIT FROM BEANO. Instead of cutting back on healthful, high-fiber foods, you can simply pair them with Beano, a product that helps reduce the amount of gas produced by such foods. Just be sure to take it with your first bite, because Beano works best if there isn't any gas in your intestines to begin with. Look for Beano in drops or tablets at your local drugstore or supermarket and follow the directions on the package.

REACH FOR LACTOSE-FREE. If you suspect that lactose intolerance may be at the root of your gassiness, you may want to switch to lactose-free dairy products (now readily available in most supermarkets) and see if it abates. Or try using products such as Lactaid, which help digest lactose by providing the lactase enzyme. You can also simply eat very small amounts of milk products at a time or with other foods to see if it helps.

SLURP MISO SOUP. A yummy fermented soybean paste, miso is a great source of fructo-oligosaccharides (FOS), indigestible dietary sugars that feed the naturally present "friendly" bacteria that facilitate digestion. If you're taking antibiotics, which wipe out these good bacteria along with the bad, eating miso could help prevent gassiness. Other foods that contain FOS include artichokes, asparagus, and fermented foods such as tempeh (made from soybeans) and sauerkraut, notes Dr. Pyke. Try eating them along with dinner and see if your gas problem evaporates.

PROVIDE PROBIOTICS. Another way to make sure you have plenty of "good" bacteria to ease your digestion is to snack on

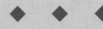

HOMEGROWN SOLUTION

◆ ◆ ◆

Blow Gas Away

If beans and other starchy foods make you gassy, simply top your dish with a sprinkling of tasty carminative (that is, gas-reducing) seeds, such as dill, fennel, or caraway. Or, for more oomph, stir in some basil, rosemary, oregano, or sage, all of which are carminative herbs.

yogurt that contains live, active cultures of *Lactobacillus acido-philus* or *L. bifidus* bacteria (check labels to be sure your preferred brand contains live, active cultures). Or pop what's called a probiotic supplement—available in freeze-dried capsules or powders at most health food stores—that contains these cultures. A typical dose is 1 teaspoon of powder (or one capsule) containing one billion microbes each of *L. acidophilus* or *L. bifidus*, taken one to three times daily on an empty stomach.

Initially, probiotics may trigger more bloating and gas. To minimize both, break open a capsule and take very small doses initially, then gradually increase the dose until your gas disappears. If this doesn't do the trick after a few days, switch brands. You may need to experiment with several, since some brands may work better for you than others, says Dr. Pyke.

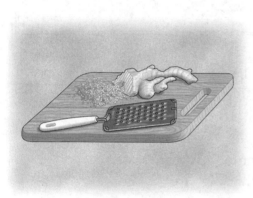

GIVE GINGER A GO. As a kid, you sipped ginger ale to soothe your achy tummy. Well, guess what? Ginger works for grownup gassiness, too. "I like to use ginger pills as a good alternative to Tums," says Dr. Pyke. Take 200 milligrams as needed, he suggests. Or enjoy the great taste of ginger tea by mixing 2 teaspoons of powdered ginger or grated fresh ginger in a cup of hot water and steeping for 10 minutes. (If you use fresh ginger, strain the tea before drinking.) Ginger-aid, anyone?

DOWN A FEW AFTER-DINNER "BRIQUETTES." Check your local health food store for activated charcoal capsules, which you can take occasionally after meals to soak up gas as well as odor. Pop 500 milligrams after meals as needed, but don't make it an everyday habit, warns Dr. Pyke, since charcoal can interfere with the metabolism of nutrients and any medications you may take. But it's great to keep on hand for those occasional bouts of gas, food poisoning, and other stomach distress.

FEAST ON FENNEL SEEDS. Those little licorice-flavored seeds you often receive after meals in Indian restaurants contain 8 percent volatile oil, which relieves gas and is an antispasmodic. They're a tasty way to settle your stomach and sidestep gas. Look for fennel seeds in the spice section of your supermarket and try chewing 1/2 teaspoon any time you feel bloated with gas.

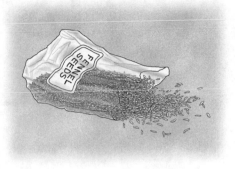

SIP STOMACH-SOOTHING TEAS. Marshmallow root and slippery elm, which, as their names imply, help coat the intestinal tract, are Dr. Pyke's favorite tummy soothers. "Both make great after-dinner teas for any kind of stomach upset," he says. You can check at health food stores or supermarkets for combination herbal teas formulated to aid digestion, or you can make your own. Simply steep 1 to 2 tablespoons of either herb in a cup of hot water for 10 minutes, then strain and drink.

HAIR LOSS

Keep Your Curls

————◦◦◦◦————

I know a woman who has started wearing her hair loosely gathered in a ponytail and pouffed up with a hair extension to camouflage the fact that her natural hair has begun thinning.

She looks lovely, even youthful—but I seriously doubt that she thinks so. Thinning or receding hair is extremely distressing, sometimes calling into question not only your appearance but also your vitality and even, in the worst cases, your identity. The crisis can leave you combing drugstores and hair salons for restorative solutions.

Make no mistake, no one holds onto their hair forever. Every day, we shed about 100 of our 100,000 scalp hairs, and whether this loss is replaced

BEAT YOURSELF OVER THE HEAD

Actually, *beat* is a little too strong a word, since this remedy involves tapping yourself on the head for a few minutes each day as a way to nudge blood to your crown to nourish hair follicles and perhaps encourage new hair growth. Jeanette Jacknin, M.D., recommends tapping thinning or balding areas of your scalp with a fine-toothed metal comb. When your scalp turns rosy, you know the blood is flowing. Repeat once or twice daily.

with new strands depends on several factors, including hormones, genetics, and age.

Like plants in a garden, each hair on your head has its own growing season. Instead of just a few months, however, the growing season for hair lasts about four years, notes Bernard Cohen, M.D., professor of dermatology at the University of Miami School of Medicine in Tampa. During this period, hair grows about 1/2 inch a month for 46 or so months, then enters a six-week resting phase. At the end of that phase, new hair sprouts from the hair follicle, pushing out the old strand—which ends up in your brush or down a bathroom drain.

As you age, however, the growth phase gets shorter, the resting phase gets longer, and new hair becomes thinner. In fact, for half of all men past age 50 and women past menopause, replacement hair never appears, leaving men with receding hairlines or bald spots, women with hair thinning all over the head and especially behind the front hairline, and both sexes feeling painfully self-conscious.

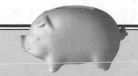

SAVE YOUR MONEY!

Don't Be an Airhead

Comb the hair-care aisle at your local supermarket or drugstore, and you'll find lots of pricey hair-thickening products (such as "volumizer" shampoos) that contain chemicals called polymers. These chemicals carry a positive electrical charge, and since hair has a negative charge, polymers stick to the hair shaft, actually coating it to make it look thicker, explains Bernard Cohen, M.D. The trouble is, by coating the hair shaft, polymers also suffocate it, preventing oxygen from reaching the follicle—and ironically, perhaps encouraging hair loss.

Avoid those volumizers, encourages Thomas Stearns Lee, N.D. Instead, check your health food store for herbal hair products that contain camphor and eucalyptus, which will dilate the blood vessels in your scalp, attract blood to balding or thinning areas, and perhaps slow hair fallout.

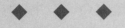

HOMEGROWN SOLUTION

◆ ◆ ◆

Sage Does It!

It may be especially, well, sage to use sage to encourage hair growth. Taken internally, this pungent culinary herb helps the body adapt to the hormonal changes that are often at the root of hair loss. Externally, to stimulate scalp circulation, Jeanette Jacknin, M.D., recommends steeping 2 tablespoons of dried sage leaves or two sage tea bags (which you can find at most health food stores) in a cup of hot water for 5 to 10 minutes. Strain, let it cool, then pour it over your hair after shampooing. Leave it on for 5 minutes, then rinse. Repeat daily. You can also add a few drops of sage extract to your favorite shampoo. (Don't use sage internally if you're pregnant or nursing.)

WHY ME?

Age-related hair loss (what doctors call androgenetic alopecia) occurs in people who have inherited higher levels of an enzyme that breaks down the male hormone (androgen) testosterone into dihydrotestosterone (DHT). When hair follicles are flooded with DHT, they sprout thinner and thinner hairs until nothing regrows, and the follicles eventually shrivel. The higher your enzyme activity and testosterone levels (in women, waning estrogen levels at menopause make testosterone more prominent), the sparser your hair.

Even before midlife, however, a host of conditions can alter—most times not permanently—your rate of hair growth and loss. For instance, shifting hormones can prompt temporary fallout. If you've just delivered a baby or stopped taking birth control pills, and your hormone levels have changed abruptly, you may be startled to see brushfuls of hair, which can continue for up to six months. Sudden shedding can also occur following a high fever or surgery, if you have an over- or underactive thyroid or iron-deficiency anemia, or if you take high-potency drugs such as chemotherapy agents or medications for high blood pressure.

If your hair suddenly starts coming out in clumps, leaving you with a perfectly round, smooth patch, and you begin losing your eyelashes, eyebrows, or hair from other parts of your body, your problem may be related to an immune disorder. In most cases, the hair regrows, although recurrent episodes of fallout are common.

Hair loss doesn't have to be related to disease, however. For instance, when you sit down to a meal, odds are that you're thinking about feeding your stomach, not your hair. But what you eat or don't eat literally goes to your head. Take protein: Skimping on this nutrient can be especially threatening to your hair—which is, after all, made up of protein. If you go on a crash diet, have an eating disorder, or simply don't get enough protein, your body will conserve it by shifting growing hairs into the resting phase. Two to three months after beginning this process, your hair will pull out easily right from the roots.

On a related note, you can also literally pull your hair out of your head—whether you're on a strict diet or not—by wearing tight hairstyles such as weaves and ponytails. Overuse of dyes, permanents, and straighteners can also weaken and thin hair.

PATCHY SUCCESS FOR THINNING HAIR

The moment you notice a pattern or rate of hair loss that's out of the ordinary, consult a dermatologist. You may simply need to switch a medication that's triggering hair loss or begin supplementing with, say, iron to correct iron-deficiency anemia, which can cause shedding.

To determine whether a medication is causing the problem, your dermatologist will go over all the medications you're taking, check your hormone and iron levels with a standard blood test, examine your hair under a microscope, and possibly even perform a scalp biopsy, during which a tiny bit of tissue is removed to look for follicle abnormalities.

If, after all that, it's determined that you have age-related hair loss, the dermatologist may suggest you take a hair regrowth medication, such as minoxidil (Rogaine). At best, these medications have sketchy success—and potent side effects. Take minoxidil, for example. The drug does stimulate hair follicles back into production and stops hair loss, but it does so in less than half of its users, and in those for whom it works, the new hair looks more like peach fuzz than the hair you're used to seeing. What's more, it must be used continually (and forever), and it interferes with hormone levels—which means you could sprout a beard! Pregnant women shouldn't use it at all.

HEALTHY HAIR IS KEY

Grim though this scenario may sound, there are many non-toxic do-it-for-your-do remedies to improve the health of your hair and perhaps even slow hair loss, minimize thinning, and help restore your lustrous locks. Give any of these a try.

FEED YOUR HAIR. While vitamins and minerals don't do a thing to jump-start hair growth in men, studies show they may prove helpful for some women. Take a two-pronged approach. First, beef up the protein content of your diet by eating plenty of chicken, fish, eggs, milk, soy, grains, and nuts, suggests Jeanette Jacknin, M.D., a dermatologist in Scottsdale, Arizona. Second, supplement your diet with nutrients that promote hair health.

Some doctors suggest a high-potency multivitamin/mineral supplement that contains the B-complex vitamins, 1,000 milligrams of vitamin C, 400 IU of vitamin E, 15 milligrams of zinc, and 1.5 milligrams of copper. Check with your doctor about taking these supplements and ask about taking iron, especially if you have hair loss following crash dieting or physical trauma.

FISH FOR THICKER HAIR. Thin, brittle hair may indicate a

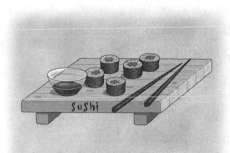

deficiency of omega-3 essential fatty acids (EFAs), which are found in cold-water fish, such as salmon, sardines, and herring. To boost the strength of your hair, you'd need to eat fish two or three times a week. Way too fishy for you? Andrew Weil, M.D., director of the Program in Integrative Medicine and clinical professor of internal medicine at the University of Arizona in Tucson, suggests buying whole flaxseeds (keep them refrigerated), grinding them up, and sprinkling 2 tablespoons a day on cereal or a salad. Plus, you can supplement with gamma-linolenic acid (GLA), another EFA, by taking either black currant oil or evening primrose oil, both of which are available in capsules or softgels at health food stores. Follow the package directions. After six to eight weeks, your hair should become shinier, stronger, and, hopefully, thicker.

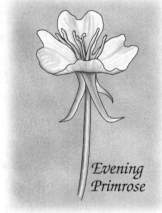

Evening Primrose

STRENGTHEN WITH HORSETAIL. This herb, also called bottlebrush, is a great source of silica, which strengthens hair (and nails), making it less likely to fall out due to wear and tear, points out Thomas Stearns Lee, N.D., a naturopathic physician in Scottsdale, Arizona. He suggests you check your health food store for horsetail capsules and take one or two with meals. You can also use the liquid extract as a hair rinse, adding 1/2 cup to 1/2 cup of water. Your hair should begin to thicken within several weeks.

There are some caveats, however. Since horsetail contains nicotine, a powerful stimulant, doses exceeding the recommended amount could cause muscle weakness, a fast or irregular heartbeat, and other unexpected discomforts. Those who have heart problems or high blood pressure or wear or use nicotine patches or gums should not use it. Also, stop taking it immediately and consult your doctor if you experience any ill effects. Horsetail is also a diuretic, so be sure to drink lots of water when you take it.

DISCOURAGE DHT. Saw palmetto, the herb most noted for shrinking enlarged prostate glands in men, appears to block the formation of DHT—maybe even as well as prescription androgen blockers. Check your health food store for saw palmetto capsules, suggests Dr. Jacknin, and take 160 milligrams twice daily.

LATHER UP WITH LICORICE. Like saw palmetto, licorice contains a chemical that may prevent testosterone from converting into DHT. To slow hair loss, Dr. Jacknin recommends using it topically. Simply add several drops of licorice tincture or extract to your favorite shampoo.

MASSAGE YOUR NOGGIN. Barbers have long known that massaging the scalp simulates circulation, feeding both oxygen and nutrients to hair follicles and perhaps stimulating hair

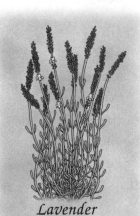

Lavender

growth. Now that you know, you should treat yourself to regular scalp massages. Dr. Jacknin suggests massaging safflower oil (an excellent vasodilator, meaning that it opens blood vessels) into your scalp for 20 minutes. Or try using bay oil (also called bay laurel) and lavender oil—both of which stimulate blood flow—daily. Add six drops of each to 1/2 cup of warm almond, soy, or sesame oil (all of which easily penetrate the skin) and massage the mixture into your scalp for 20 minutes, then wash it out with shampoo to which you've added three drops of bay oil.

BRING ON THE HEAT. Not hot water, mind you, but red

pepper, which contains capsaicin, the substance in chile peppers that gives them their fiery bite. It's an excellent warming stimulant, meaning that it improves blood flow to any area it touches. And when the oil is combined with rosemary oil (an herb long used to keep hair lush), the mixture may just help your hair regrow, says Dr. Jacknin. She suggests adding one or two drops of red-pepper (cayenne) oil to 1 ounce of rosemary oil in a clean, small bottle, massaging your entire scalp with the mixture for at least 20 minutes, then washing your hair with shampoo to which you've added five drops of rosemary oil per ounce of shampoo. Lather up every day.

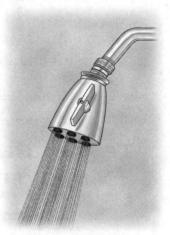

USE THE RIGHT SHAMPOO. A buildup of sebum—the fatty, DHT-laced oil produced by the sebaceous glands of the skin to protect your scalp from drying—can shrivel hair follicles and contribute to hair loss. To keep your tresses thick and relatively sebum-free, Dr. Lee suggests shampooing daily with a product that contains polysorbate (which cuts through the oily stuff as well as any accumulation of mousse, gels, or styling sprays that may be plugging your hair follicles) and coconut oil (which helps strengthen and protect hair).

HANGOVER

Remedies for a Bleary Brain

❦

Who among us hasn't celebrated a bit too spiritedly on some special occasion, only to awaken the next day feeling somewhat, well, under the weather. I recall one New Year's Eve in Montreal when that literally was the case: The French champagne hit me so hard that in the morning, even the sound of sleet beating against the window—*mon dieu!*—was unbearable.

Typically, darker-colored drinks, including red wine, brandy, bourbon, tequila, and dark rum, are more likely to cause hangovers than lighter-colored drinks. The former contain congeners—tiny impurities such as methyl alcohol and aldehydes created during the fermentation process—which are thought to

---

A BARTENDER-TESTED RECIPE FOR HANGOVER RELIEF

One favorite hangover remedy recommended by bartenders is to simply drink hot water laced with honey, which contains 40 percent fructose—a sugar known to speed the body's metabolism of alcohol by 25 percent. For the same reason, James A. Duke, Ph.D., suggests munching on dates, which contain 30 percent fructose.

---

be responsible for a hangover's miserable symptoms. In fact, studies show that these congener-laden drinks are three times more likely to cause hangovers than clear, filtered drinks, such as white wine, vodka, or gin.

Champagne, however, is another matter. Although it's pale, the bubbly can do you in (I'll attest to that!) simply because it's bubbly. Carbonation speeds alcohol absorption, so, for example, drinks such as Scotch and soda or rum and Coke (both dark drinks plus bubbles) are doubly lethal.

WHY ME?

The severity of a hangover can vary depending on factors aside from the type of alcohol you're drinking. If you drink regularly, for instance, your tolerance increases because your body makes more of the enzymes that metabolize the toxic by-products of alcohol. On the other hand, if you drink infrequently, your tolerance for any kind of alcohol is probably pretty low—and the chance that your hangover will be a doozy is probably pretty high.

If you're allergic to yeast, unfiltered beer can leave you with a crushing headache. So can wine, if you're sensitive to sulfur

THE BEST PARTY FAVOR?

A tiny vial of standardized ginkgo extract gets the vote from some herb experts. The seeds of this Asian herb contain an enzyme that may help speed the body's metabolism of alcohol. In fact, the Japanese are so convinced of the herb's protective powers that they serve ginkgo seeds at cocktail parties so guests don't leave with a hangover, says James A. Duke, Ph.D., president and CEO of Duke's Herbal Vineyard in Fulton, Maryland, and a former specialist in medicinal plants for the USDA. Want to try ginkgo before your next celebration? As long as you aren't taking other medication, check your health food store for standardized extract and follow the directions on the label.

PUT THE CRIMSON LADY TO WORK

Many people swear by a Bloody Mary—tomato juice seasoned with a splash of vodka and dashes of Tabasco, Worcestershire sauce, and red pepper—to cure a bloody awful hangover. And the crimson lady may actually work, but probably not for the reason you think. It's not the vodka, which will actually delay relief, but the red pepper that does the trick. It contains capsaicin, a potent ingredient that helps stop the production of substance P, which promotes both inflammation and pain. Try a pinch in a glass of tomato juice (which, as a bonus, is loaded with the electrolytes you may have lost if you vomited), suggests Linda White, M.D. Just be sure you make it "virgin" (that is, sans the alcohol).

dioxide, a preservative added to many wines to keep them fresh, or to the histamines in dark grape skins. If you mix different types of alcohol—such as grain alcohol and wine or beer—you tend to feel more hung over in the morning, although it's unclear why. And finally, drinking on an empty stomach tends to be a one-way ticket to tipsy-land.

HANGOVER HELPERS

The best way to help yourself *prior* to an evening of tippling is to fill your belly with food to offset the booze. Drinking on a full stomach goes a long way toward preventing a hangover because the food you've eaten—especially greasy or starchy food, according to some people—lines the stomach and slows the absorption of the alcohol. If you really want to bypass a hangover, however, the experts at the National Headache Foundation suggest that you eat honey on a cracker or piece of toast before or after drinking. Honey contains as much as 40 percent fructose, a sugar known to speed the metabolism of alcohol.

Let's say you have a hangover already. Your first impulse—to grab a couple of pain relievers and wash them down with an econo-size cup of Joe—is a real no-no. Aspirin and ibuprofen are stomach irritants that can further aggravate a belly already aboil with extra gastric acid produced in response to the alcohol. And acetaminophen can actually enhance alcohol's toxicity in the liver, which is already working overtime to rid you of the poison you imbibed the previous night, and perhaps even cause liver damage.

As for the cup of Joe, it isn't dangerous, really—it's simply too dehydrating, especially since alcohol also dries you out.

In fact, one of the best things you can do on "the morning after," says James Schaefer, Ph.D., professor of anthropology at Union College in Schenectady, New York, who has studied the behavioral and physiological effects of alcohol, is to drink at least one very tall glass of water to rehydrate and wet that dry mouth—and remove yourself from the bathroom (which is hopefully not where you slept).

As soon as you can haul your sorry self to the kitchen or out the door to the store, you can try these additional hangover helpers.

PUT YOUR HEAD ON THE ROCKS.
Put some crushed ice in a plastic bag (or grab a bag of frozen peas) and hold it against your head to help shrink the swollen blood vessels that are causing the throbbing. Some experts also recommend placing your feet in a tub of warm water at the same time. Although the remedy's medicinal benefits are hazy, it's bound to feel wonderful.

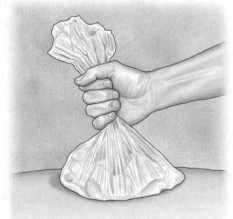

FEED YOUR HANGOVER. Eating food of any kind the morning after a bit too much Beaujolais can help to ease a hangover, assures Stephanie Brooks, R.D., a registered dietitian and San Francisco–based nutrition consultant. By eating, you'll replace any electrolytes (salts such as sodium and

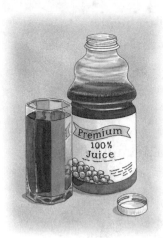

potassium) you lost if you vomited. If your tummy is still tender, chug a sports drink, which packs lots of electrolytes. Or, if you find the citrus in sports drinks irritating, reach for a vegetable juice such as tomato, carrot, or celery, all of which are loaded with potassium and sodium. If you want something warm and soothing, chicken soup or plain broth will boost your electrolytes.

SIP WHITE WILLOW TEA. Like coffee or any other caffeinated drink, black tea can constrict your blood vessels and chase away a throbbing headache, but it can also be dehydrating. White willow bark tea has no caffeine, which means it will rehydrate you. Plus, it contains salicin, which is similar to the pain reliever in aspirin. The only difference between the two, says Linda White, M.D., a pediatrician in Golden, Colorado, who has written extensively on herbal remedies, is that willow bark is easier on the stomach than aspirin. Buy some powdered white willow bark tea at a health food store, then follow the package directions. Drink three cups a day. Avoid the herb if you're allergic to aspirin, though, and never mix the two or use white willow with alcohol.

BURN YOUR TOAST. That shouldn't be too tough, given the bleary state of your brain. The idea is to ingest the carbon in the burned bread to help soak up any congeners in your system. Of course, if the thought of eating singed anything makes you want to toss your cookies (again), you can simply head to a health food store and pick up some activated carbon tablets. The carbon lines the stomach and small intestine, supposedly trapping the toxins and preventing them from entering your bloodstream.

Follow the package directions. (For best results, you should really take the tablets before you begin drinking and while you're imbibing as well as afterward.)

DETOX WITH DANDELION. This pesky little garden weed may actually be the perfect little hangover helper. It not only stimulates the liver, which may speed alcohol metabolism, it's also a gentle diuretic that may help reduce puffiness without flushing out those all-important electrolytes. Check health food stores for dandelion root in tincture form and take 30 to 60 drops three times a day, suggests Dr. White. Check with your doctor first, though, if you're taking diuretics or potassium supplements.

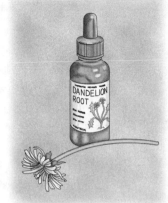

TAKE YOUR VITAMINS. The entire B complex—crucial for nervous system functioning—tends to be depleted after drinking, says Dr. White. To replenish your supply, pop a supplement that contains 50 milligrams of each B vitamin. She suggests that you also take 100 micrograms of folic acid (another B vitamin) and—as long as you don't have stomach or kidney problems—1,000 milligrams of vitamin C (to help break down and remove alcohol from your system). Add a multivitamin/mineral supplement that contains 15 milligrams of zinc (which also assists the enzymes that break down alcohol).

Headaches

Put Pain in the Past

———— ❖ ————

Taking the family for a drive through rolling, sun-dappled hills dripping with lilac blossoms may be an idyllic way for many people to while away a gorgeous spring afternoon. For my mom, though, it was usually a trip straight to migraine hell. The up-and-down motion, changing light, and perfumed air often turned her green with nausea and triggered a gradually worsening headache that frequently became so intense that she would say her hair hurt.

If you get migraines, as my mom did, your pain is felt as a gradually worsening throbbing on one side of your head or behind your eye that's caused, in part, by blood vessels widen-

Get Fewer Migraines with Feverfew

The herb feverfew should really be renamed "migrainefew." Studies show that taking feverfew in capsule form daily can reduce the frequency and potency of migraines. Just be sure you search the health food store for standardized capsules that contain parthenolides, the constituent in feverfew that appears to affect serotonin levels—and ward off migraines. Follow the label directions.

ing (dilating) and pressing on nerve endings. Nausea and sensitivity to light, sound, and odors are often part of the equation. In addition to migraine pain, sinus headache pain falls into this category, as does the pain of cluster headaches (so called because they usually occur in groups)—a particularly excruciating type of headache that sufferers (mostly men) say feels as though a spike is being driven repeatedly through one eye.

If you get chronic "tension" headaches—the most common type—your pain starts with aching muscles at the back of your neck and travels to the top of your head, where you may feel a squeezing sensation, as if you're wearing a hat that's several sizes too small. Despite its name, this type of headache isn't caused by chronically coiled muscles but by the release of pain- and inflammation-causing brain chemicals triggered by stress, anxiety, and poor posture. If you frequently have tension headaches, you probably wake up with them and may have them for a week or even longer.

MAKE YOUR HEAD MINTY FRESH

Peppermint isn't just for keeping your breath fresh. In fact, studies show that if you rub peppermint oil—a proven anesthetic—on your forehead, you may be able to relieve the pain and reduce the sensitivity associated with tension headaches. What's more, if you use the oil daily, you may even be able to sidestep future headaches. Simply mix peppermint oil (available at any health food store) with an equal amount of rubbing alcohol and apply no more than a couple of drops to your forehead and temples. Wait 15 minutes, then massage the area for 3 minutes. Repeat three times a day.

WHY ME?

No matter what type of head pain you feel, researchers now believe that all severe headaches result from a complex, underlying nervous system disorder that may start in the brain stem and cause a cascade of chemical events throughout the head and body. An emerging theory is that in some people, nerve cells in the trigeminal nerve, which runs from the brain stem to your jaw and other parts of your face, become overly excited by stress and other stimuli. The nerve cells then release proteins, causing nearby blood vessels to swell and activate pain receptors. Irritation of the trigeminal nerve may also be responsible for the "aura"—the shimmering lights or flashing spots—that many people with migraines experience before the pain hits.

FIGHT BACK

Unfortunately, many medications prescribed for headaches have drawbacks. Corticosteroids, for instance, can cause osteoporosis—dangerous thinning of the bones—and leave you vulnerable to fractures. Other drugs can increase the risk of heart attack and stroke.

The good news is that nondrug treatments have proven hugely successful in relieving headaches—especially in women, perhaps because they have more mechanisms for pain relief, theorizes Karen Berkley, Ph.D., professor of neuroscience at Florida State University in Tallahassee. Women also tend to be more open to experimentation than men are, she says—and the key to relieving headache pain in either gender is a willingness to try different approaches. Here's how to get started.

DIVIDE AND CONQUER. In this age of highly advanced medicine, we often assume that a therapy has to be just that—highly advanced or technical—in order to be effective, but that's simply not the case when it comes to headache pain. Just keeping blood sugar levels steady by eating multiple meals throughout the day provides relief for half of all people with migraines.

WATCH WHAT YOU EAT. About a third of all headache sufferers get relief simply by avoiding foods known to trigger headaches. Of the 100 or more troublemakers, the worst offenders include red wine; hot dogs; chocolate; fermented foods such as soy sauce; foods that contain the flavor enhancer monosodium glutamate (MSG); and those that contain the amino acid tyramine, such as aged cheese and preserved meats. But headaches can also be caused by hidden food allergies, and they can be prevented just by eliminating the most common allergenic foods, such as corn, wheat, eggs, soy, peanuts, or milk, that cause them. "Eliminating dairy products in particular helps resolve many of my patients' headaches in a month," reports Suzanne Lawton, N.D., a naturopathic physician in Tigard, Oregon.

JOT IT DOWN. To identify your triggers, keep a headache diary. Jot down anything that appears to be a trigger, including foods, activities, sleep changes, stressful events, what point you're at in your menstrual cycle, and even the weather. Then try to eliminate as many as you can.

CHILL OUT. If you're in the grip of a headache, place a cold cloth at the base of your skull and put your feet in a tub of warm water, advises Christy Lee-Engel, N.D., a naturopathic physician and assistant dean at Bastyr University near Seattle. According to folk wisdom, this old-time remedy pulls blood out of the swollen blood

WHEN TO DIAL THE DOC

• • • • • • • • • • • • •

Consult your doctor if you have three or more headaches a week or feel you must take a pain reliever every day. Also, even if it's just a one-time occurrence, dial your doc if you have any of the following, which may indicate an underlying disorder that requires further attention.

• A sharp, abrupt, severe headache
• A headache accompanied by fever, stiffness, rash, mental confusion, seizures, double vision, weakness, numbness, or difficulty speaking
• A headache after a head injury, even if it's a minor fall or bump and especially if the headache gets worse
• A chronic, progressive headache that worsens after coughing, exertion, straining, or sudden movement
• Onset of new headache pain after age 40

vessels in the head and moves it toward the feet.

REACH FOR WHITE WILLOW. Long before that little Bayer aspirin bottle became a medicine-cabinet staple, Native American medicine men dispensed the bark of the white willow tree for pain relief. Willow contains salicin, which is similar to the painkilling substance used to make aspirin. But the old-fashioned remedy may be even better, says Alexander Mauskop, M.D., director of the New York Headache Center in New York City, since it won't upset your stomach the way aspirin can. At the first sign of pain, drink a cup of white willow tea or take 3 to 5 milliliters of liquid extract (both are available at health food stores; to make tea, follow the package directions). Avoid the herb if you're allergic to aspirin, though, and never mix the two or use white willow with alcohol.

HAVE A CUPPA CHAMOMILE TEA. Relaxing, antispasmodic chamomile can calm migraine-associated queasiness as well as ease the stress associated with tension headaches. "Have a cup or two at the first hint of pain," suggests Dr. Lawton, "and use two tea bags to maximize its potency and effectiveness." Don't use chamomile if you're allergic to ragweed.

OR TRY VALERIAN. If chamomile doesn't do the trick, valerian, a stronger sedative herb, may be effective, Dr. Lawton says. As long as you're not taking any medications, check your health food store for valerian tincture, then, at the first twinge of pain, add 15 to 30 drops to a cup of water and drink. Just be sure to hold your nose—this herb smells like stinky feet!

MEDICATE WITH MOCHA JAVA. Caffeine constricts blood vessels, which can ease your head pain and even delay or dampen a migraine. If you drink caffeinated beverages regularly, however, your blood vessels will grossly overdilate when it wears off, triggering the last thing you need—a whopper of a headache. "The first thing I suggest is weaning yourself off your daily fix," says Dr. Lee-Engel. Then, the next time you feel a headache coming on, you can head to a Starbucks for a cup or two of dark roast.

GIVE SINUS HEADACHES THE STING. "For headaches triggered by allergies that swell the sinuses and cause blinding pain, nothing works better than stinging nettle tea," observes Dr. Lawton. The herb contains a compound that's similar to serotonin, the brain chemical that regulates blood vessel dilation, and is most potent in the bulk herb, which you can buy at health food stores. Add 1 heaping teaspoon to a cup of hot water, steep for 10 to 15 minutes, and strain. "You should get relief in 5 to 20 minutes," she says. Breathe in the tea's vapors as you sip, and their ability to help your sinuses release the fluid that's making them swell will speed relief.

FORGET IBUPROFEN. If you're plagued with headaches, you may already have discovered the hard way that popping analgesics for relief results in anything but. Ibuprofen, aspirin, and other nonsteroidal anti-inflammatory drugs (NSAIDs) work by constricting your blood vessels. When their effects wear off, however, the vessels typically overdilate, leaving you with even more pain than you had before. Soon, you're taking larger and larger doses, getting less and less relief, and possibly winding up with daily "rebound" headaches. As if that weren't enough, prolonged use of NSAIDs can lead to ulcers and possibly interfere with the absorption of nutrients, including tryptophan—an amino acid the body uses to make serotonin.

MIND YOUR MINERALS. Specifically, pay attention to magnesium and calcium, both of which tend to be lacking in people who have migraines. When that dynamic mineral duo is combined with riboflavin (a B vitamin shown to crush head pain) and the herb feverfew (see "Get Fewer Migraines with Feverfew" on page 248), "it helps ward off severe head pain in half my patients," says Dr. Mauskop. "In fact, those who take a formula called MigraHealth, which combines all these ingredients, have either fewer headaches or milder episodes." Look for MigraHealth at drugstores.

CONSIDER COENZYME Q$_{10}$. "Next to magnesium, this nutrient may be the most promising nondrug headache therapy around," says Dr. Mauskop. In fact, studies show that people who took CoQ$_{10}$ daily experienced 60 percent fewer headaches than when they weren't taking it. Look for supplements at health food stores and drugstores and follow the label directions.

PICK DANDELION. This unassuming herb helps the liver metabolize estrogen and may ease migraine pain associated with fluctuating hormone levels, says Dr. Lee-Engel. Plus, dandelion is rich in magnesium, which is often lacking in people with migraines. Check your health food store for dandelion capsules and take 400 to 500 milligrams a day throughout your cycle. You can also pick some fresh dandelion leaves from a chemical-free lawn and toss them into a salad. If you're taking diuretics or potassium supplements, check with your doctor before using dandelion.

RUB AWAY A MIGRAINE. A study at the University of Miami School of Medicine Touch Research Institute revealed that when participants had a 30-minute massage twice weekly for five weeks, migraine pain decreased, and the duration of the headaches was shortened by 80 percent. Massage not only feels simply delicious, it also boosts blood flow, removes pain-causing lactic acid from muscles, and promotes the release of natural painkilling substances. It also inhibits the release of hormones called catecholamines, which contribute to pain.

PRACTICE MINI–TENSION TAMERS. The moment you feel yourself tensing up, close your eyes and take several deep, cleansing breaths, inhaling deeply through your nose and exhaling through your mouth. As your lungs fill and deflate, imagine that you've locked your worries—deadlines, concern about a family member's illness, unpaid bills—inside a suitcase tied to a hot-air balloon. Then, in your mind's eye, watch as the balloon lifts your worries up, up, up—and away.

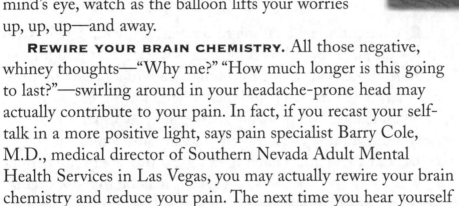

REWIRE YOUR BRAIN CHEMISTRY. All those negative, whiney thoughts—"Why me?" "How much longer is this going to last?"—swirling around in your headache-prone head may actually contribute to your pain. In fact, if you recast your self-talk in a more positive light, says pain specialist Barry Cole, M.D., medical director of Southern Nevada Adult Mental Health Services in Las Vegas, you may actually rewire your brain chemistry and reduce your pain. The next time you hear yourself begin an internal moan, repeat the following statement instead: "I have a biological predisposition for headaches, and right now, I'm going to focus on things that can help relieve the pain."

ADD ACUPUNCTURE TO YOUR ARSENAL. When the National Institutes of Health evaluated the benefits of acupuncture (inserting hair-thin needles at certain points on the body, supposedly to release blocked energy), relief from chronic headache pain was near the top of the list. Interested in giving it a try? Ask your doctor for a referral to a reputable acupuncturist.

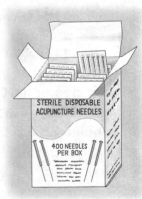

STERILE DISPOSABLE ACUPUNCTURE NEEDLES

400 NEEDLES PER BOX

HEARTBURN

Douse the Fire

———◦◦◦———

I once considered late-night dinners at my favorite restaurant the ultimate reward for a long day's work—that is, until heartburn turned this heavenly indulgence into a hellish punishment that ruined my sleep and made the following day seem that much longer. You probably know this type of post-meal misery—one minute you're eagerly tucking into a plate of zesty lasagna, and a few hours later, you've got a five-alarm fire behind your breastbone that not even a whole roll of Tums can douse.

STICK IT TO HEARTBURN

Continually chewing gum stimulates saliva that neutralizes acid and may even protect the esophagus, studies show. Look for brands that contain sodium bicarbonate, a stomach settler, and chew a stick or two after meals.

WHY ME?

The burn in heartburn is caused by stomach acid that backs up (refluxes) into your esophagus, the passageway from your mouth to your stomach. The backup occurs because the valve (called the lower esophageal sphincter, or LES) between your esophagus and stomach becomes irritated and fails to close properly, allowing acid and sometimes other stomach contents to migrate north.

What sets it off? Tomato-based dishes (like my beloved lasagna), coffee (decaf as well as caffeinated), citrus fruits, onions, garlic, chocolate, wine, and beer are all prime LES irritants. But overeating or gobbling any food can worsen your misery, since the less thoroughly food is chewed and broken down by saliva, the more stomach acid is needed to digest it, and the more burning you'll feel when your stomach contents back up.

Bending over from the waist or lying down soon after eating, wearing tight waistbands, or even having excess abdominal fat can also force open the LES and send you into heartburn hell. Plus, everyday, garden-variety stress can induce heartburn because it impairs the nerves that control the wavelike muscle contractions that move food through your esophagus.

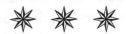
DOUSE THE FLAMES

Given our through-the-roof stress levels and fondness for jumbo portions and caffeine fixes, it's no wonder heartburn medications are the most widely sold drugs on the planet. The downside is that popping antacids as if they were after-dinner mints or living on acid blockers such as famotidine (Pepcid) can cause constipation, diarrhea, and headaches. Even worse, when their effects wear off, your stomach amps up acid production, creating more heartburn. A better approach is to reduce your triggers (ease off coffee, ditch those tight jeans, eat smaller meals, chew slowly, and avoid post-meal naps) and try one of the following nondrug methods when the searing starts. If you're receiving medical treatment for heartburn, have a talk with your doctor first.

SWALLOW ALOE VERA. The juice (not the gel, which is for external use only) from this succulent desert plant can take the sting out of heartburn by coating the esophagus and keeping stomach acid where it belongs, says Anil Minocha, M.D., chief of gastroenterology at Southern Illinois University School of Medicine in Chicago. He suggests drinking 1/2 cup of aloe juice (which you can find at health food stores) once or twice a day between meals.

TAKE TURMERIC. The spice that gives curry its distinctive flavor can also help break down fatty food—a leading heartburn trigger—and reduce acidity in the stomach. Get some empty gel capsules at the drugstore, fill them with turmeric powder straight from your spice rack, and take three capsules every day after dinner, suggests Dr. Minocha. You can also find turmeric capsules at health food stores.

SIP SLIPPERY ELM. The saliva in your mouth makes this

herb slimy, so it soaks up excess acid and soothes any inflammation in your esophagus on the way to your stomach, says Dr. Minocha. Mix 1 teaspoon of powdered slippery elm bark (available at health food stores) into 1/2 cup of boiling water, let it cool slightly, and sip as a tea two to four times a day.

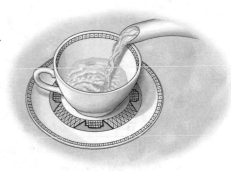

TRY PAPAYA. To reduce acid reflux and soothe indigestion and gassiness, drink a cup of papaya juice laced with 1 teaspoon of organic sugar (available at health food stores) and two pinches of cardamom, which, like papaya, aids digestion and reduces gas and cramping.

GRAB SOME LEMON AID. Lemon balm, or melissa, is a time-honored relaxant that can help soothe your jangled nerves and any heartburn you may have as a result. Steep 2 to 3 teaspoons of leaves (which you can find at a health food store or simply snip from your garden) in a cup of hot water for 10 minutes, then strain and sip one to three times a day.

GET BITTER. Add 1 teaspoon of gentian root tincture (available at health food stores) to a cup of water and drink it 15 minutes before eating. Gentian is a powerful bitter herb that will increase saliva and enzyme production, stimulate digestion, and quash post-meal heartburn.

PEPPERONI PIZZA PROTOCOL

Fans of pizza delivery, take heart. Studies show that a post-meal session of progressive muscle relaxation (alternately tensing and releasing one group of muscles at a time, starting with your feet) and deep belly breathing may help you dig into fiery foods such as pepperoni pizza without feeling the burn afterward. Plus, you'll have fewer reflux episodes in the future. You can learn this technique from videotapes or ask your doctor for a referral to a stress-management center.

NIBBLE LICORICE. Chewing two 380-milligram tablets of deglycyrrhizinated (DGL) licorice (which you can find at health food stores) 20 minutes before each meal can calm indigestion that triggers acid backup It may also help heal an inflamed esophagus.

BABY YOUR BELLY. Eat dinner at least 3 hours before bedtime, then take a leisurely 5- to 10-minute stroll to aid digestion. When you hit the sack, settle down on a wedge-shaped pillow, which will prop up your entire torso, rather than a stack of pillows under your head that can compress your belly. Finally, lie on your left side. In that position, your stomach is lower, so acid is less likely to back up.

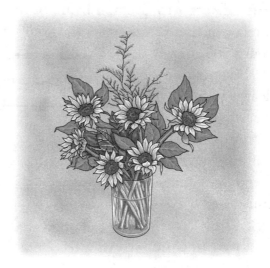

HEMORRHOIDS

The Itch You Can't Mention

Most of us would sooner discuss a messy family feud than talk about—ahem—hemorrhoids. Yet half of the adult population has these itchy, sometimes achy, swollen veins that can bulge around the anus or inside the rectum. That includes everyone from pregnant moms (I can testify to that!) and weight lifters to cab drivers, cashiers, and computer jockeys.

WHY ME?

Some experts believe that the veins surrounding the anus and inside the rectum are prone to prolonged swelling because they lack the valves present in most veins that shunt blood back to the heart. When these veins are exposed to pressure—such as straining during a bowel movement or pressure on the lower abdomen from pregnancy, childbirth, sitting or standing for

---

GO NUTS

Not with the itching, but with nutmeg, a time-honored Ayurvedic remedy for curbing constipation and hemorrhoids. Just add 1/4 teaspoon of ground nutmeg to a glass of warm lemon water (an astringent that will shrink blood vessels) and drink it twice daily.

SIP TO STOP
BLEEDING

Hemorrhoids staining the toilet water red? Simply mix a few ounces of cranberry juice with an equal amount of pomegranate juice and drink it between meals. Both fruits are hemostatics, which help stanch bleeding.

long periods of time, or heavy lifting—they dilate and remain that way, engorged with blood. This causes them to bulge and sag.

The external hemorrhoids that form around the anus (the itchy kind) are usually hard, tender to the touch, and easy targets for irritation—from wiping, for instance, which can make them bleed.

The soft, internal hemorrhoids that form inside the rectum are normally painless and barely noticeable, unless straining during a bowel movement causes bleeding. If they slip down out of the anus, however, and develop clots, they can become extremely painful.

SHRINK THOSE SUCKERS

If your hemorrhoids become very painful or bleed persistently with very dark red blood, consult your doctor immediately. You may need to have them removed with a laser or tied off with rubber bands—a painless office procedure that literally cuts off the circulation to the bulges so they shrivel. In most cases, however, you can easily manage these prickly unmentionables with the following noninvasive remedies.

ROOT 'EM OUT. Check your health food store for powdered elderberry root, which contains vessel-strengthening bioflavonoids. Mix it with warm water to make a paste, smear it on a piece of gauze, and hold it against your hemorrhoids for 10 minutes once or twice daily.

FILL UP ON FIBER. Adding fiber to your diet is the best way to soften stools and reduce straining, which in turn can eliminate hemorrhoids, says Anil Minocha, M.D., chief of gastroenterology at Southern Illinois University School of Medicine in Chicago. Load up on crunchy veggies, hearty whole grains and legumes, and oranges and pineapple, which are brimming with vein-strengthening bioflavonoids. Swear off white bread, bagels, pasta, and rice, which slow both digestion and elimination.

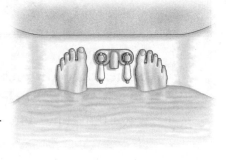

TRY PSYLLIUM. Studies show that the fastest, most effective way to get the fiber necessary to help shrink hemorrhoids is to mix 2 heaping tablespoons of a commercial psyllium powder, such as Metamucil, which you can find at any drugstore, into a large glass of water and gulp it down daily. Be sure to drink plenty of water throughout the rest of the day as well. Psyllium is a super source of mucilage, a gummy fiber that literally swells up with water and thus helps make stools comfortably mushy.

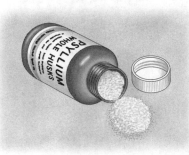

SHRINK THEM IN A SITZ. A simple sitz bath—sitting in enough water to cover your nether regions—can ease both constipation and hemorrhoids. Add a cup of witch hazel (an astringent herbal liquid available at drugstores and health food stores) to warm water, then sit and soak. The warmth stimulates circulation to keep the blood moving, and the witch hazel shrinks blood vessels. Try it for 20 minutes both morning and night (unless you're pregnant, in which case you should apply ice packs four times a day, for 10 minutes at a time, instead).

TUCK IN AN ASTRINGENT. Saturate a small square of tissue

TWEAK YOUR TOILET TECHNIQUE

Squatting in the woods may not be tops on your list of ways to relieve yourself, but if it were, you might have fewer hemorrhoids, says Anil Minocha, M.D. Sitting on a modern toilet, which forces your body into a sharp right angle, cuts off the downward movement of feces in the colon and makes you strain. In contrast, squatting is gravity assisted, making straining unnecessary. To simulate squatting while you're on the toilet, place your feet on a footstool and bend forward as far as possible.

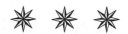

with witch hazel gel, which you can purchase at a health food store, and tuck it between your buttocks to tighten the distended veins.

SHORE UP WITH HORSE CHESTNUT. The leaves, bark, and seeds of the horse chestnut tree contain aescin, a compound that helps block enzymes that weaken veins even when applied externally. "Plus, dabbing horse chestnut tea onto hemor-

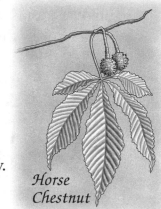

Horse Chestnut

rhoids can be soothing as well as strengthening," says Jerry Gore, M.D., medical director of the Center for Holistic Medicine in Riverwoods, Illinois. First, make some horse chestnut tea (available at health food stores) according to the package directions, then soak a small, soft cloth with the cooled liquid and apply it after each bowel movement.

HIGH BLOOD PRESSURE

Stop the Silent Killer

———◦◦◦———

I once thought the only people with high blood pressure were those who were reckless with the saltshaker, coating every morsel of every meal with the white grains. Not anymore. An astounding 60 million Americans have high blood pressure, and although many, like one of my close relatives, keep their shakers in the cupboard, their "pressures" still climb sky-high.

WHY ME?

Salt does boost blood volume, making the heart work harder to pump all that blood and increasing the pressure on the walls of the blood vessels

---

FIND A FURRY FRIEND

Just 10 minutes spent with a pet can lower your blood pressure. In fact, if you have borderline hypertension, there's even a holdover effect: If you spend time with Benji or Tiger before work, you may be less reactive to blood pressure–raising stress on the job.

SNACK ON CELERY

Crunching your way through just four stalks a day could ease down your blood pressure. A component in celery (3-n-butyl phthalide) serves as a diuretic and vasodilator and helps relax the muscles lining the blood vessels.

as it courses through. It turns out, though, that salt is only one factor in the development of high blood pressure. Other dietary and lifestyle factors—such as a high-fat diet, obesity, and a highly stressful life—also contribute, because they narrow arteries. Since smaller arteries mean that the blood has less room in which to move, the pressure on the vessel walls increases, and the arteries weaken. When this happens, you're a prime candidate for a heart attack, stroke, and/or kidney failure. Your risk is greatest if you smoke, abuse alcohol, have a family history of high blood pressure, or are male or African-American.

The really scary part, though, is that this book may be the only warning you get. High blood pressure, or hypertension, is dubbed the silent killer because it often goes undetected until it's too late. In fact, you may not know your arteries are in distress unless you get a blood pressure reading, which consists of two numbers: The top number (systolic reading) is a measurement of the pressure within the arteries when your heart's pumping. The bottom number (diastolic reading) measures the pressure between beats. Anything above 140/90 on three separate readings means you have high blood pressure, but experts say you should start worrying if you have readings higher than 120/80, because blood pressure can quickly shift into the high, dangerous range.

DIALING IT DOWN

Many people with high blood pressure take prescription diuretics to help their bodies eliminate sodium, thus reducing blood volume and blood pressure. The problem is, some diuretics tend to flush out potassium and other vital minerals along with sodium. Besides, Harvard researchers have found that a low-fat, plant-based diet such as the DASH (Dietary Approaches to Stop Hypertension) diet can lower blood pressure as well as, if not better than, the most potent prescription drugs— with none of their side effects, such as constipation or sexual dysfunction.

Consult your physician about your options. Nondrug remedies (such as herbal diuretics, which don't flush out potassium and other vital minerals) and lifestyle changes may be enough to keep borderline hypertension from going over the line, or, at the very least, help you lower dosages of prescription meds. Here's where to start.

DASH FOR IT. Following the DASH diet—that is, eating 8 to 10 servings of fruits and vegetables and 3 servings of dairy foods, limiting saturated fat, and consuming less than 2,000 milligrams of salt daily—for a month could shave off up to 11 points off your top number and 5 points off the bottom, and the beneficial effects start kicking in after two weeks. After two months, your blood pressure could return to normal—especially if, as studies have shown, you reduce your salt intake to less than 1,200 milligrams a day.

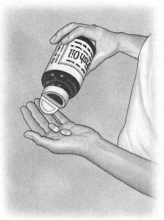

GO FISH. Omega-3 essential fatty acids, which are found mainly in salmon, tuna, and other cold-water fish, can help lower blood pressure—but you need about 5 grams (5,000 milligrams) a day for the best effect. To reach your quota, Darin Ingels, N.D., a naturopathic physician and director of New England Family Health in Southport, Connecticut, suggests that you check with your doctor about taking fish-oil capsules along with 400 IU of vitamin E to offset any fishiness. Check your drugstore or health food store for both—or opt for 1 to 3 tablespoons daily of flaxseed oil, also available at health food stores. Both fish and flax may help inhibit inflammatory reactions that can cause arteries to narrow. Since they both thin the blood, however, don't use them if you take aspirin or prescription blood thinners.

POP COENZYME Q$_{10}$. This antioxidant, available at health food stores, makes arteries less vulnerable to constriction. Stephen T. Sinatra, M.D., a cardiologist and director of medical education at Manchester Memorial Hospital in Hartford, Connecticut, reports that people who took 100 milligrams a day were able to cut their doses of blood pressure medications in half.

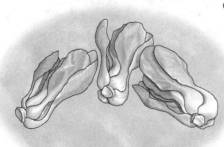

GET YOUR MINERALS. Calcium and magnesium, in particular, help reduce the tension on artery walls and relax the muscles that control blood vessels so blood flows freely—the keys to lowering blood pressure. Feast on magnesium-rich navy, pinto, and kidney beans and calcium king bok choy to get what you need.

TAKE A DIP. Just be sure it's guacamole, since avocado is packed with potassium, a mineral that helps keep all the other minerals in balance and is vital for lowering blood pressure, says Jeremy Appleton, N.D., chairman of the National College of Naturopathic Medicine in Portland, Oregon.

DINE ON DANDELION. The greens are an excellent diuretic that won't flush out potassium and are in fact rich in the mineral. Don't like the idea of munching from your lawn? Ask your doctor if you can substitute three or four cups of dandelion tea—which you can find at health food stores—a day, suggests Dr. Ingels. Don't even think of combining it with medication, though, especially diuretics or potassium supplements.

HOLD HANDS. Touch lowers the stress hormone cortisol, which constricts blood vessels and bumps up blood pressure. To try this antidote, simply get in close touch with your loved ones today!

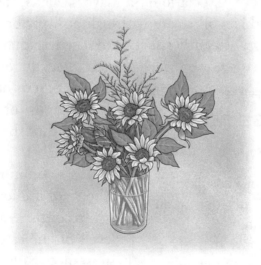

HIGH CHOLESTEROL

Keep It on the Level

⊰⦿⊱

My friend Marie could be a poster gal for the American Heart Association. She savors salads, stays slim with daily runs, and lets off steam with pals at lively book club meetings. Yet she was recently shocked to discover that her total cholesterol level had shot up since her last checkup. Since her mother took potent heart medication for most of her life, Marie worried that she faced the same fate.

It's a common concern. About 98 million Americans—a third of us!—have unhealthy levels of cholesterol, the waxy substance made in the liver that attaches to proteins to travel through the bloodstream as lipoproteins.

THE SWEETEST TREAT

A frothy cup of hot chocolate made with pure cocoa powder (or an ounce of dark chocolate with a high cocoa content) does more than stave off winter's chill: Cocoa is rich in flavonoids, which have been shown to lower LDL and raise HDL.

Low-density lipoprotein (LDL) is the "bad" cholesterol that can cling to artery walls and set the stage for heart attacks. High-density lipoprotein (HDL) is the "good" cholesterol that sweeps the gunk out of the bloodstream. LDL plus HDL (along with other blood fats, such as triglycerides) equal your "total cholesterol." The idea is to minimize LDL and maximize HDL—but unfortunately, many of us inadvertently do the opposite.

WHY ME?

A number of out-of-your-hands factors can make LDL levels rise and HDL levels fall—including loss of estrogen at menopause, diabetes, a thyroid disorder, or, as with Marie, a genetic predisposition to hold onto excess cholesterol in the bloodstream. Yet, as one expert put it, "Genetics may load the gun, but lifestyle habits like a fat-laden diet pull the trigger."

Smoking lowers HDL levels by 15 percent, while animal foods from beef to butter are loaded with saturated fat and drive up LDL levels, as do the trans fatty acids in prepared foods such as doughnuts and deep-fried chicken. And starchy, sugary foods don't just raise triglycerides, which are associated with unhealthy total cholesterol levels, they lower HDL, too.

THE WAY TO GO LOW

A healthy cholesterol profile is one in which total cholesterol is below 200 mg/dl (milligrams per deciliter of blood), LDL is

---

WARD OFF VAMPIRES—AND HIGH CHOLESTEROL

Allicin, the active component in garlic, quashes cholesterol-producing enzymes. Taking garlic in enteric-coated capsules (which you can find at health food stores) may be more effective than eating it, since the allicin isn't destroyed by stomach acid. Take two capsules daily.

REACH FOR RED

According to a study at the University of California, Davis, drinking three to six glasses of red wine a week lowers LDL levels, possibly due to its relatively high concentration of saponins. These plant compounds—believed to bind to and prevent the absorption of cholesterol—are 10 times more abundant in red grapes, especially those in red zinfandel, than in white. You could just eat the grapes, but alcohol seems to release saponins and may also raise levels of estrogen, an HDL booster.

If you have elevated triglycerides (which may be boosted by alcohol's high sugar content) or diabetes, if you're pregnant, or if alcoholism runs in your family, stick to the other red drink—unsweetened cranberry juice. Three glasses a day could raise your HDL level by 10 percent after three months.

lower than 129 mg/dl, HDL is above 40 mg/dl, and, most important, the ratio of total cholesterol to HDL is below 5. The best way to get there? That depends on your profile.

More than 15 million Americans take cholesterol-lowering drugs called statins (atorvastatin, or Lipitor, is the leading prescription medication in the United States). These drugs help block the production of cholesterol in the liver, so they're a tremendous boon to people with very elevated cholesterol levels. But the drugs can also leave you with everything from headaches and muscle weakness to a failing liver.

Consult your doctor to see if you need cholesterol-lowering medication. If you have borderline or mildly elevated cholesterol, though, you may be better off turning to nondrug therapies and making lifestyle changes—or, to get your cholesterol levels as low as possible, doing both in combination with medication. Limiting saturated fat to no more than 10 percent of your total calories, for instance, may help you reduce LDL and your statin dosage. Plus, if you combine a low-fat diet with 45 minutes of aerobic exercise three times a week, you may lower your LDL by a whopping 20 points in just three months. Here are more drug-free ways to go low.

GO FOR OATS. The soluble fiber in oats clears out excess cholesterol better than any other type of fiber. In fact, eating about 1/3 cup of dried oats daily can lower your LDL by more than 5 percent after just one month.

SIP SOY MILK. Soy contains isoflavones, estrogen-like compounds that can lower LDL by 10 to 15 percent, says Michael Miller, M.D., director of the Center for Preventive Cardiology at the University of Maryland Medical Center in Baltimore. You need 25 to 30 grams (about 2 cups) of soy milk daily to reap the benefits.

SWITCH TO FISH. Trading cholesterol-raising steak for salmon, which is filled to the gills with cholesterol-lowering omega-3 essential fatty acids (EFAs), just three times a week could slash your cholesterol by nearly half, say some studies. Not big on fish? Take 2 tablespoons of flaxseed oil daily (try drizzling it over your salad) to get an equivalent amount of EFAs, says Melissa Stevens, R.D., a registered dietitian and nutrition program coordinator for preventive cardiology at the Cleveland Clinic in Ohio. If you are taking aspirin or blood thinners, check with your doctor first.

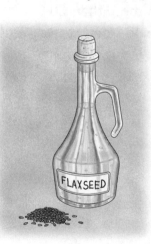

STOCK UP ON STEROLS. The best way to dress steamed veggies is with 2 tablespoons of a margarine-like spread such as Benecol or Take Control. These spreads contain plant sterols, substances that have been shown to block cholesterol from being absorbed, thus lowering total cholesterol by 10 percent and LDL by nearly 15 percent. Or simply take 200 to

250 milligrams of phytosterols in capsule form three times a day with meals. Most supermarkets carry the spreads; check health food stores for capsules.

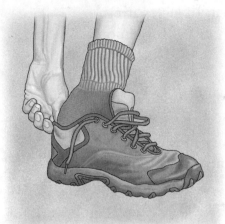

STEP IT UP. Researchers at Duke University in Durham, North Carolina, have found that people who walk a total of 12 miles a week have bigger HDL molecules that are better at clearing out bad cholesterol than their punier cousins.

SUGAR IS NICE. For mildly elevated cholesterol, new research indicates that a waxy substance called policosanol, which is derived from sugar cane, may help lower LDL as well as or better than statins and may raise HDL, too. Darin Ingels, N.D., a naturopathic physician and director of New England Family Health in Southport, Connecticut, recommends taking no more than 20 milligrams daily in capsule form (available in health food stores and from the Internet). Talk to your doctor first if you're taking a statin drug or have diabetes.

Hot Flashes

Turn Down the Heat

———————

Nothing broadcasts the change of life more noticeably than having a hot flash. As my friend Dina, a nurse-midwife who frequently lectures to new doctors, told me, "I break out in a sweat, I turn beet-red, my mascara smudges…" And her composure in front of her young charges? "It ends up as wrecked as my makeup."

Dina isn't the only one sweating hot flashes. About 75 percent of women in the United States experience them as their periods come to an end and menopause begins. Flashes can begin as early as age 40 or as late as 53. They can be as light as a little glisten on the upper lip or as heavy as a full-blown drenching, and they can come on occasionally or occur hourly, day or night (when they're called night sweats).

WHY ME?

Hot flashes are a by-product of fluctuating estrogen and progesterone levels. The flux interferes with the vasomotor nerves that control your body temperature, and this causes your blood vessels to widen suddenly, turning you red and sweaty. To compensate for the hormone loss, your pituitary gland begins to

overproduce luteinizing hormone (LH). The more abruptly your estrogen drops and the more LH is produced, the more severe your hot flashes.

TURN DOWN THE HEAT

Hot flashes typically occur for about five years and stop altogether two to four years after your period ends, as your body adjusts to its new hormone levels. In the meantime, however, you don't have to walk around with a smudged face or resort to potentially dangerous hormone replacement medications such as Prempro, the widely prescribed estrogen/progestin combo that was recently found to increase the risk of breast cancer, heart attacks, and even Alzheimer's disease. With dietary changes, exercise, and a few simple, nondrug remedies, you can not only cut the number and severity of your hot flashes, you can do so without jeopardizing your overall health.

To start, avoid vessel-dilating foods such as caffeine, alcohol, and hot or spicy dishes; take a multivitamin with 400 IU of vitamin E (which has been found to cut hot flashes); exercise regularly (walking and other forms of exercise decrease the amount of circulating LH and increase levels of feel-good brain chemicals called endorphins, which nosedive during hot flashes); and use these additional tricks for dialing down the heat.

FILL UP ON PHYTOS. Women in Asia get far fewer hot flashes than Western women, possibly because they eat a plant-based diet brimming with phytoestrogens, which bind to estrogen receptors in the body and reduce overall estrogen levels. To mimic their phyto-dense diet, load up on soybeans, which contain isoflavones, the most potent phytos. In fact, studies show that eating 50 milligrams of soy a day— roughly equivalent to 1 1/2 cups of soymilk—could slash the frequency of your hot flashes in half. Chickpeas, lentils, and flaxseed oil (try 1 table-spoon a day) also pack plenty of these beneficial compounds. Women who have been diagnosed with breast or ovarian cancer should not load up on phytoestrogens.

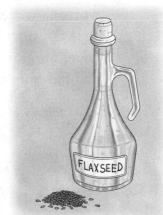

TRY BLACK COHOSH. In one study, most women who took black cohosh daily for three months had lower LH levels and 70 percent fewer hot flashes than those who didn't take it. For the best results, use RemiFemin, a widely tested commercial black cohosh supplement available in most health food stores, advises Maida Taylor, M.D., associate clinical professor of obstetrics, gynecology, and reproductive sciences at the University of California, San Francisco. Follow the package directions.

COME OVER TO RED CLOVER. According to two small studies, this isoflavone-rich herb reduces the number and severity of hot flashes by nearly half. The studies involved Promensil, a commercial preparation available in health food stores, but you can also take the herb as a tincture according to the label directions. Don't take red clover in any form if you have a history of breast cancer.

TURN TO MOTHERWORT. This herb's Latin name means "lion's ear," which is fitting since motherwort is a ferocious mood tamer and a powerful phytoestrogenic herb favored by women's healers to quell hot flashes and night sweats. Mix 25 drops of tincture (available at health food stores) into a cup of water and drink it two to four times a day. Avoid motherwort if you have heavy periods.

SIP SOME SAGE. At the first hint of a flash or night sweats, drink some sage tea, suggests Carol Leonard, a certified nurse-midwife and chair of the New Hampshire Council of Midwifery in Hopkinton. To make the tea, steep 1 tablespoon of dried sage (available at health food stores) in a cup of hot water for 10 minutes, then strain. Sage is what's called a hormonal stimulant and is often used to minimize menopausal discomforts such as hot flashes and dizziness, but don't use it if there's any chance you could be pregnant.

IMPOTENCE

When You're Not Up to Snuff

————◆◇◆◇◆————

We can thank former senator and Viagra pitchman Bob Dole for bringing impotence out of the bedroom and into mainstream conversation. Just because the issue is openly discussed, though, that doesn't mean it's any less distressing. When a man has erectile dysfunction (ED)—and most men over 40 have, at one time or another, experienced what's defined as the inability to maintain an erection long enough for intercourse—it's a two-person problem. As one female friend put it, "When the tool doesn't work, the project is stalled."

WHY ME?

Men over 50 experience erectile problems three times more frequently than men under 30, most often due to a

---

PUMP IT UP

According to one study, erections improved in 80 percent of participants who performed exercises that improve blood supply to the penis, buttocks, and upper leg muscles, such as squats and leg lifts, for three months. Only 74 percent of men who took Viagra had similar results. Ask a trainer to devise a regimen of such exercises for you for just that purpose.

No More Blazing Saddles

In the ninth century, horseback riding was nailed as an ED culprit. Today, cycling (both moving and stationary) claims that dubious distinction—especially if the bicycle seat compresses the arteries and nerves that feed the penis. If you've noticed numbness, stop cycling for six weeks and purchase a wider, padded seat or a style that has a hole in the middle. Then point the seat downward when you return to the saddle, and hop off every 10 minutes or so to encourage blood flow.

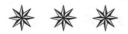

physical problem rather than a psychological one (despite how much we hear about it, "performance anxiety" plays only a small role, experts say). Circulatory problems head the list, because when blood doesn't flow into the penis, engorgement can't happen, and erections are no-shows.

Among the many factors that can narrow arteries and blood vessels and/or affect nerves that control blood flow are high blood pressure, diabetes, smoking, obesity, and many common medications, including those for high blood pressure (such as beta-blockers), antidepressants, and even antihistamines.

PUT AN END TO ED

Before you decide to stock up on an erection-enhancing drug, such as sildenafil (Viagra), and possibly render your bank account as depleted as your love life, consult your doctor for help in determining the underlying cause of your ED. If it's stress related, you can see a therapist or psychologist to defuse your anxiety and/or calm your nerves. If it's accompanied by declining sexual interest, you may be able to use—with your doctor's guidance, of course—supplements of testosterone or DHEA (dehydroepiandrosterone, which the body uses to make testosterone). You can also stop smoking, step up your exercise routine, and eat a plant-based diet that minimizes fat, meat, and salt—all strategies that will protect your blood vessels and keep blood pumping to all your organs, including the all-important organ in question.

Finally, you can experiment with nondrug erection enhancers that, unlike drugs, address underlying circulatory problems and are cheaper and relatively free of side effects. Their only drawback? They generally take longer than Viagra's record of 30 minutes to kick in—but the wait could well be worth it. Start with the following suggestions, then see what you think.

GRAB SOME GINKGO. "As an all-around blood booster, ginkgo has more going for it than any other natural aphrodisiac," says Chris Melitis, N.D., dean of natural medicine at the National College of Naturopathic Medicine in Portland. "It can improve erections and guard against heart attacks." In fact, studies show that ginkgo may be especially helpful for reversing weak erections in men taking fluoxetine (Prozac), sertraline (Zoloft), or other selective serotonin reuptake inhibitors for depression. As long as you're not taking other medications, check your health food store for standardized products and follow the label directions. If you take ginkgo daily, erections could return in a month.

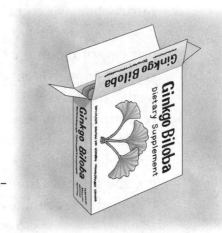

TRY ASIAN GINSENG. This herb improves blood flow to the penis and may increase testosterone levels to boost libido and encourage erections. What's more, ginseng is an adaptogen, which means it helps defuse the effects of stress on the body. "If stress is at the root of your impotence, this herb may be just the sparkplug you need," says Dr. Melitis. As long as you don't have high blood pressure, check your health food store for a standardized product, then take it according to the label directions. Give it a few weeks to work.

POP MUIRA PUAMA. In one French study, researchers found that more than half of men who took this Brazilian herb (nicknamed "potency wood") daily for two weeks had improved erections, possibly because the sterols it contains may help stimulate chemicals responsible for both erections and pleasure, says Dr. Melitis. As a bonus, muira puama can also lower blood pressure. Check your health food store for a supplement, then follow the label directions.

SCARF ARGININE. The body converts this amino acid into nitric oxide, which helps to widen blood vessels, thus allowing blood to flow freely to the penis. Beans and peanut butter are just two of the many foods that contain arginine, but to be sure you get enough, consider taking a supplement (available at health food stores). A third of men who take it notice erections returning within just 2 hours, notes Dr. Melitis. Or, as long as you don't have high blood pressure, try ArginMax, a widely available combination supplement that includes arginine, ginkgo, and ginseng. Studies show that it improves erections in nearly 90 percent of men who try it.

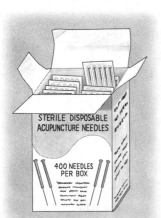

STERILE DISPOSABLE
ACUPUNCTURE NEEDLES

400 NEEDLES
PER BOX

GO FOR YOHIMBINE. Available only by prescription, this extract from the bark of the African yohimbe tree has been shown to rival Viagra by encouraging erections within an hour. The prescription form is less toxic than regular yohimbine, which can cause headaches and anxiety attacks and raise blood pressure. Ask your doctor about giving it a try.

TRY NEEDLE THERAPY. Studies have shown that twice-weekly acupuncture treatments relieved impotence in nearly 40 percent of men in just one month. Ask your physician to recommend a reputable, licensed acupuncturist.

INSOMNIA

Drift Off to Dreamland

———◆———

I found myself "sleepless in Pennsylvania" for some time a while ago, and I sampled nearly all of the usual quick-fix solutions, from sipping warm milk to popping drugstore "PM" medications and even prescription sleeping pills. The fact that I was extremely worried that I'd never again get enough shuteye didn't help matters, I'm sure—but I couldn't help myself.

If you're among the 20 to 40 percent of people (most of them women) who can't fall asleep, stay asleep, or get enough sleep to feel refreshed, you no doubt understand my concern. But as I can attest, worrying only leaves you frustrated, tense, and more wide awake than ever, while sleeping pills can leave you groggy the next day.

If you really want to get a good night's sleep, experts say, you're better off changing your

> ### OIL UP
>
> Rubbing warm, organic sesame oil on your scalp and the soles of your feet before bed is one of the simplest—and most pleasant—sleep potions, says Vasant Lad, M.A.Sc., director of the Ayurvedic Institute in Albuquerque.

sleep-wrecking daytime habits and thoughts—including worrying about sleeplessness.

WHY ME?

Many physical conditions—including everything from menstrual cramps and sheet-drenching night sweats to arthritis and side effects of medications such as decongestants—can lead to insomnia. But by changing daytime behaviors and thoughts, Harvard researchers found, most cases can be reversed. This makes behavior modification more effective than any knockout pill on the market—especially if you nudge it along with a key alternative treatment or two.

TAKE THE SLUMBERLAND EXPRESS

Here are some nifty ways to drift off to dreamland without being sidelined the next day.

NO MO' STIMULANTS. "Insomnia can be blamed on a slew of things that keep the body and mind agitated 24/7," says Ted Zeff, Ph.D., an insomnia specialist in San Francisco. If you want to get to sleep—and stay asleep—cut out caffeine after 6:00 P.M. (make that noon if even a spoonful of cappuccino yogurt revs your engines), skip the nightcap (alcohol may make you sleepy, but it will wake you up later), and pass up the late-night news.

GET A ROUTINE. Start going to bed at the same time every night and getting up at the same time every morning (aim for 7 to 8 hours of sleep), even on weekends.

LULL YOURSELF WITH LAVENDER

A bedside essential oil diffuser that mists the room with sweet-smelling, calming lavender may help you sleep longer and more soundly. You can buy diffusers from natural products companies and some health food stores.

This will set your sleep clock (circadian rhythms) so your body will know when it's time to go to sleep.

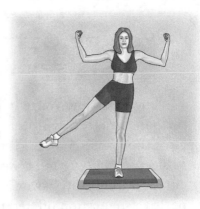

WORK OUT EARLY. Exercise can release tension and help you sleep more soundly, but it will keep you too stimulated if you exercise within 3 hours of bedtime. Working out 5 hours before you hit the sack is ideal, says Dr. Zeff.

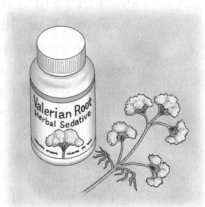

PLAN YOUR BATH STRATEGI-CALLY. Soaking in a warm bath for 30 minutes raises your body temperature, which then drops and makes you drowsy 2 hours later, points out Gregg Jacobs, Ph.D., assistant professor of psychiatry at Harvard Medical School. The best time for a good, sleep-inducing soak? Two hours before bedtime.

TALK IT OUT. "Talking aloud to yourself at day's end, acknowledging your anxieties and concerns, can help you release the emotions that are bothering you so they won't bother your sleep," says Dana Ullman, M.D., advisor for the council of the Alternative Medicine Center at Columbia University College of Physicians and Surgeons in New York City. Keeping a bedtime journal can also help.

POP HERBAL VALIUM. Valerian root's active components, called valepotriates, appear to work in a way similar to diazepam (Valium). Its only downsides are that the tea and capsules smell like dirty socks, and, as with many substances that relax you, there is a possibility of becoming reliant on it. As long as you're not taking any other medications, take it according to package directions.

SAVOR EVENING OATS. Oats have long been used to soothe the nerves and treat insomnia, and adding milk further invites drowsiness, since it's loaded with tryptophan, the amino acid necessary to make the brain chemical serotonin, which controls sleep patterns. If you'd rather sip your oats, try some oatstraw tea. Get the tea and the herbal sedatives dried chamomile, skullcap, and catnip at a health food store, then mix equal parts of each and steep 1 heaping teaspoon in 1 cup of hot water for 20 minutes.

HOPS TO IT. Hops is a time-honored sleep-inducing herb used to make "dream pillows" because exposure to air increases its sedative effect. Stuff some dried leaves (which you can find at a health food store) into your pillowcase and use the rest to make a tea by steeping 1 to 2 teaspoons in a cup of hot water along with equal parts of lemon balm and valerian root. Studies show that drinking a cup of this concoction 15 minutes before retiring works directly on the central nervous system and could help you nod off within a half-hour.

INTERMITTENT CLAUDICATION

Walk Away from Pain

———◦◦◦———

Not long ago, a new woman joined my walking group. She appeared fit and was highly motivated. By the time we'd walked about three blocks, though, she'd invariably develop a calf cramp and begin limping. She'd stop for a few minutes until her cramp eased and then begin again, but the same thing would happen after walking a few more blocks. Soon she dropped out of the group altogether.

It wasn't until later that I learned that her cramps were linked to intermittent claudication (IC)—a symptom that's associated with hardening of the arteries and is shared by 12 million Americans over age 50—and that if she'd only found a way to stay with the group, her cramping might have gone from intermittent to nonexistent.

WHY ME?

The name *intermittent claudication* comes from the sporadic nature of the cramping and a reference to the Roman emperor

Claudius, who had a limp. It's most likely to develop if you smoke; have high blood pressure, high cholesterol, or diabetes; or are obese. All of these factors can cause a buildup of plaque (fatty cholesterol deposits) on the interior walls of the arteries that supply blood to the lower body. As a result, your arteries narrow, making it tougher for your legs to get oxygen when they need it most—when you're moving.

Yet that's the very best way to manage IC—by moving (i.e., walking) regularly. Walking forces blood flow to the smaller vessels of the legs, bypassing the clogged ones. Plus, it trains your leg muscles to use oxygen more efficiently. In fact, if you don't walk regularly, the condition can worsen, you'll limp more—and you'll double your risk of heart disease and stroke.

LOSING THE LIMP

Of course, you can't walk away from IC without making other lifestyle adjustments. Quitting smoking, losing weight, and eating a low-fat, fiber-rich diet can keep it from worsening. Don't try to do so alone, however; consult your doctor if you have calf cramps that start when you walk and stop when you rest. You may need tests to measure blood flow to your legs and determine if the arteries to your heart are similarly clogged.

Depending on the results, you may be advised to take a cholesterol-lowering drug such as a statin. No matter what the finding, though, you can control the pain and remain active with these non-drug methods.

STEP TO IT. Studies show that a regular walking program improves IC as effectively as clot-busting medications and surgical procedures that open arteries. Just be sure to get your doctor's okay to walk for 45 minutes to an hour three to five days a week. When you walk, use this start-and-stop strategy: When you set out, walk to a point just beyond where you feel the first twinge of pain, then rest before starting again. The next time out, try to make it to the nearest telephone pole beyond the spot where you stopped previously before you take a break. Each time the pain strikes, gradually lengthen the distance you walk before resting. Soon you'll be covering more ground with less pain. In fact, within three months, you could double your walking distance.

CREATE A STINK. A compound in garlic called allicin aids arterial blood flow, so load up on the smelly bulb whenever you can. Or, to make sure you get enough often enough, take garlic daily in capsule form (available at drugstores and health food stores).

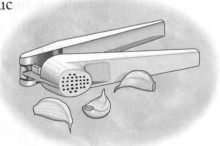

FISH FOR OMEGA 3'S. Cold-water fish, such as salmon and tuna, are excellent sources of omega-3 essential fatty acids, which may help reduce cholesterol in the arteries.

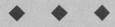

HOMEGROWN SOLUTION

◆ ◆ ◆

Pocket the Purslane

The next time you're on your knees weeding, save the purslane. This leafy green botanical is a rich source of alpha-linolenic acid, a plant-based omega-3 fatty acid that may help reduce cholesterol in the arteries—and perhaps prevent leg cramps when walking. Try steaming it like spinach.

Not much of a fish lover? Take 1 to 3 grams (1,000 to 3,000 milligrams) of fish oil in capsule form (available at health food stores) daily—but ask your doctor first, especially if you're taking aspirin regularly or use blood-thinning medications, since fish oil also thins the blood.

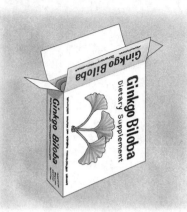

GIVE 'EM GINKGO. A slew of studies suggest that this well-known blood-thinning herb could take the pain out of your walking program. The dose used in the studies was 120 milligrams twice daily. Look for standardized products at drugstores and health food stores. Just be sure to get your doctor's approval first if you're taking aspirin or blood thinners.

POP CARNITINE. This amino acid, abundant in red meat and dairy products, helps deliver oxygen to muscles. Check your health food store for carnitine supplements, then take 250 to 500 milligrams twice daily. You may need to take up to 1 gram (1,000 milligrams) to increase your walking distance by 75 percent. "This amount is about twice as high as normal recommendations, so talk with a nutritionally oriented doctor before supplementing," suggests Ronald Steriti, N.D., Ph.D., a naturopathic physician in Naples, Florida.

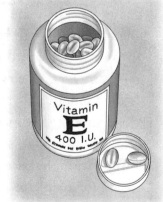

REACH FOR E. Taking 400 IU of supplemental vitamin E a day makes plaques less sticky and therefore less likely to glom onto arteries and gum up blood flow to the legs. Allow four to six months for the effects to kick in.

Irritable Bowel Syndrome

Stop the Spasms

❧

Wheat may be the staff of life, but for me, just a few mouthfuls can trigger symptoms that feel like the kiss of death—or close to it, anyway. If you have irritable bowel syndrome (IBS), you know what I mean. The searing abdominal pain, crampy constipation, and/or explosive diarrhea can be as embarrassing and depressing as they are debilitating—especially if you're forced to bolt to the bathroom during a lunch meeting with your boss or midway through your best friend's wedding.

WHY ME?

If you've had symptoms of irritable bowel syndrome for three months or more—plus mucus in the stool, gas, sudden urgency, or straining—you probably have what's called a hypersensitive digestive tract. In other words, your colon spasms at the slightest irritation—from foods you're allergic to or intolerant to (wheat and milk are the most notorious); fatty and gas-forming foods; stimulating foods such as coffee, tea, and chocolate; hormone imbalances (the menstrual period is a prime time for IBS flare-ups); or even emotional upsets. The spasms either move the contents of the colon along too slowly (causing constipation) or too quickly (causing diarrhea). To make matters worse, the nerves in the digestive tracts of people with IBS are also hypersensitive, so even normal contractions from digesting a meal can make you double over with gut-stabbing pain.

CALM YOUR COLON

Sure, you can turn to commercial antispasmodic drugs, but like most medicines, they can have significant side effects, such as blurred vision and dry mouth. Many people with IBS can find relief without resorting to medication. Here's how.

CHECK FOR FOOD TRIGGERS. Two-thirds of those with IBS are allergic to or have an intolerance for at least one food, and almost half find relief by keeping a food diary, identifying their triggers, and eliminating the offenders. In my case, switching from foods made with wheat to oat bread and rice cereals made a huge difference. Other people find that eliminating caffeine, dairy products, foods sweetened with sorbitol and xylitol (including chewing gum), and raw veggies staves off symptoms. Eating smaller meals can also reduce the intestinal load—and colon spasms.

CHOOSE ARTICHOKE LEAF EXTRACT. In one study, people with IBS who took capsules of artichoke leaf extract twice daily for six weeks were able to significantly reduce their crampy constipation and diarrhea. If you prefer, you can take liquid extract. Both forms are available at health food stores; follow the label directions.

FIGHT IT WITH FENNEL. This licorice-flavored herb assists digestion and reduces gas and bloating. Plus, its antispasmodic properties make it one of the best weapons to fight IBS, says Anil Minocha, M.D., chief of gastroenterology at Southern Illinois University School of Medicine in Chicago. He recommends munching 1 teaspoon of 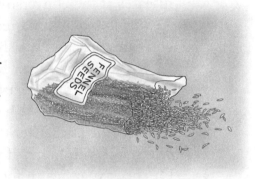 fennel seeds (available at supermarkets and health food stores) or sipping fennel tea three times a day after meals. For the tea, boil 1 teaspoon of seeds and one piece of fresh ginger in a cup of water for 5 to 10 minutes, then strain before drinking.

POP PEPPERMINT. This refreshing antispasmodic herb not only wards off painful gas but may also help control an overgrowth of yeast in the gut that can bloat your belly like a hot-air balloon and cause excruciating IBS pain, says Dr. Minocha. Take one or two capsules of enteric-coated peppermint oil (available at any health food store) three times a day after meals, whether or not you have symptoms.

MASSAGE IN THE MINT. To ease constipation, lie on your back and place a drop or two of peppermint oil on your abdo-

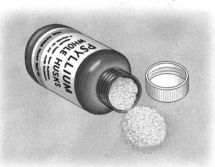

men. Press your palms firmly into your stomach and massage for 5 to 10 minutes in a clockwise motion to mimic the direction that food moves when passing through the digestive system, suggests Dr. Minocha.

TRADE RAW FOR ROASTED. Raw fruits and vegetables are notorious gas promoters in people with IBS, but you can still get your fiber (which will also ease constipation) and nutrients by roasting or grilling fresh produce, says Gary Gitnick, M.D., chief of the division of digestive diseases at the University of California, Los Angeles, School of Medicine. Try roasted red peppers tossed with grilled eggplant and pineapple and splashed with ginger dressing. Mmmm!

REACH FOR RICE. Rice helps reduce diarrhea, protects the mucous lining of the gastrointestinal tract, and reduces IBS symptoms in a jiffy. When you boil rice, just add 2 extra cups of water to the pan. After the rice is cooked, strain the liquid, sweeten it with honey if you like, and sip it throughout the day. Or check your health food store for rice bran oil extract—called gamma-orysanol—in capsule form, then take 100 milligrams three times a day.

BULK UP. Bulking up the stools with fiber supplements such as psyllium or flaxseed (both of which are available at health food stores) can reduce the severity of IBS-related colon spasms. Each morning, add a heaping tablespoon of the powdered form of either fiber to a full glass of water, stir to thicken, and down the mixture on the spot. Chase it with another glass of water, then be sure to drink 8 to 10 full glasses of water throughout the day.

ITCHY SKIN

Stop Scratching—Naturally

———◦◦◦◦◦———

Whenever I'm sitting on the couch with my daughter and the cushions start jiggling, I know that the maddening itch on her legs has flared, and she's furiously scratching like a hound with fleas. "It's like having poison ivy that never goes away," she moans.

If you've ever had an intense itching episode, also called hives or pruritis, you know that it's impossible to take a hands-off approach. The catch-22 is, of course, that the more you scratch, the more you aggravate the irritation and increase the likelihood of infection.

WHY ME?

Itchy, red welts appear as a result of the body's release of

HYPNOTIZE YOUR ITCH

People with atopic dermatitis who undergo hypnosis to reach a deeply relaxed state in which they are open to suggestions about achieving calm, itch-free skin are able to reduce their discomfort and scratching by a significant 60 percent after just two months, says Philip Shenefelt, M.D. Ask your dermatologist about hypnosis or any method of stress management that involves deep relaxation and encourages you to focus on calming your skin.

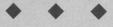
histamines—inflammatory chemicals that cause swelling and redness in response to (here's the tricky part) a mind-numbing array of triggers, including plants, perfume, pet dander, soaps, cleaners, nickel in pierced earrings, artificial fingernails, and even sunburn. My daughter's hives crop up periodically in association with atopic dermatitis, or eczema—a stubborn itch that usually occurs in people with a history of allergies and is easily aggravated by indoor heat, scratchy fabrics, and harsh detergents.

Other causes of lingering itching include a hormone imbalance involving the thyroid, liver, or kidneys, and even emotional upsets.

DITCH THE ITCH

An incessant, angry itch sends most people racing to the medicine chest, but long-term use of hydrocortisone cream can thin and discolor the skin. Antihistamines such as diphenhydramine (Benadryl) can dry out your skin—and the drier it is, the more you'll itch. Your best bet is to avoid increasing the irritation by forgoing long, hot showers, for instance, using soap-free body cleansers, and rinsing your clothes twice to protect your skin from harsh or scented chemicals. And instead of sharpening your nails, reach for one of these remedies.

SOAK IN OATMEAL. "When mixed with water, the gluten in oats turns into a gooey mass that cools and moisturizes ravaged skin," says Philip Shenefelt, M.D., associate professor of the division of dermatology and cutaneous surgery at the University of South Florida in Tampa. Pour one to two handfuls of ordinary oatmeal into an athletic sock, tie the top, and drop it into a tub of cool water. While you're soaking, you can use the sock to sponge your itchy spots. Or check your drugstore or health food store for colloidal oatmeal (the kind intended for soaking, so it won't gunk up the drain), then follow the package directions.

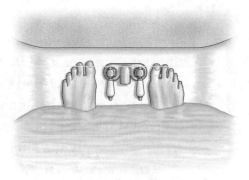

SEAL IN H$_2$O. After your soak, lock moisture into your skin by smearing chamomile cream, calendula lotion, or comfrey ointment (all available at health food stores) directly onto the itchy area. These herbs have anti-inflammatory properties that will help relieve your discomfort, says Jeanette Jacknin, M.D., a dermatologist in Scottsdale, Arizona. You can even keep these emollients in the fridge for instant relief whenever itching flares.

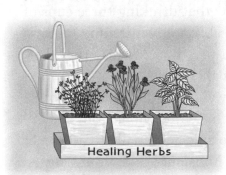

Healing Herbs

CHILL OUT WITH CHILIES. Capsaicin cream, made from the red-hot component in chile peppers, stimulates nerve endings and helps convert a maddening itch to a more tolerable sting. "Capsaicin is a form of 'chemical scratching,'" says Dr. Shenefelt. "You get the same sensation as scratching, but without injury to your skin." Look for capsaicin cream at drugstores. Wash your hands thoroughly after using it, and don't use it on areas of broken skin or near your eyes.

LICK IT WITH LICORICE. The glycyrrhizin in licorice works like a topical steroid to reduce inflammation, but it doesn't thin the skin. Simmer 2 tablespoons of ground, dried licorice root (available at health food stores) in 2 cups of water for 15 minutes. Then strain the liquid, let it cool, and apply it to your eczema. Or check your health food store for glycyrrhetinic acid cream and apply it to itchy areas three or four times a day.

TREAT IT WITH TANNINS. The angrier your rash, the more you need a natural astringent, such as witch hazel, mullein, or plain old tea. The tannins in these botanicals help constrict tissues and control inflammation, says Dr. Shenefelt. The simplest relief? Squeeze out a cooled tea bag and slap it on your itch.

SIP OOLONG TEA. Studies show that drinking three cups of oolong tea a day (one after each meal) improves itching in many people with eczema. Researchers suspect that the tea's polyphenols may suppress allergies.

OIL UP. Swallowing 3 to 6 grams of evening primrose oil (which contains gamma-linolenic acid) daily may correct a fatty acid imbalance and reduce any itching and redness associated with eczema, says Dr. Shenefelt. Or take 3 to 6 grams of flaxseed oil, which the body converts to inflammation-fighting omega-3 essential fatty acids. You can also try a flaxseed compress: Simply grind flaxseed (which, like evening primrose oil and flaxseed oil, you can find at health food stores) to make a paste, apply it to a piece of gauze, and hold it against your rash. Since flaxseed oil can thin the blood, don't take it if you're taking aspirin or prescription blood thinners.

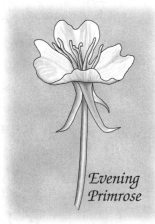
Evening Primrose

LARYNGITIS

Hoarse No More

I have a friend who is normally quite the chatterbox, both on the job (she's a choir director) and off. When she has laryngitis, though, and her larynx (the organ at the top of the windpipe that contains the vocal cords) is inflamed, she can force out only a few syllables, and her lilting soprano is reduced to a squeak. The only upside: I can finally get a word in edgewise!

WHY ME?

A full-throttle yell from the bleachers, a bout with the flu, and inhaling pollen, fumes, or secondhand smoke can inflame the mucous membranes of your larynx to the extent that you can barely rasp out a whisper. Heartburn that causes excessive backflow of acid into the esophagus and throat may cause contact ulcers on your vocal cords, while excessive

GORGE ON GINGER

The next time your throat feels the slightest bit sore, you may want to feed it some stir-fry spiced with ginger. The herb is used the world over to help relieve laryngitis.

ON-THE-SPOT RELIEF

Stretch Your Neck

If you carry tension in the shoulder and neck area, you could be stressing your vocal cords and impairing your voice. To loosen the muscles surrounding your voice box, Murray Grossan, M.D., suggests gently turning your neck to the right and left while you're standing in a warm shower, with the flow of water directed onto the back of your neck.

talking can cause callus-like nodules on them. Both can squelch your voice. Telemarketers, in fact, suffer so much wear and tear on their vocal cords that they are nearly twice as likely as less talkative types to report having hoarseness.

SPEAK EASIER

For those times when your lips move but no words come out, don't force it; even whispering can place undue stress on your vocal cords. Give your voice a vacation, guzzle plenty of water, resolve any heartburn, and avoid the drying effects of caffeine, alcohol, cold medicines, and overheated rooms. Then, instead of sucking on mint or mentholated commercial cough drops, which may only irritate your sore cords, sip the time-honored singer's remedy (hot water with a teaspoon of honey or lemon juice) and give these kinder, gentler methods a go.

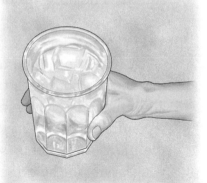

SKIP THE SALT. Treating a sore throat with a saltwater gargle is like rubbing your eyes when they're inflamed, says Murray Grossan, M.D., a consultant in the department of otolaryngology at Cedars-Sinai Hospital in Los Angeles. Instead, boil some water in a pot, remove it from the stove, and lean over it so your head is close enough to inhale the rising steam but not close enough to be burned. Then stick out your tongue and breathe in the vapors. You can even add a few drops of eucalyptus oil to the water to help thin mucus and increase healing blood flow to your inflamed larynx. Look for the oil at health food stores.

SOOTHE WITH HERBS. If you simply must gargle, Eric Jones, N.D., a naturopathic physician in Seattle, suggests using a widely available herbal tea blend: licorice root, marshmallow, and slippery elm, all of which amp up mucus production to coat the vocal cords. Make the tea according to package directions and let it cool, then gargle with 1/2 cup and swallow the other half. Avoid licorice if you have high blood pressure, though.

SAVOR MALLOW AND MULLEIN. These two herbs contain gel-like fiber that helps coat mucous membranes to ease irritation. Look for either herbal tea at your local health food store and sip it throughout the day.

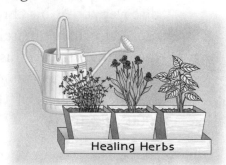
Healing Herbs

SIP HOREHOUND TEA. Don't like mallow or mullein? James A. Duke, Ph.D., president and CEO of Duke's Herbal Vineyard in Fulton, Maryland, and a former specialist in medicinal plants for the USDA, suggests sipping horehound tea to increase mucus production and ease irritation. Simply add some lemon, licorice, the natural sweetener stevia, and 1 to 2 teaspoons of dried horehound (available at health food stores) to a cup of boiling water, steep for 10 minutes, and strain. Skip the licorice if you have high blood pressure.

STICK WITH LICORICE. To soothe your inflamed throat, chew on sticks of licorice (a noted inflammation fighter)—not

Twizzlers, mind you, but the sugar-free type found in health food stores. Don't try this remedy, however, if you have high blood pressure.

CALL ON CLEAR-EASE. Search your health food store for Clear-Ease tablets. They contain papaya and pineapple enzymes, which help reduce inflammation and swelling of the vocal cords and may restore your voice, says Dr. Grossan. Simply tuck a tablet between your cheek and gum and let it dissolve.

TRY THE ALEXANDER TECHNIQUE. This simple movement therapy was founded by F. M. Alexander, an actor who discovered that his chronic laryngitis and raspy voice were caused by undue muscle tension. He developed specific movements that restored his voice by creating greater ease and freedom of movement. For more information, contact the North American Society of Teachers of the Alexander Technique at (800) 473-0620.

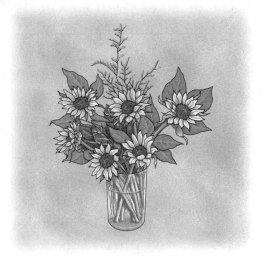

LOW LIBIDO

Fan the Flames of Desire

———◆◆◆◆◆———

I have a friend who has a closet full of sexy lingerie, a CD player stacked with sultry tunes, and a table lined with fragrant candles. But they're all collecting dust because for her, as for many women, the flames of desire have gone out.

Despite the numerous sexual images bombarding us from television and movie screens and the pages of countless magazines, lack of desire is quite common. In fact, in one national survey, more than 85 percent of women seeking routine gynecological care reported low libido as their leading concern.

WHY ME?

If you're coping with kids, work, household chores, or a stressor such as a death in the family or a move, you may be

PASSION FRUIT

For a fruity alternative to chocolate—the classic aphrodisiac—try sticky dates drenched in Indian spices, suggests Vasant Lad, M.A.Sc., director of the Ayurvedic Institute in Albuquerque. His recipe: Soak 10 fresh dates in a jar of ghee (clarified butter), then add 1 teaspoon of ginger, $1/8$ teaspoon of cardamom, and a pinch of saffron. Refrigerate the dates for at least two weeks, then eat one daily.

Good and Sexy

Need an instant libido lifter? Take a whiff of Good and Plenty licorice candy, or slice up some cucumbers and inhale their aroma. When women sniffed either of these, their vaginal lubrication—and libido—increased more than with any other scent tested, according to studies from the Smell and Taste Treatment and Research Foundation in Chicago. The first runner-up? Banana nut bread. There's something about food…

too tapped out even to light a candle. If you've reached menopause, desire can dwindle because your body is producing less testosterone, the hormone that sparks desire in both men and women. Plus, menopause can slow the output of estradiol, the hormone that keeps the vagina lubricated, and this can make penetration painful.

Other libido killers include depression as well as the widely prescribed medications called selective serotonin reuptake inhibitors, such as fluoxetine (Prozac) and sertraline (Zoloft), used to treat it; birth control pills; blood pressure drugs; and underlying problems such vaginal infections, endometriosis, and low thyroid levels. And we haven't even touched on the desire-dampening emotional issues such as marital problems or a poor body image from weight gain.

REVIVING DULLED DESIRE

Restoring libido may require a blend of physical, psychological, and relationship strategies, says Sandra Leiblum, Ph.D., director of the Center for Sexual and Marital Health at the Robert Wood Johnson Medical School in New Brunswick, New Jersey. The best place to start is with a simple gynecological checkup to determine your hormone levels. You may also need couples counseling to help resolve conflict and reconnect with your partner.

At the end of the day, however, you may simply need to start being more aware of doing things that can enhance desire, such as eating whole fresh fruits and veggies and protein to increase your overall vitality and cutting back on energy-zapping caffeine, alcohol, and fatty and sugary foods. Also, depending on what's at the core of your lowered libido, you may want to try one or more—or even all—of the following natural arousal enhancers.

DOWN AN HERBAL APHRODISIAC. In Victorian times, women who wished to fan the flames of desire sipped the discreetly named Lydia Pinkham's Compound, which featured sarsaparilla, a testosterone-like herb. The compound also contained fenugreek, an estrogenic herb that may help relieve vaginal dryness. Women's health herbalist Susun Weed, of the Wise Woman Center in Woodstock, New York, recommends checking your health food store for herbal formulas that contain these herbs.

GET GINKGO. According to researchers at the University of California, San Francisco, ginkgo (which enhances blood flow) reversed sexual problems in 84 percent of men and women who were taking libido-lowering antidepressants—with no adverse side effects. As long as you're not taking other medications, look for a standardized product at your health food store and follow the label directions.

SCARF ARGININE. Almonds are a highly prized aphrodisiac in India, perhaps because they contain arginine, an amino acid necessary for the production of nitric oxide, which promotes blood flow to the genitals. In fact, it's now widely included in modern-day sex-enhancing products such as ArginMax, a dietary supplement available in most health food stores that contains arginine along with ginseng (an herb touted for energy enhancement) and ginkgo. Women with low libido who took ArginMax for a month reported increased desire.

STRIKE A SEXY POSE. Yoga-based squats and lunges help nudge blood flow to the pelvis and clitoris and may calm your mind and boost your body image, points out Katherine Susan Kellogg-Spadt, director of sexual medicine at the Pelvic Floor Institute at Graduate Hospital in Philadelphia. Ask your friends to recommend a yoga class or instructor near you.

TURN ON YOUR MIND. In studies comparing sildenafil (Viagra) with a placebo (dummy pill), women with low libido who took the placebo reported arousal levels equal to those of women who took the prescription drug. Using any sexual enhancer can help you feel sensual by simply focusing your mind on sex, says Dr. Leiblum. Once your mind is turned on, your body follows. Take a half-hour at least three times a week to get your mind off meal planning, meetings, and soccer games and turn it to what makes you feel sexy. Treat yourself to sensual pleasures such as dance lessons, a pedicure, a massage, or even reading a steamy novel.

LUPUS

Outsmart a Sneaky Disease

Soon after my friend Linda made a stressful move to a major city, she developed a puzzling array of symptoms that included sore joints and a sunburn-like rash on her nose and cheeks. It was the fact that ordinary sunlight suddenly made her squint in pain, however, that prompted her doctor to suspect lupus, a chronic autoimmune disease in which immune cells turn traitorous and attack healthy cells in the skin, joints, muscles, brain, kidneys, and connective tissues all over the body. But as Linda was undergoing tests for lupus, her symptoms disappeared as suddenly and mysteriously as they had arrived.

Lupus can be crafty, as its name (which means "wolf" in Latin) implies. One minute, its symptoms rage; the next, they slink off. The most common form of this hide-and-seek disease is systemic lupus erythematosus (SLE), which causes more widespread problems than discoid lupus erythematosus (DLE), which attacks mainly the skin and is marked by disk-like rashes.

WHY ME?

No one knows why women develop lupus 10 times more frequently than men do. Doctors suspect an imbalance of female (estrogenic) and male (androgenic) hormones as well as infections and heredity. This much seems clear, though: Sunlight, a virus, and intense stress can send your immune system into hyperalert, prompting it to attack your own tissues. Interestingly, consuming alfalfa in any form, from sprouts to tea, can also be a trigger. The culprit? L-canavanine, an amino acid that sets the stage for attacks.

STAVE OFF SYMPTOMS

Whether your lupus is active or inactive, the idea is to stop flare-ups and keep symptoms bearable. To that end, you may need to take drugs to reduce inflammation, including corticosteroids and nonsteroidal anti-inflammatory drugs such as ibuprofen—but you may also be able to minimize your dosages and remain flare-free. Talk to your doctor about using the following nondrug strategies for giving this very sneaky disease the slip.

WEAN YOURSELF OFF WIENIES. Meat and other animal-based, high-protein foods such as dairy products and eggs provide your body

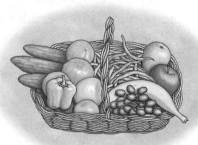

with arachidonic acid, which is used to make pro-inflammatory biochemicals that contribute to pain. Going vegan (that is, eschewing meat, dairy, and eggs) may relieve you of your symptoms, says Pamela Houghton, N.D., a naturopathic physician in Seattle.

GO FISH. Protein from land-based animals may enhance inflammation, but trout, salmon, and other cold-water fish contain beneficial omega-3 essential fatty acids that squelch it, notes Dr. Houghton. If a fishy diet isn't to your taste, and you're not taking blood thinners, take 1 gram (1,000 milligrams) of fish oil daily in capsule form. Or 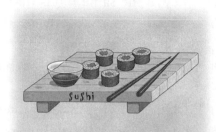 try 1,000 to 2,000 milligrams of evening primrose oil, which packs gamma-linolenic acid, another natural anti-inflammatory. Check your health food store for both—and be patient, since you may not see benefits for two months or more.

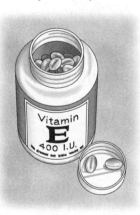

ENERGIZE WITH E. Vitamin E is an antioxidant that helps fight damage to organs caused by inflammation, and people with DLE tend to be deficient in it. To make sure you're getting plenty, take a multivitamin supplement daily and snack on E-rich sunflower seeds whenever you can. To quickly clear up inflamed skin, you may want to take an additional 400 IU of mixed tocopherols (types of vitamin E that are available 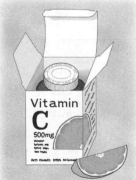 in drugstores and health food stores) twice a day, suggests Jeanette Jacknin, M.D., a dermatologist in Scottsdale, Arizona.

ADD SOME C. Vitamin C, a powerful antioxidant, helps keep lupus inactive even as it helps reduce pain. If citrus fruit sparks flare-ups, and as

The Worst Foods for Lupus?

They're the same foods that spark allergies and other autoimmune diseases—dairy, wheat, citrus, sugar, caffeine, and preservatives, says Glenn Rothfeld, M.D., clinical assistant professor of medicine at Tufts University School of Medicine in Boston. Once you eliminate these offenders (along with foods in the nightshade family, such as potatoes, eggplant, and green peppers, which can aggravate joint pain), your symptoms may go underground. To identify potential troublemakers, ask your doctor to test you for levels of IgG, the antibody that's released during delayed allergy reactions.

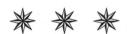

long as you don't have stomach or kidney problems, talk to your doctor about taking 1,000 milligrams of vitamin C in tablet form three times a day.

BET ON BROCCOLI. Not only are these mini-trees chock-full of powerful anti-inflammatory vitamin C, they also contain indole-3-carbinol, a chemical that may help rebalance hormones in women with lupus.

TALK YOURSELF RELAXED. People with SLE appear to have a heightened immune response to stress, which raises blood levels of the stress hormone cortisol and worsens their symptoms. The simplest way to de-stress? Monitor your negative self-talk, says Roberta Horton, program and research coordinator in the division of rheumatology at the Hospital of Special Surgery in New York City. She suggests that if you notice yourself thinking, "The weather's warm, my lupus will flare all summer, and I'll never get out of the house," you should counteract it with, "I'll cover up with a long-sleeved shirt and a hat, limit time in the sun, and pace myself by doing cool indoor activities like going to the movies."

MEMORY LOSS

Stop "Senior Moments"

On a recent stop at a local ATM, I completely forgot the access number I've had for a decade. I was panic-stricken that I might be in the early stages of Alzheimer's—a dreadful disease that my dad developed at an early age.

It's easy to fear the worst when you forget important numbers, make embarrassing verbal slips, or can't remember why you went into a room. In most cases, however, forgetfulness isn't a symptom of disease but merely a by-product of being both distracted and depleted.

EXERCISE À DEUX

While any physical exercise enhances blood circulation and therefore memory, studies show that activities such as tennis that require moving in sync with a partner and responding to each other's movements are the best way to keep your brain on its toes. Regular dancing, in fact, lowered the risk of Alzheimer's among older people by a whopping 76 percent in one study.

WHY ME?

If you're a woman, you may be both distracted by dueling demands and experiencing a sharp decline in hormones that can occur following childbirth or a hysterectomy or as you near menopause. Estrogen enhances memory in a number of ways, helping nerve cells to grow in complexity and increasing connections between them. That's why when it nosedives, retrieving information may take longer.

Chronic stress also worsens brain fog. It depletes the adrenal glands, which take over the production of estrogen at menopause. If they're producing just a trickle of estrogen, you may have more obvious—and distressing—"senior moments." Worse, ongoing stress actually destroys neurons in the hippocampus, the brain's memory headquarters.

Other factors specific to memory loss in women include low levels of thyroid hormone and the tendency to skip meals. "When your blood sugar drops, thinking and remembering go out the window," says Elisa Lottor, N.D., Ph.D., a naturopathic physician and psychologist in Santa Monica, California.

BOOST YOUR BRAIN

If you have difficulty performing the steps of a familiar task such as serving a meal, are confused about time and place, have forgot-

ON-THE-SPOT RELIEF

Double Your Memory, Double Your Fun

Chomp some Doublemint and you'll ace that real estate exam! British researchers have found that chewing gum improves memory, possibly because it raises the heart rate, which in turn boosts the delivery of glucose and oxygen to the brain and creates a surge in insulin, which may be key to recall.

ten the names of the president or close family members, or your memory lapses are getting worse, ask your doctor for an evaluation. You may need tests to determine your thyroid levels and/or detect circulatory disorders.

In many cases, however, forgetfulness can be reversed nonmedically by keeping your blood sugar levels stable. One way to do this is by grazing on several small meals featuring complex carbohydrates and protein, such as apple slices smeared with peanut butter. The following memory-enhancing methods will also help.

REMEMBER YOUR ANTIOXIDANTS. Estrogen mops up oxygen damage to brain cells caused by free radical molecules, says Claire Warga, Ph.D., a midlife health psychologist in New York City.

When your body's estrogen wanes, she suggests turning to plant estrogens that do double duty as natural antioxidants. "People with high levels of antioxidants tend to score better on memory tests," she says. To improve your memory, feast on antioxidant-rich fruits and veggies, such as oranges, grapefruit, broccoli, and carrots. Also consider taking a daily antioxidant supplement that includes 1,000 milligrams of vitamin C and 400 IU of vitamin E.

PICK BLUEBERRIES. According to early animal studies at Tufts University in Boston, eating ¹/₂ cup of antioxidant-rich blueberries a day may help sharpen memory. Is your market fresh out of blueberries? Go for strawberries and spinach, both of which have nearly the same memory-restoring effects.

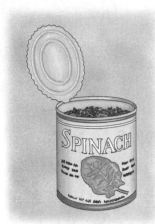

SLURP SOY. As estrogen dwindles, so does acetylcholine, a brain chemical used by memory cells to communicate with each other. To make up for the loss, stock your diet with lots of high-protein foods (such as soy foods, eggs, and lean meat) that contain choline, a component of lecithin used to make acetylcholine. Or opt for 2 tablespoons of lecithin (which you can find at health food stores) sprinkled on your cereal. By midday, you should notice the fog lifting and your recall becoming crystal clear. Still another choice is soy-extracted isoflavone tablets (55 milligrams) taken twice daily, which research from the University of California, San Diego, has shown to help verbal recall. If you're at risk for breast cancer, however, check with your doctor before supplementing, since isoflavones may have an estrogenic effect on tissues.

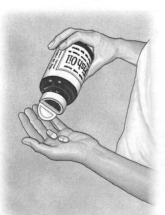

FISH FOR FOCUS. Cold-water fish, such as salmon and sardines, are the richest sources of docosahexaenoic acid (DHA), a type of omega-3 essential fatty acid that helps to promote cell-to-cell communication, improve focus, and possibly reverse memory loss. Not keen on fish? As long as you're not taking blood-thinning medications, check your health food store for fish-oil capsules that contain DHA and take 1 to 3 grams (1,000 to 3,000 milligrams) daily.

GO FOR GINKGO. This herb helps to clear the cobwebs because it shunts more blood to the brain. As long as you're not taking other medications, take 120 to 240 milligrams a day of a standardized product. Better yet, check your health food store for ginkgo in formulas that include huperzine A, an herbal extract of Chinese moss that appears to help maintain healthy levels of neurotransmitters, the brain chemicals that help memory cells communicate with each other.

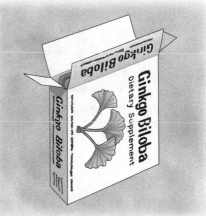

POP PS. Phosphatidylserine (PS) is a fatty substance made from soybean oil that researchers at the Memory Assessment Clinics in Bethesda, Maryland, believe may resemble the nutrient in the brain that helps sharpen focus and enhance recall. "The only known side effect is a positive one—improved mood—and PS seems to work especially well when combined with ginkgo," says Dr. Lottor. Check your health food store for both. The suggested dose of PS is 100 milligrams three times daily; give it several weeks to work, she adds.

MENSTRUAL PROBLEMS

Go with the Flow

⬥

Most people don't call periods "the curse" anymore, but many women often do feel as if they're under a wicked spell each month. One woman I know suffers viselike cramps that keep her couch-bound for a day or two every month, while another has periods that arrive cramp-free but with a flow so heavy that it gushes straight through super tampons and jumbo napkins—and ruins her best slacks.

WHY ME?

It's actually quite common for periods to go haywire, especially once you hit your forties—the perimenopausal years—when your hormones themselves go haywire.

SHINE A LIGHT ON IT

According to a small study conducted at the University of California, San Diego, women with irregular menstrual cycles who sleep with a light shining in their eyes have shorter cycles. If your periods are irregular, get a timer for your bedside lamp and set it to go on after you're snoozing.

During this time, you may start producing too much estrogen, which builds up uterine tissue, or too little progesterone, which keeps this buildup in check and controls ovulation—the main period regulator. You may also have excessive levels of prolactin, a hormone that prevents the liver from clearing excess estrogen. All of this can turn a previously light flow into a deluge.

Flooding and cramps can also occur if you're overproducing a hormone called prostaglandin F_2 alpha. Some women naturally produce an excess of this hormone, but a high-fat, low-nutrient diet can raise levels, too.

Finally, underlying medical conditions can trigger period problems. A leading cause of flooding is fibroids, noncancerous uterine tumors that plague up to 40 percent of women over age 35 and disrupt the uterine contractions that expel menstrual flow. There are also others, including endometriosis, a condition that occurs when uterine tissue migrates outside the uterus and attaches to other organs within the pelvic cavity; too little thyroid hormone; and iron deficiency.

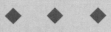

HOMEGROWN SOLUTION

◆ ◆ ◆

Just for Ladies

To help regulate heavy flows, chop up a tablespoon of lady's mantle leaves (their folds resemble a pleated coat), steep them in a cup of boiling water for 10 minutes, and strain. Drink one or two cups a day for two weeks prior to your period. Or take lady's mantle tincture according to the label directions for two weeks prior to menstruation, and your period may be lighter when it arrives. It may take two months or more to see benefits. Both forms of the herb are available at health food stores.

LIGHTEN UP

If you routinely soak through a pad an hour on your heavy days or have pain that interferes with daily functioning, clots larger than a quarter, or periods that last twice as long as they once did, consult your doctor. Otherwise, you might consider holding off on the pain relievers for a month or two and trying a few of these equally effective yet gentler remedies—not one of which will upset your stomach.

TRY VITEX. Also known as chasteberry, this herb helps regulate periods, lightening a very heavy flow, says Tori Hudson, N.D., a naturopathic physician and director of A Woman's Time clinic in Portland, Oregon. Take 30 to 60 drops of chasteberry tincture (which you can find at health food stores) daily. You should see results in four to six months.

GIVE IT THE RASPBERRY. Red raspberry leaf is a highly prized uterine tonic that helps to stem heavy bleeding, spotting between

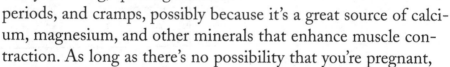

Healing Herbs

periods, and cramps, possibly because it's a great source of calcium, magnesium, and other minerals that enhance muscle contraction. As long as there's no possibility that you're pregnant, Carole Leonard, a certified nurse-midwife and chair of the New Hampshire Council of Midwifery in Hopkinton, suggests drinking at least two cups of raspberry leaf tea daily. Look for prepackaged tea at a health food store and prepare it according to the package directions.

DOWN JAMAICAN DOGWOOD. Folks on the "friendly isle" use this West Indian herb to poison fish. When used in humans, however, this muscle relaxant/sedative kills cramps "better than any remedy I

LIP SERVICE

Pressing on the center of your top lip just under your nose for 1 minute every 15 minutes several times a day during days of heavy flow can help stanch flooding, says certified nurse-midwife Carole Leonard.

know," says Judy Lyn Patrick, N.D., a naturopathic physician who specializes in women's health in Tucson. She recommends taking Jamaican dogwood in capsule form (available at health food stores) according to the label directions.

GO WITH GINGER. This tangy root dampens production of troublemaking prostaglandin F2 and lightens menstrual flow. Stir 1/4 to 1/2 teaspoon of powdered ginger into a cup of hot water and drink it daily, suggests Dr. Hudson.

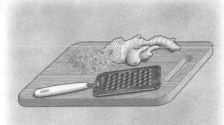

RUB IT IN. Natural progesterone creams such as ProGest help to block excess estrogen and can lighten menstrual flow in some women, says Christiane Northrup, M.D., director of the Women to Women clinic in Yarmouth, Maine. Apply 1/4 to 1/2 teaspoon of cream (which you can find at drugstores and health food stores) to smooth, hairless skin twice a day for three weeks prior to menstruation. Stop during the week of your period.

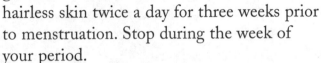

NUTS TO YOU! Studies show that 1/4 cup of soy nuts or a tablespoon of flaxseed (both available at health food stores)—perhaps swirled into a smoothie—can help regulate the menstrual cycle if you're skipping periods. Just be sure to "go nuts" every day.

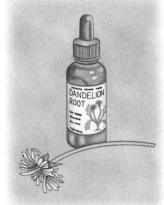

DIG INTO DANDELION. It's brimming with iron, which you may be lacking if you're flooding every month. Ironically, iron deficiency may actually open the floodgates, while eating iron-rich foods may help to close them. To be sure you're getting plenty, mix 20 drops of dandelion tincture (available at health food stores) into a glass of orange juice and sip it throughout the day, every day. The vitamin C in the juice will enhance absorption of the iron. If you're taking diuretics or potassium supplements, check with your doctor before using dandelion.

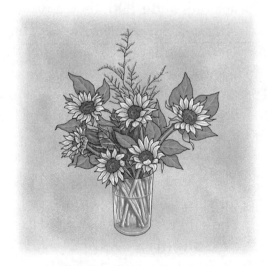

FISH FOR RELIEF. Cold-water fish, such as salmon and tuna, contain essential fatty acids that help lower levels of prostaglandin F_2, which contributes to flooding and cramps, and boost levels of prostaglandin F_3, which relaxes the uterine muscle. Not big on fish? Take 1 to 3 grams (1,000 to 3,000 milligrams) of fish oil (available at health food stores) daily. Studies show that fish oil can cut cramps—and ibuprofen use—by half, but don't use it if you take aspirin or prescription blood-thinning medication.

MIDLIFE BLAHS

Rediscover Your Joy

———————⧓⧓⧓———————

I'm fond of the 1989 movie *Shirley Valentine*, which is about a woman who finds herself feeling weary, bored, and dumpy in her middle years, so she takes off to a Greek isle. There she sheds her self-doubts and daily doldrums (as well as her clothes, in a memorable skinny-dipping scene) and reconnects with an exuberant love of life and her real self, both of which she had lost during many years of raising kids and caring for her husband.

Many of us in our fourth and fifth decades are Shirley wannabes, feeling as though

> ## SAGE ADVICE
>
> Sage's botanical name—Salvia—comes from the Latin word *salvare*, which means "to cure." For centuries, this relaxing yet gently stimulating herb has been used as a remedy by distressed, middle-aged women. Brew a cup of sage tea (you can find it in any health food store) according to the package directions, add warm milk and honey, and inhale deeply while you sip. Avoid sage if there's any chance you could be pregnant.

we've been buried alive under mountains of "other-directed" responsibilities and longing to have passion and meaning in our lives once again. Some women experience this feeling as a midlife crisis, while many simply feel stale, as if, as one expert put it, "nothing flips their skirt" anymore.

WHY ME?

A better question in this instance might be, "Why not me?" Reaching the stage where you shift from being "other-directed" to "self-directed" once again is not only perfectly natural, it's absolutely necessary for further growth—even though it involves the sometimes scary work of relinquishing old roles, refocusing on new goals, and reconnecting to your real self. "I call those the 3 Rs of midlife, and it's vital to carve out time for them to unfold," says Linda Edlestein, Ph.D., a Chicago psychologist who specializes in midlife issues. If you don't, you could wind up becoming bitter, resentful, and/or prone to anxiety, depression, migraines, and irritable bowel syndrome.

BEATING THE BLAHS

Here's the good news: You don't have to run off to Greece to renew your energy or improve your self-esteem. You probably don't need an antidepressant. Heck, you don't even need a big chunk of time—just 5 minutes traveling to what's been called "the land of self" (perhaps while sitting on a park bench at lunch) may be enough, provided you go there regularly.

In those snatches of time when you attend solely to yourself, you'll learn to discard thoughts and behaviors that no longer fit your true self, and as you feel more solid—more you—you'll find the strength to face life's inevitable losses, such as children leaving home, parents passing on, or former dreams not achieved. Here's a mini-map to the "land of self."

AWAKEN YOUR SENSES. "Use the sights, sounds, smells, and feel of the world around you to help you remember what makes you feel fully alive," advises Kathleen Behony, Ph.D., a psychologist in Virginia Beach. Some suggestions: Sink your fingers into the soil and plant an herb garden, taste exotic street fare at an outdoor ethnic food market, or listen to Japanese flute music.

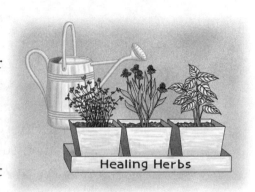

Healing Herbs

REDO YOUR DREAMS. Midlife blahs often stem from the harsh realization that you're not going to fulfill the dreams you once had, so why bother? says Dr. Edlestein. But finding a spin-off of that dream can give you the same excitement in a different way. Maybe you won't hike around the world, but you can venture into undiscovered parts of your favorite city or learn a foreign language. Recast your dreams, preserving the pieces of former passions as best you can.

SWEEP OUT YOUR PSYCHE. "It's vital to get rid of old grievances, resolve parental issues, and toss out outmoded ideas of getting older—especially notions about how you should look as you age—that clutter your psyche and weigh on your spirit," says Elisa Lottor, N.D., Ph.D., a naturopathic physician and psychologist in Santa Monica, California. One suggestion: Take a compassionate look at yourself in the mirror, identifying five things you love about your face and body (your bow-shaped lips, perhaps, or your tapered fingers or delicate ankles). Record them in a journal, then repeat this phrase: "I have grown into a richly textured person who is not defined by appearance. My beauty radiates from the inside out."

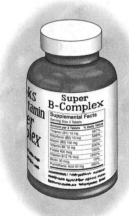

LEARN SOMETHING NEW. To ease the transition to a newer, truer self, learn something new that feels true to who you are about to become or want to become. Join a yoga class or book group. Begin meditating. Start training to walk or run a local 3-mile race. Learning something new, taking on new roles, and regaining a measure of control over your life and body are the keys, says Dr. Edlestein.

GIVE YOUR MOOD A B-OOST. When life feels stale, Mother Nature offers refreshment in the form of nutrient-rich foods, especially those abundant in B vitamins, such as whole grains, leafy greens, poultry, and fish, says Dr. Lottor. Vitamin B_6, for instance, helps convert the tryptophan found in foods (including turkey) into serotonin, a natural mood booster. She also suggests taking a twice-daily vitamin supplement that supplies all of the Bs.

GO GA-GA OVER GABA. "I find that many midlife women respond favorably to GABA [gamma-aminobutyric acid], a natural calming chemical made in your brain that plays a role in producing serotonin and 5-HTP [5-hydroxytryptophan], another serotonin booster," says Dr. Lottor. Ask a natural health–oriented doctor about this supplement.

NAIL FUNGUS

Go Barefoot Again

———◦◦◦◦———

When sandal season arrives, my friend Lily is strictly a no-toes-bared kinda gal. She keeps her tootsies under wraps because she's often plagued by onychomycosis, a fungal condition that's caused by a cousin of the athlete's foot fungus. It feeds off the tough keratin protein in nails, thickening them, turning them yellowish-brown, and sending out a room-clearing odor. Eventually, the nails crumble and separate from the nail bed, and it's not a pretty sight.

Lily, like many people who are nailed by nail fungus, spends long hours on her feet

> ## THE GENTLE GRAPEFRUIT
>
> One excellent treatment for nail fungus is tea tree oil, but some folks find it harsh. If you're one of them, don't get discouraged—try grapefruit seed extract, another strong antifungal that's available in health food stores. Apply two drops twice daily directly to your problem nails, avoiding the surrounding skin.

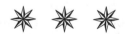
(she's a chef), so the skin of her feet is more prone than, say, a desk jockey's to tiny breaks, which allow this nasty fungus easy entry. But the bug also targets folks who have circulatory problems, diabetes, or depressed immune systems, and those whose feet perspire excessively. Tight-fitting shoes and long-distance running can also make you vulnerable.

WHY ME?

You can pick up nail fungus just as you might athlete's foot—by going barefoot in moist, public places such as locker rooms. Once it hitches a ride on your nails, the bug thrives in hot, damp environments, making airtight shoes the ideal breeding ground. Over time, the fungus can spread to other toenails and the skin surrounding them. It can even lead to ingrown nails and wincing pain when you walk, setting you up for inflammation and a secondary bacterial infection to double your misery.

As if that isn't bad enough, the fungus can also settle in those other, more noticeable nails on your fingers. Typically, this occurs in women who continually immerse their hands in water, or those who pick up the bug from unsanitary manicure implements (ironic, isn't it?). Their fingernails thicken and take on an unsightly yellowish-green appearance, and the damage can make everyday activities, from writing to applying makeup, acutely painful.

NAIL THAT FUNGUS

If the fungus has invaded your nail bed, has spread to multiple nails, or causes you significant pain, see a podiatrist or dermatologist. Likewise, seek medical treatment at the first hint of a nail infection if you have diabetes. In other, more moderate cases, however, you may want to consider your options.

Pricey antifungal drugs and nail lacquers can leave you with troublesome side effects ranging from stomachaches to rashes. The following nondrug remedies may help squelch a mild infection just as effectively—and certainly more gently.

PAINT ON TEA TREE. Trade that ruby red polish for tea tree oil, and you'll have toenails my friend Lily would envy—but patience is key, says Andrew Weil, M.D., director of the Program in Integrative Medicine and clinical professor of internal medicine at the University of Arizona in Tucson. Tea tree oil, available in health food stores, is an excellent treatment for nail fungus, he says, but it can take two to three months for the infection to clear from fingernails and three times that long from toenails (since they're thicker). Apply two drops of oil twice daily, dabbing it all around the perimeter of the nail.

MAGNIFY THE RESULTS. Studies have shown that when tea tree oil is paired with butenafine hydrochloride—an herbal/drug combo sold in drugstores and from the Internet—it cures 80 percent of toenail fungus.

DUNK THEM. Soaking your toes in tinctures of fungicidal plants is a soothing way to knock out the nail bug with zero side

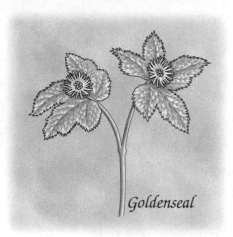
Goldenseal

effects, says Daniel DeLapp, N.D., associate professor of dermatology at the National College of Naturopathic Medicine in Portland, Oregon. He suggests mixing several drops of tincture of black walnut hulls, thyme, pau d'arco, spilanthes, goldenseal, and oregano (which you can get at health food stores) in a quart of warm water, then soaking your nails twice daily. Dry your feet thoroughly, then sprinkle with sage powder (also available at health food stores), a mild antiperspirant, before donning clean cotton socks.

APPLY OREGANO STRAIGHT UP. Dilute 1 part oregano oil (available at health food stores) in 4 parts vegetable oil and swab your nails with the solution daily. It may take nine months to a year to kill all the spores and completely destroy the fungus while the nail regenerates, warns Alan Christianson, N.D., a naturopathic physician in Scottsdale, Arizona.

TRY VICKS. That smelly gunk that your mom rubbed on your chest to treat a cold may also rub out nail fungus, says syndicated columnist Peter H. Gott, M.D., an internist in Lakeville, Connecticut, who claims that Vicks VapoRub cleared up his own nail fungus problem. It won't work for an advanced infection that has turned your nails hard and yellow, he says, but if you're in the early stages and want to try this remedy, trim the affected nail as short and as far back toward the cuticle as possible (be careful not to nick your skin). Then apply Vicks twice a day to the nail, the cuticle, and the toe or finger and rub it in well.

NAUSEA

When Your Urge Is to Purge

———◆◆◆———

 once tried deep-sea fishing off the coast of Florida, but all
I managed to catch was a tuna-size case of seasickness. My
stomach lurched each time the boat rolled over a wave, and suffice it to say, there were many waves. I counted the seconds until
my companions voted to turn the cabin cruiser around and call it
a day.

Most likely, you've experienced that queasy, "please-let-
this-be-over" sensation,
whether from the motion of a
swaying boat or a twisty car
ride, a bout of the flu, or
something disagreeable that
you ate or drank. The room
spins, your stomach flip-flops,
your throat tightens, you salivate, you sweat—and you both
fear and pray that you'll vomit
to put an end to your misery.

POST-OP RX

Taking several deep breaths when
coming out of surgical anesthesia can
quell queasiness caused by the anesthetic. The reason: The vomiting and
respiratory centers are neighbors in the
brain, and when the brain is focused
on taking deep, controlled breaths, it's
less focused on nausea, say researchers
at the University of Connecticut
Health Center in Farmington.

HOMEGROWN SOLUTION

◆ ◆ ◆

Snip and Sip

The emerald leaves of the basil plant contain an aromatic, camphor-bearing oil that makes a pleasant-tasting anti-nausea tea. Simply steep 1 teaspoon of the leaves in a cup of boiling water for 15 minutes, then strain and sip.

WHY ME?

If something you ate or drank—such as tainted deli salad or too many margaritas—is at the root of your nausea, the mechanism is fairly straightforward: Your irritated digestive tract signals your brain that a toxin's on board. Your brain responds by triggering queasiness and other symptoms to shut down your appetite so you won't ingest another morsel that could worsen the irritation. Finally, vomiting helps to purge the toxic substance.

When you become nauseated while in a car or a rocking boat, however, it's because the balance center in your inner ear receives mixed signals. Your body is still, but the fluid in your inner ear is sloshing around. The confusion that results trips those awful symptoms we know as motion sickness.

Sometimes hormonal shifts—most notably during the first trimester of pregnancy and during your period—can make you sick to your stomach. Other triggers include side effects of drugs such as anesthetics, migraine headaches, unpleasant sights or smells, or even something dreadful that you fear in the pit of your stomach (having blood drawn or attending a tax audit comes to mind).

SIDESTEPPING THE SPINS

When nausea sneaks up on you, sometimes the quickest way to get relief is simply to give in to the urge to purge and get it over with. If you're not at the purging point (or would prefer not to get there), however, powerful—and pricey—anti-nausea drugs aren't your only answer. In fact, natural, even folksy remedies such as my mom's (she advocates taking the fizz out of warm cola by dumping it back and forth between two glasses, then drinking the sugary syrup to help settle your stomach) may work as well as drugs like dimenhydrinate (Dramamine) without making you drowsy. Here are more nausea remedies used by moms—and natural-oriented doctors—the world over.

GO FOR GINGER. This pungent root has proven in countless studies to be more effective at curbing queasiness than most conventional meds,

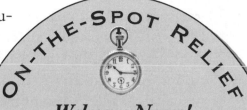

ON-THE-SPOT RELIEF

Welcome News!

If you're stuck on a bus or plane when that telltale lump of nausea rises in your throat, quickly reach for a newspaper—and sniff it four or five times in a row! It may sound ridiculous, but it's a quick fix for queasy stomachs, says Anil Minocha, M.D., possibly because of a chemical in newspaper ink. (And if it doesn't work, you can always fold the paper to fashion a motion sickness bag).

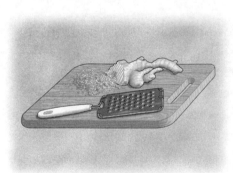

including the scopolamine patch sold for motion sickness. The dried powder—which you can find at any supermarket or health food store—works best, says Anil Minocha, M.D., chief of gastroenterology at Southern Illinois University School of Medicine in Chicago. Stir 1 teaspoon into a cup of hot water and drink. If that doesn't do the trick, take another 1/2 teaspoon of ginger. You can also chew soft, crystallized ginger candy, munch on gingersnaps, or drink ginger ale (check labels to find products that include real ginger).

BET ON BARLEY. If dining out on hamburgers at the local

greasy spoon led to nausea, sipping barley water is the ideal "dessert." This bland grain contains catechins, which help quell the queasies. Boil a small handful of pearl barley (which you can find in supermarkets) in 1 quart of water for an hour. Strain the liquid, then add 1/2 cup of it to 1/2 cup of warm milk. Try to eat the cooked barley, too, since it may help counter any accompanying indigestion and diarrhea.

SPICE THINGS UP. In traditional Indian medicine, common spices are used to quiet a roiling stomach. Try eating 1/2 cup of plain yogurt to which you've added 2 pinches of cardamom and 1/2 teaspoon of honey, suggests Vasant Lad, M.A.Sc., director of the Ayurvedic Institute in Albuquerque. Simply chewing cardamom seeds works, too, he says, as does sipping a tea made by steeping 1 teaspoon of cumin seeds or ground cinnamon and a pinch of nutmeg in a cup of hot water for about 10 minutes.

USE YOUR NOSE. If the thought of drinking even mild tea makes you want to lose your lunch, try dipping a cloth into a brew made with chamomile, fennel, or peppermint and placing it on your stomach. The warmth will settle tense digestive muscles, while simply inhaling the aroma of any of these carminative (stomach-settling) herbal teas—all of which are available at supermarkets and health food stores—may have a calming effect on your rebellious belly.

PRESS HERE. At the first twinge of nausea, press the point along the crease of your inner wrist at the base of your thumb for 20 seconds. Release, then press for another 20 seconds. Repeat on the opposite wrist.

OSTEOPOROSIS

Keep Walking Tall

Many people, my mom included, mistakenly believe that losing height and becoming hunchbacked is a natural consequence of getting older, much like going gray. But while 25 million Americans, most of them women, do develop osteoporosis, a condition involving thinning of the bones that can result in a tendency for fractures and a hunched posture, becoming brittle boned and shrunken isn't an inevitable part of aging. It need not happen to you.

WHY ME?

It's true that some people carry the osteoporosis gene, which means they're unable to absorb bone-building calcium. Others are more prone to losing bone mass because they have small, thin bones to begin with or take bone-thinning

PASS ON THE SALT

Salt drains your body of calcium. In fact, cutting out salty foods (such as fast food and packaged foods, like soup, salsa, cheese, and condiments) and reducing your sodium intake to about 1,700 milligrams daily is just as beneficial as supplementing with 900 milligrams of calcium daily, says Robert Heaney, M.D., professor of medicine at Creighton University Medical Center in Omaha, Nebraska.

SOAR LIKE SUPERMAN

Dianne Daniels, an exercise physiologist in San Diego, recommends this exercise for strengthening the hips, spine, and wrists: Lie face-down on the floor and extend both arms in front of you alongside your head (á la Superman in flight), then lift them as high as you can while keeping your feet on the floor. Pause, then lower your arms slowly. Repeat 15 times. As your strength becomes ever more super, you can up the ante by adding hand weights, starting with 1-pounders.

steroids for arthritis or other conditions. For many of us, though, osteoporosis is largely a lifestyle disease, the result of consuming too few calcium-rich foods, too many calcium drainers (including caffeine, salt, bubbly drinks, and high-protein foods), and not exercising regularly (both strength training and weight-bearing activities such as walking stimulate bone growth). These factors are important past age 35 and become crucial after menopause.

After 35, the natural process of "bone remodeling"—tearing down old bone and building new bone—changes, and you begin losing bone faster than you're making it. The trend accelerates as estrogen levels dwindle during menopause, since estrogen limits calcium loss in urine and boosts its absorption in bones. The same thing happens if you've had your ovaries removed.

This means that if you haven't banked sufficient quantities of calcium by menopause and aren't depositing ample new amounts (by taking the bone-building steps mentioned earlier), your bones may thin to the point where simply bumping into a counter can cause a hip fracture. Even if your bones don't break, by age 60, the vertebrae in your spine can begin to collapse, leading to a shrunken, stooped posture.

None of this is inevitable, though. Nondrug methods can

delay bone loss or stabilize the situation so that you can continue to walk tall, no matter what your age.

STEPS TO A STURDY SKELETON

First things first: Ask your doctor to schedule a painless bone scan called DEXA (dual-energy x-ray absorptiometry) that measures the thickness of your bones and detects whether bone is breaking down faster than it's being rebuilt. Then, no matter what your test reveals, follow these measures. Building bone is never a bad thing.

EAT YOUR CALCIUM. Food (as opposed to supplements) is the best source of calcium because it probably contains other undiscovered bone-building factors, but you needn't be a devotee of dairy foods to benefit. A slew of other foods— black-eyed peas, sardines, cabbage, broccoli, bok choy, herbs such as dandelion and nettle, and calcium-fortified orange juice and apple juice, to name just a few—are brimming with this mineral, says Susan L. Greenspan, M.D., professor of medicine at Beth Israel Deaconess Medical Center in Boston. Be sure to eat at least two servings of calcium-rich foods every day.

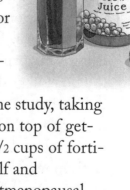

POP SUPPLEMENTS FOR INSURANCE. In one study, taking 1,000 milligrams of calcium in supplement form on top of getting 750 milligrams from foods (such as about 2¹/₂ cups of fortified O.J.) helped to reduce bone loss by nearly half and increased the thickness of the lower spines of postmenopausal women. The most absorbable form of supplemental calcium is calcium citrate, which can be pricey and must be taken on an

TEA GETS AN A+

Drinking even a single cup of black or green tea a day may preserve bone density (especially if you sip it daily for 10 years), according to studies that looked at the tea-drinking habits of women ages 65 to 76. In contrast to coffee, which increases calcium loss in urine, the natural phytoestrogens in tea may help bones remain thicker by boosting calcium absorption as natural estrogen decreases during menopause.

empty stomach. If you opt for calcium carbonate, take it with food. No matter what the form, divide your doses for better absorption.

LIGHTEN UP. Exposing your skin (without sunscreen) to 30 minutes of sunlight a day helps your body synthesize vitamin D, which aids calcium absorption. If you live in a northern climate where sunshine is limited in winter, be sure to take 700 to 800 IU of vitamin D in supplement form daily. In one study, women past age 60 who took that amount of vitamin D along with 500 milligrams of calcium citrate twice daily had nearly half the number of broken hips compared with women who didn't take supplements. Plus, their spines actually thickened, notes Judy Lyn Patrick, N.D., a naturopathic physician who specializes in women's health in Tucson.

GO NUTS. Roasted soy nuts contain phytoestrogens called isoflavones, which may take up where human estrogen leaves off (by boosting calcium absorption in the bones) as it dwindles during menopause. In fact, 1/2 cup packs 167 milligrams, which is four to eight times more than other soy products. But skip ipriflavone pills, which provide a synthetic version of soy isoflavones. They may help inhibit cells that break down bone, but they may also encourage growth of cancer-causing cells.

PAINFUL INTERCOURSE

Reignite Intimacy

———◆◆◆◆◆———

Matters of the bedroom are hardly hush-hush anymore, yet many women remain mum about making love when the act causes more pain than pleasure. It's no wonder, then, that few of us know how prevalent it is—and how preventable.

Painful intercourse (technically called dyspareunia or difficult mating) occurs in up to 60 percent of women at one time or another and is usually easily treated, says Willard F. Harley Jr., Ph.D., a clinical psychologist specializing in relationship issues in St. Paul, Minnesota. If the underlying causes aren't addressed, however, it can set you up for complications and more pain, which can turn you off to sex altogether. And nobody wants to think—much less talk—about that!

WHY ME?

Perhaps the most common cause of painful intercourse, says Dr. Harley, is a dry vagina triggered by insufficient arousal; waning estrogen levels before, during, or after menopause; or the use of drying medications such as antihistamines. Simply assuring

FORGET SITUPS— DO PELVIC PUSHUPS

The stronger your pelvic muscles, the more responsive they are— and the more pleasure (and less pain) you may have during sex. Kegel exercises—the equivalent of pelvic floor pushups—are designed to tone the muscles down below. Here's what you do: First, to identify the muscles, imagine holding back gas or squeezing around a penis, suggests Anne Marie Cosby, a licensed physical therapist specializing in women's health in San Francisco. When you squeeze, pull the muscles upward, keeping your buttocks and inner thigh muscles relaxed while breathing deeply. Contract for a count of 10, then release for a count of 10. Repeat several times daily.

arousal and using personal lubricants can restore moisture, as well as sexual pleasure, in most cases. But even if vaginal dryness is severe, prescription estrogen creams and suppositories may work wonders.

Other possible causes of pain during intercourse include allergic reactions to condoms or soaps, vaginal or bladder infections, pelvic inflammatory disease, herpes blisters, endometriosis, fibroids, vaginal scarring from childbirth or surgery, and even a tipped uterus. None of these problems—even the more serious ones—has to be a barrier to pleasurable sex, and the sooner you address them, stresses Dr. Harley, the sooner you can enjoy intimacy again.

TRADING PAIN FOR PLEASURE

Intercourse need never hurt. If you feel acute pain at penetration or during deep thrusting, or if you experience bleeding or other symptoms, such as itching, burning, or a foul-smelling discharge after intercourse, consult your doctor. If your discomfort is mild, however, you may simply need to vary your routine just a bit for a not-to-be-missed payoff. Here's how.

DON'T FORGET FOREPLAY. If you aren't sufficiently aroused, insertion of the penis will cause friction and irritation that can worsen each time, says Luigi Mastroiani Jr., M.D., chair of obstetrics and gynecology at the University of Pennsylvania Medical Center in Philadelphia. Plus, your vagina may not engorge or lengthen internally, which can also make for painful intercourse. The best lubricant is a woman's vaginal secretions that flow when she's been aroused during kissing or cuddling—and the best sex occurs when they're present. So don't rush the foreplay; it definitely serves a purpose!

E IS EXCELLENT. Studies show that taking vitamin E—up to 600 IU daily for just a month—could help you become moist again.

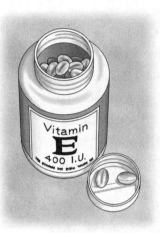

Check with your doctor to see if this dose is okay for you.

GET SLICK. Vitamin E may work as well topically as it does orally. Simply insert a capsule directly into your vagina for lubrication (the casing will dissolve naturally). Or check your drugstore for a water-based personal lubricant, such as GyneMotrin, Astroglide, or Replens, which draws moisture to the vaginal walls so they plump up and are better able to withstand friction. In fact, Replens helped reduce vaginal

GET THE KINKS OUT

Just as a physical therapist can work out the knots in a tense back, a myofascial trigger point specialist for pelvic pain can use steady pressure (from outside the body and inside the vagina) to release tension in the muscles of the vagina, pelvic floor, buttocks, and hips. This often eases penetration or even makes it possible in the first place. To find a qualified, reputable myofascial trigger point therapist who specializes in women's health, contact the American Physical Therapy Association at (800) 999-2782.

dryness in 80 percent of women in one study—but only after they used it three times a day for at least a month. So be patient.

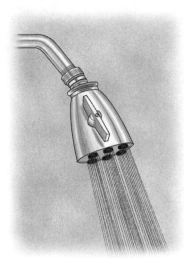

STOP SCRUBBING. Another common cause of painful intercourse is burning or irritation of the vulva (the opening of the vagina) caused by frequent soapy washings, says Maia Chakerian, M.D., a pain management specialist in Los Gatos, California. You shouldn't use anything on your vulva that you wouldn't put in your eyes, she warns. In other words, avoid bubble baths, body washes, and douches. Even soaps and products claiming to be gentle and nonallergenic can be irritating. If you feel burning or irritation, just rinse with plain water and blot dry. Consult your doctor if the irritation persists for more than a few days.

CLIMB ON TOP. If your uterus is naturally tipped, you may feel as though your partner's penis is bumping into it during sex. To avoid painful collisions, place a pillow beneath your buttocks or between your legs to alter the angle of entry. Better yet, make love in the woman-on-top position so you can control the depth of penetration.

LEARN TO OPEN UP. In many women, the vaginal muscles tighten involuntarily in response to prior pain, fear of pregnancy, or other issues. The result is vaginismus, a condition that makes insertion of a penis or even a tampon extremely painful. You can condition your muscles to stay loose during penetration simply by inserting your fingers and moving them in ever-widening circles, says Dr. Harley. To start, lubricate your finger, insert it slowly into your vagina, and move it gently in wider and wider circles. Remove your finger, then repeat five more times. Do this every day. When inserting one finger feels comfortable, use two, then three, and so on until you've reached the approximate width of an erect penis.

PREMENSTRUAL SYNDROME

Manage the Misery

———◦◦◦———

For years, I belonged to that group of women—a whopping 75 percent of all females who menstruate—who feel as if aliens take over their bodies, minds, and emotions for one miserable week out of every month. These aliens do crazy things: They rant at their partners, weep at sappy commercials, and gobble chocolates by the handful.

The "alien," of course, is premenstrual syndrome (PMS)—that total body/mind takeover that also triggers breast tenderness, fatigue, headaches, sleeplessness, and a host of other bothersome symptoms.

CHASTE IT AWAY

Studies show that extracts of chasteberry (also called vitex) cut PMS symptoms by more than half. One explanation is that the herb reduces both estrogen and prolactin (in fact, as its name implies, chasteberry was originally thought to limit sexual desire). Look for liquid extract at health food stores, then take it according to the label directions. Give it three cycles for the benefits to kick in.

WHY ME?

Some experts theorize that a dip in available serotonin—the brain chemical that normally helps to regulate appetite, mood, sleep, and pain—may be to blame. Others speculate that an imbalance in estrogen and progesterone levels (too much estrogen, too little progesterone) prevents your brain from sending out the chemicals that help control mood and pain. Supposedly, this estrogen-progesterone imbalance may also precipitate an overload of the hormone prolactin, which prevents the liver from sweeping out excess estrogen, leaving you with tender breasts, throbbing headaches, and other miseries.

TAKE CONTROL

If your mood swings and irritability are severe and debilitating, don't hesitate to consult your doctor. You may be among the 10 percent of women with premenstrual dysphoric disorder (PMDD), an extreme form of PMS that can strain relationships and seriously interfere with daily activities. If your symptoms are less serious, though, that doesn't mean you can't take them seriously—and do something about them.

To start, avoid stimulating, stress-inducing foods such as fat, alcohol, sugar, salt, and caffeine (drinking more than two cups of coffee a day worsens PMS symptoms), which overwork your liver and throw off your hormonal chemistry. Then try the following measures to further neutralize that alien creature—or, at the very least, turn her into a sweet, G-rated E.T.

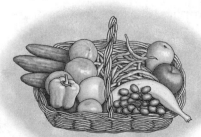

HOLD THE MEAT, HOLD THE DAIRY.

Animal fats contain arachidonic acid, which reduces the liver's ability to metabolize hormones and may encourage the production of prostaglandins, which are linked to bloating and mood swings. Eating a high-fiber, low-fat, vegan (no meat, no dairy) diet, on the other hand, significantly limits water retention, pain, and other PMS complaints.

GORGE ON SOY. Like chocolate, soy contains magnesium, which stabilizes mood, normalizes the metabolism of blood sugar, and reduces water retention and bloating. Some researchers speculate that a deficiency of the mineral may be behind the classic PMS craving for chocolate. Unlike chocolate, however, soy isn't fattening and won't give you that short-lived "sugar high." Try dousing your Cheerios with soy milk or whipping up a special soy milkshake every day during the week prior to your period.

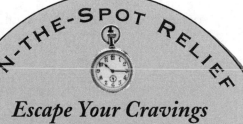

BET ON B. Studies indicate that foods high in vitamin B_6 (such as brown rice, bananas, chicken, and tuna) may reduce PMS-related mood swings, breast tenderness, and bloating. Vitamin B_6 is needed to make serotonin and boost magnesium. In fact, when these two nutrients are taken together daily in a balanced supplement, women feel less moody and anxious in general. Since high doses of vitamin B_6 have been associated with nerve damage in some people, check with your doctor before supplementing.

Go green. One cup of greens such as broccoli, bok choy, or kale contains about 200 milligrams of calcium, a nutrient that may be a key to the PMS riddle. "A calcium deficiency could be central when you consider that women [in one study] who boosted their intake of this mineral had half the number of symptoms as they had before," says Nadine Taylor, R.D., a registered dietitian and chair of the women's health council of the American Nutraceutical Association in Birmingham, Alabama. The dose used in the study was 400 milligrams three times a day. To be sure you get enough, supplement with calcium citrate—the most absorbable form.

Turn to burdock. Women with PMS crave sugar because blood sugar levels dip a week before their periods, so the brain requires more fuel. Giving in to sugar cravings invariably leaves you feeling headachy, fatigued, and moody, so the next time you're jonesing for a fistful of Oreos, brew up some burdock tea, suggests Susan M. Lark, M.D., director of the PMS Self-Help and Menopause Center in Los Altos,

---

BABY YOUR BACK

The yoga position known as the child's pose is deeply relaxing, massages the pelvis, and uncoils a tense, achy back. To perform it, kneel with your buttocks resting on your heels. Bend at the hips and let your torso fall forward so it rests on your thighs (place a pillow on your thighs if you need to) and your forehead touches the floor. Relax your arms and hands alongside your body, with your palms facing upward and your fingers pointing toward your feet. Breathe slowly and deeply. Hold the pose for as long as you like.

California. You can buy it prepackaged at a health food store, then just make it according to the package directions. Burdock helps squelch cravings and minimizes bloating, too.

STEP ON IT. Studies show that walking for at least 45 minutes at a time three times a week will result in fewer and less severe PMS symptoms, possibly because the activity boosts blood flow, nutrient absorption, and levels of feel-good brain chemicals called endorphins even as it reduces fluid retention.

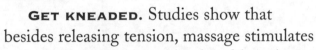

GET KNEADED. Studies show that besides releasing tension, massage stimulates blood and lymph circulation and reduces bloating and annoying achiness in the small of your back. If you have a massage once a month just before your period, incorporating aromatic herbal oils (especially geranium, a hormone balancer, or bergamot, a tension releaser), may enhance the effect. Look for both oils at health food stores.

PSORIASIS

Beat the Plaque Attack

A woman with whom I shared a dorm room in college had psoriasis that flared so badly at exam time, she went through bottles of flesh-colored foundation to camouflage the silvery scales that appeared on her knees when she was stressed. If you, like my former roomie, are among the three million American men and women who have psoriasis, you may be itching to discover what's behind your recurring flare-ups.

GO FOR ALOE

In one study, aloe gel helped improve itchy lesions in more than 80 percent of participants with psoriasis. For the best results, coat your lesions with aloe gel (either scooped straight from the plant or purchased at a health food store) three times a day for one month.

WHY ME?

Unfortunately, scientists still aren't entirely sure what causes psoriasis. They can tell us only that this autoimmune (and probably hereditary) condition involves overexcited T cells, or immune cells, that trigger an overgrowth of skin cells. Like widgets spewing from a revved-up conveyer belt, the dead skin cells pile up in scaly plaques on the knees, elbows, scalp, and other sites instead of being shed. Nutritionally oriented doctors believe the psoriatic pileup stems from allergies, nutritional deficiencies, too much animal fat in the diet, or a buildup of toxins in the liver. But most doctors agree that hyped-up emotions and other forms of stress set the plaque attack in motion, as can dry air, cigarette smoking, and too much or too little sun exposure.

SLOUGH AND SOOTHE

Sunlight in appropriate doses remains a mainstay of conventional treatment for psoriasis because it helps the body make vitamin D, which slows skin cell reproduction. It isn't foolproof, though: Too much sun can worsen plaques and set you up for skin cancer, as can some of the light-activating drugs and coal tars that are often used in light therapy.

Fortunately, there are a number of safe, natural methods that help tame T cells and put the brakes on the rapid overgrowth of skin cells so that you may need less UV exposure. Relief starts with consuming more veggies and fewer dairy foods and meats (animal fat spurs inflammation and toxic waste buildup) and drinking eight glasses of water a day to flush out toxins. There are also many herbs and nutrients that tamp down the inflammatory process and many nonmedical, noninvasive therapies that relieve the itch, thus making mild to moderate plaques less

LIGHTEN UP

Studies show that worrywarts with psoriasis heal more slowly during UV light therapy than their more carefree colleagues. The next time you're bathing in light, try listening to stress-reduction tapes that feature meditation and visualization. If you visualize smooth, scale-free skin while inhaling deeply through your nose, your lesions could clear up three times faster.

pesky. What follows are the best of the bunch.

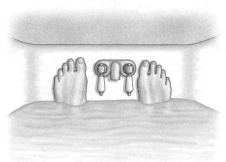

GET AGITATED. A bathtub with a water-agitation attachment or a freestanding Jacuzzi or whirlpool will help soak off dead skin and relieve the itching, says Jeanette Jacknin, M.D., a dermatologist in Scottsdale, Arizona. To soften really thick lesions, add 1 to 2 pounds (two boxes) of baking soda to the water.

DUNK IN DEAD SEA SALTS. According to research from the Dead Sea Mor Clinic in Ein-Bokek, Israel, soaking in a special blend of salts scooped from the Dead Sea clears 90 of psoriatic lesions in a majority of patients. You can buy the salts from the Internet, then soak for at least 45 minutes three times a week.

DOUSE WITH CIDER. To take the sting out of irritated lesions, splash apple cider vinegar on scaly areas and leave it on for 1 minute before rinsing, suggests Dr. Jacknin.

RUB IT IN. Bathe your plaques twice daily, pat them dry, and immediately rub in layer after layer of petroleum jelly or vitamin E oil. Within a week, at least 80 percent of your problem will disappear, says David Cohen, N.D., a naturopathic physician in New York City.

PEANUTS, ANYONE? To soften hand or foot lesions, soak in a bath laced with Epsom salts, pat your itchy areas dry, and massage them with warm peanut oil. Then cover the oil with a paste made with baking soda and castor oil, don white cotton gloves or socks, and hop into bed. Your scales should soon melt away.

SUNBATHE SENSIBLY. If you have mild psoriasis, and you can get a half-hour of natural sunlight daily (slathering unaffected areas with sunscreen) at least three days a week, your lesions may start to heal within six weeks, says Mike Cronin, N.D., a naturopathic physician in Scottsdale, Arizona. But do your sunning outdoors, not in a tanning booth.

TRY MILK THISTLE. According to Dr. Cronin, milk thistle helps the liver eliminate leukotrienes, which are responsible for inflammation and the deregulation of skin cell growth. The suggested dose is 120 to 175 milligrams of standardized extract in capsule form or 1/2 teaspoon of liquid extract twice daily. Check health food stores for milk thistle combined with other liver tonics (such as burdock, yellow dock, red clover, or sarsaparilla) in tea, capsule, or liquid form, then follow the label directions.

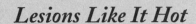

ON-THE-SPOT RELIEF

Lesions Like It Hot

Counterintuitive though it may be, if you apply an over-the-counter cream containing capsaicin—the ingredient that gives chile peppers their bite—to your lesions, your skin will be less irritated, since capsaicin helps tamp down chemicals that transmit pain and itching. Wash your hands well after using the cream, and don't get it near your eyes or apply it to broken skin, warns Jeanette Jacknin, M.D. Capsaicin creams are available at most drugstores.

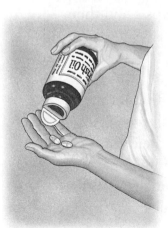

STRIKE OIL. People with psoriasis tend to have low levels of omega-3 essential fatty acids, which help to squelch inflammation-causing arachidonic acid. To rebalance your acids, limit animal fats in your diet and take 4 to 6 grams (4,000 to 6,000 milligrams) of fish oil daily in capsule form, divided into three doses, says Bradley Bongiovanni, N.D., a naturopathic physician in Atlanta. That's a lot of fish oil, so get your doctor's okay first, especially if you take aspirin or prescription blood thinners.

RASHES

Ditch the Itch

━━━◦◦◦◦━━━

I'd like to say that I haven't had a rash since my diaper days. The truth is, though, that I often wind up with red, blistering bumps after a run-in with poison ivy in my garden and a sprinkling of red dots on one knee—a "heat rash"—whenever I wear shorts on hot, sticky days and sit for long periods with one leg crossed over the other. Ooh, they're itchy. Ugh, they're unsightly. Yet I count myself incredibly lucky that I can at least identify my culprits—and perhaps avoid them the next time out!

WHY ME?

Pinning down the culprit behind a rash isn't always so easy when you consider the dozens of suspects you come into contact with daily. The list includes detergents; cat dander; nickel in rings, earrings, and zippers; latex and

WHEN TO DIAL THE DOC

• • • • • • • • • • •

A rash accompanied by wheezing, dizziness, or fever (or any other symptom, really) is potentially very serious. You could be having a life-threatening allergic reaction caused by inflammatory histamines released by your body's mast cells, so you should seek medical help immediately.

rubber in protective gloves, balloons, and waistbands; hair, shoe, and clothing dye; and the worst offender—fragrances, which are found in everything from detergents to lotions. If you're susceptible, any one of these offenders can leave a rash (sometimes with raised, angry welts) at the point of contact.

You can also get a blotchy rash in response to stress and an itchy, hive-like rash with bumps the size of quarters from taking penicillin, certain pain relievers, and other medications or from eating nuts, chocolate, shellfish, strawberries, or foods that contain additives or preservatives. In some cases, a rash can be a symptom of a fungal infection, toxic shock syndrome, or an underlying disease such as lupus, psoriasis, or meningitis. Finally, there are the rashes that fall into the "heaven knows what" category.

BEAT BIKINI BUMPS

To keep your bikini line from looking like a minefield of razor bumps and infected hair follicles, use shaving gel, leave it on for a few minutes, then shave using a wet razor—all of which will allow more water to soften the hair for a closer shave and less chance of ingrown hairs. Afterward, smooth on a cream with alpha hydroxy acids (AHAs), which can reduce ingrown hairs and minimize the bumps, suggests J. Michael Maloney, M.D., a Denver-based dermatologist. Follow this with a vitamin C–based cream to reduce redness. You can also ice the area or spritz it with water in which you've dissolved two aspirin tablets and a drop of glycerin to reduce redness and swelling.

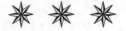

GET THE RED OUT

No matter how annoying your rash is, resist running pell-mell to the medicine chest in search of hydrocortisone cream. Instead, spend some time trying to ID your suspects so you can avoid them (and the need for any kind of cream) in the future. For instance, if you think your rash may be related to something you're eating, keep a food diary for a week, then see your doctor for a skin test to confirm any suspects you come up with. In the meantime, check out the following rash remedies. They can provide relief even if you haven't a clue yet about what's getting under your skin.

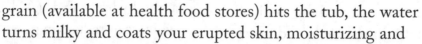

FEEL YOUR OATS. Forget the fancy aromatherapy bubbles and sink into a cool, slimy colloidal oatmeal bath for 5 to 30 minutes, suggests Sharol Tilgner, N.D., a naturopathic physician and director of Wise Acres Education Center in Eugene, Oregon. When this finely ground grain (available at health food stores) hits the tub, the water turns milky and coats your erupted skin, moisturizing and reducing the itch. You can also mix colloidal oatmeal with a bit of water to form a paste and apply it directly to the rash.

A GEM OF A REMEDY. If you've been bushwhacked by poison ivy and live in the eastern United States, look for another plant—jewelweed—to treat it. Simply squeeze the juice from the stem and slap it onto the affected area. The jewelweed can help keep the irritating urushiol oil in poison ivy from binding to your skin and spreading, says Beth Burch, N.D., a naturopathic physician in Gresham, Oregon. A few drops of jewelweed extract, which you can find at

HOMEGROWN SOLUTION

◆ ◆ ◆

Season, Don't Scratch

For a rash of unknown origin, simply chew a fresh oregano leaf (a strong antiseptic), spit it into your hand, and slather it on your rash, suggests Sharol Tilgner, N.D. If you prefer a less primitive method of application, use a few drops of oregano oil, available at health food stores.

health food stores, will work, too. To keep a reserve handy, mix a few drops of the extract with water and freeze the solution as ice cubes to use on any itchy spots that might crop up.

SOOTHE IT. A good Rx for any itchy rash is to mix up a paste with 3 parts baking soda and 1 part water or witch hazel (an astringent), then dab it directly onto your skin. Or simply scoop some gel from an aloe leaf, mix it with a drop of peppermint oil, which also relieves pain, and smear it on the affected area.

ADD FAT. If you've erupted in a red, bumpy rash on your forearms and thighs, it could be a telltale sign that you're lacking essential fatty acids—the kind found in fish, flaxseed, and evening primrose oils—which help keep skin lubricated, supple, and smooth. Jeanette Jacknin M.D., a dermatologist in Scottsdale, Arizona,

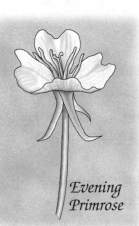

Evening Primrose

suggests taking 1 teaspoon or 500 milligrams of flaxseed oil, evening primrose oil, or fish oil (all of which you can find at health food stores) three times a day. You can also apply evening primrose oil directly to your rash. If it's progressed to the point where the skin is cracking, you should see healing within a week or two. People who take aspirin or prescription blood thinners should not take flaxseed oil or fish oil.

Restless Legs Syndrome

Wriggle No More

❧───────❦❦❦───────❧

I once attended a weekend retreat where one woman kept popping up to pace the room during the evening seminars. I learned later that sitting still made her legs feel jumpy—almost as if she had ants crawling inside them. Moving around helped her stamp out the icky, uncomfortable sensation.

Creepy-crawly sensations and an irresistible urge to wriggle your legs are the hallmarks of restless legs syndrome (RLS), a condition that typically acts up in the early evening and doesn't dissipate until near dawn. This slowly progressive (and probably inherited) condition affects about 15 percent of all Americans over age 50. While it isn't super-scary or life-threatening, it may be debilitating: The sensations can make it tough to attend a lecture, movie, or concert; watch TV; read a book; and, worst of all, get a decent night's sleep.

WHY ME?

Scientists aren't sure what's behind the odd twitching of RLS. It may be caused by a glitch in a brain protein that affects the uptake of iron, which in turn causes misfiring of nerve signals to the legs (and sometimes to the thighs and arms). It could be a result of a deficiency of dopamine, a brain chemical that helps to regulate the nervous system. In fact, a leading drug used for RLS is actually a dopamine substitute approved to treat Parkinson's disease, a serious neurological condition.

GIVE IT A GOOD, SWIFT KICK

When you have the irresistible urge to move, make that movement count, says health educator Jill Gunzel. Forceful, dramatic movements seem to get rid of the twitchies most rapidly. Try marching for eight steps, kicking your legs in front of you for four (left leg, right leg, left leg, right leg), then kicking them behind you for four. End by rising on your toes four times. Repeat the sequence as often as necessary.

SIDESTEP THE SENSATIONS

Just because RLS doesn't as yet have an identifiable cause or a specific drug approved to treat it, that doesn't mean you can't calm your jumpy limbs. Start by discussing your symptoms with your doctor and having your blood tested for levels of iron, folic acid, and vitamin B_{12}, all essential nerve nutrients. You may need to boost your intake of iron and avoid alcohol, antihistamines, ice cream (yes, all flavors), and especially caffeine, all of which rob your body of those nerve nutrients you so desperately need.

To further tame the twitchies, try one or more of the following therapies, all guaranteed to help you both sit and sleep.

EXERCISE BEFORE BED. Strenuous exercise actually worsens RLS, but studies show that moderate activity—say, walking for 30 minutes three or four times a week just before turning in—can reduce twitching and greatly enhance sleep. The same is true for stretching the muscles in the backs of your legs just before bed. The only downside: It takes about four months for the benefits to show up.

GET AMPLE MINERALS. To make sure your nerves get the nutrients they need to function properly, take a high-potency multivitamin/mineral supplement that contains zinc and folic acid, suggests Andrew Weil, M.D., director of the Program in Integrative Medicine and clinical professor of internal medicine at the University of Arizona in Tucson. He also recommends taking a calcium/magnesium supplement at bedtime to help calm nerves and muscles. Ask your doctor about the dose that's right for you.

LULL THOSE MUSCLES. Any activity that increases muscle relaxation may also decrease the frequency and severity of RLS episodes, but the key is finding what works for you, says Mark J. Buchfuhrer, M.D., an RLS and sleep disorders specialist in Downey, California. Try soaking in a warm bath, massaging your legs, or alternating between hot and cold compresses.

WRAP 'EM UP. Many people with RLS find relief when they use

THE BEST BAND-AID

An elastic exercise band is a great tool for minimizing the creepy-crawlies during long car or plane trips, says health educator Jill Gunzel. Simply loop a band (which you can find at sporting goods stores) around the ball of your foot and pull the ends with both hands while raising your foot about 8 inches off the floor. Hold, then lower. Repeat five times before switching to the other foot. Just don't break out the band when you're driving!

an elastic sports wrap (available at sporting goods stores) to compress their legs, which warms and relaxes them, notes Dr. Buchfuhrer. For the same reasons, you may get relief by wearing compression panty hose designed for people with varicose veins.

DISTRACT YOURSELF. Be sure you have a distraction method—such as knitting, doing a crossword puzzle, or even balancing your checkbook—at the ready whenever you have the urge to wriggle, says Jill Gunzel, a health educator at the Restless Legs Foundation in Rochester, Minnesota. Many people with RLS find that using a hand-held DVD player or game that challenges the brain is the ticket when they're trapped in cars or planes and can't get up to walk off the wiggles.

RUB-A-DUB-DUB. When you're confined in a movie theater, concert hall, or church—and a hand-held game is out of the question—try rubbing your hands together or massaging your shoulders. The sensation will produce a counter-stimulus to override the uncomfortable sensations in your legs, says Gunzel. The jumpy feeling will return as soon as you stop rubbing, but the strategy may help you get to the end of the flick.

SAVE YOUR MONEY!

Tonic Isn't a Tonic

Some experts may recommend tonic water as a remedy for restless legs, but according to Mark Buchfuhrer, M.D., it's nothing but a waste of a buck. Quinine, the active ingredient in tonic water, is an old-time remedy for leg cramps, possibly because it relieves excessive nerve firings. There's no evidence that it works for the creepy-crawlies, though. If you do try dosing with tonic water, and it works, you can rule out RLS, says Dr. Buchfuhrer.

RINGING IN THE EARS

Deaden the Din

———◦◦◦———

Years of working as a chef, surrounded by whirring blenders and screaming coffee grinders, have left my friend Linda with a low but insistent roar in her ears—an always-there hiss that she likens to the persistent chirp of "zillions of cicadas." It's a lovely image—but an extremely annoying and surprisingly common problem.

One out of four people have tinnitus (from the Latin word *tinnire*, meaning "to ring"), a catchall term doctors use to describe abnormal ear noises that typically sound like a high-pitched hiss or low-

DROWN OUT THE RACKET

Can't sleep because of all the noise in your ears? Turn on the shower. The constant cascade of water will mask ear noise, and the steady, even drumming of the shower will soothe your frazzled nerves and lull you to sleep.

pitched roar. Tinnitus isn't a disease but a symptom caused by damage to the hairs that surround the auditory cells of the inner ear. These hairs trigger the auditory (hearing) nerve to send sound to the brain, and when they become bent or broken—by persistent loud noise such as the kind Linda was exposed to, for instance—they move about in a state of irritation, sending sound randomly and continuously.

WHY ME?

Aside from loud noise, tinnitus can originate from normal, age-related hearing loss, which usually begins around age 60. It can also result from decreased blood supply to your hearing centers due to heart disease and high blood pressure. Long-term use of many medications can trigger tinnitus, including aspirin and other anti-inflammatories; antibiotics; diuretics; quinine-derived drugs; and drugs for anemia, high or low blood pressure, diabetes, migraines, thyroid problems, earwax buildup, ear infections, allergies, and temporomandibular disorder (TMD). Tinnitus can also be a symptom of Meniere's disease, a condition caused by excess fluid in the inner ear, or even a B vitamin deficiency.

TURN DOWN THE VOLUME

There is no cure for tinnitus. With a little help, however, your brain can learn to ignore the "zillions of cicadas," just as it

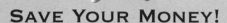
does the incessant hum of your refrigerator, assures Brian Freidenberg, Ph.D., coordinator of tinnitus research at the Center for Stress and Anxiety Disorders at the State University of New York in Albany.

If your tinnitus is very severe or becoming worse, and/or you're having trouble understanding speech, make an appointment with an ear specialist, or otolaryngologist. The doctor can fit you with a device that emits white noise or a vibration that harmonizes with your ear sounds and helps sharpen your hearing while blocking out the phantom crickets and buzzers.

Not ready to resort to a hearing aid? Try these lower-tech tricks to tame your tinnitus.

MAKE YOUR OWN NOISE. Silence only makes those cicadas sing louder! Turn on static between FM radio stations, purchase a tabletop machine that mimics natural sounds such as rolling surf or falling raindrops, or play background music all the time. "If you're not bothered by tinnitus, it doesn't exist," says Dr. Freidenberg.

PLUG YOUR EARS. Moviegoers sitting in surround-sound theaters are exposed to noise intense enough to destroy hair cells. "I tell everyone to wear earplugs during action movies, as well as when attending concerts and nightclubs," says Dr. Freidenberg. If you operate machinery or are often exposed to any noise loud enough that you have to shout to be heard, wear

ear protection. If you listen to headphones, dial down the volume. Repeated exposure to loud sounds can further damage the hairs in your inner ears and make your tinnitus worse.

KEEP BLOOD VESSELS FLEXIBLE. Eating a low-fat diet and exercising at least 30 minutes a day will not only aid your cardiovascular system, it'll also help keep the tiny blood vessels leading to your hearing centers flexible. That's important, stresses Michael D. Seidman, M.D., director of neurotologic surgery at Henry Ford Hospital in Detroit, since those tiny vessels can spasm when exposed to loud noises, cutting off blood flow to the ears and resulting in tinnitus. Also, avoid blood vessel constrictors such as alcohol, caffeine, and nicotine and cut back on salt and sugar, which have the same effect.

GET YOUR Bs. If your tinnitus is caused by a deficiency of B vitamins, taking a B-complex supplement can minimize your symptoms, possibly by improving function of the nerves in your ears, says Dr. Seidman. Look for a formula that includes thiamin, niacin, and B_{12}. Avoid individual B supplements, since large amounts of some B vitamins—particularly thiamin—can cause nerve damage.

MAXIMIZE MINERALS. Meats and shellfish are rich in zinc, a mineral that may minimize age-related tinnitus and hearing loss. The recommended dose is 15 milligrams a day. In addition, if you work or play around noisy equipment, ask your doctor about taking 250 milligrams of supplemental magnesium as well—or just feast regularly on green veggies, whole grains, nuts, and beans, all of which are great sources—suggests Dr. Seidman. Low magnesium levels may constrict inner ear arteries and lead to tinnitus.

POP PERIWINKLE. Vinpocetine, which is made from the extract of the periwinkle plant and sold in health food stores, promotes blood flow and may ease tinnitus triggered by antibiotics, says Dr. Seidman. He suggests taking 20 milligrams daily. Just one caveat: Vinpocetine is a blood thinner, so don't take it if you regularly use aspirin or a prescription blood-thinning medication.

TALK SHOP. When you're the only one around who's "hearing things," you can feel pretty isolated. Join a tinnitus support group for the sheer camaraderie—and to pick up proven tips for coping with ear chaos. To find a group in your area, contact the American Tinnitus Association at (800) 634-8978.

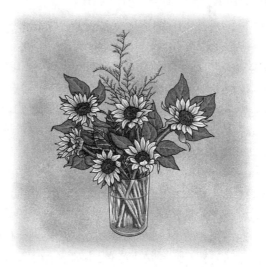

ROSACEA

Stop Seeing Red

———◄◦◦◦►———

I've been known to blush rather easily. Not when I hear a bawdy joke, mind you, but when I drink hot coffee, eat spicy nachos, sip Bordeaux, exercise strenuously, or simply come in from the frosty air. I've learned that my quick-to-turn-crimson cheeks may put me at risk for rosacea, an inflammatory skin condition involving the blood vessels of the face. Rosacea affects 13 million adults, most of them fair-skinned women between the ages of 30 and 60—like me.

WHY ME?

Doctors believe that people with rosacea have "twitchy," reactive blood vessels, a chronic bacterial infection caused by microscopic skin mites, and/or an ulcer-type infection that affects the blood vessels. Any one of these can precipitate leakage of blood from the vessels, triggering low-grade

SWITCH SPICES

By simply trading spices—using cumin mixed with oregano instead of red pepper or paprika—when you cook, you can minimize flushing without sacrificing flavor.

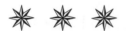
inflammation that may gradually progress from blush-like episodes to permanent ruddiness marked by red, spidery-looking, "broken" blood vessels and, in some cases, tiny, red, pus-filled pimples.

Depending on its cause, rosacea is usually treated with topical antibiotics to squelch the infection and subsequent inflammation, sulfur agents such as permethrins (Elimite) to kill the skin mites, or an antifungal gel.

BEAT THE BLUSH

There's no need to make a mad dash for the drugstore—especially if your rosacea is mild or occasional like mine. Surveys conducted by the National Rosacea Society indicate that simply avoiding triggers helps curb 96 percent of flare-ups. They also suggest that the best way to begin is by limiting the big three vessel dilators: sun, red wine, and heat in all its forms, from spicy or piping-hot foods to steamy showers. You'll also need to steer clear of things that sting, such as products containing ethyl alcohol, witch hazel, menthol, peppermint, eucalyptus oil, or clove oil. And babying your skin is vital—no harsh or scented soaps or rough washcloths allowed!

If you follow the above advice, you may be able to keep flushing flare-ups to a minimum—without even a modicum of medication. Then, when redness flares, here's how to strike back.

SLICK ON SILYMARIN. You can use cover-up lotions to try

to camouflage your redness, but studies show that preparations containing silymarin and vitamin E can actually help reduce redness—even if you have long-standing rosacea. Silymarin is a component of milk thistle that may help squelch free radical–generated inflammation, while vitamin E is an antioxidant that may reduce swelling, says Gail L. Nield, M.D., a dermatologist in Woodbridge, Ontario, Canada. If you use it when your face is merely pink, it could prevent it from progressing to the red stage. Look for silymarin-based preparations such as Rosacure on the Internet.

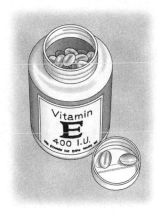

TONE UP. All the dilation that occurs when you flush can leave your blood vessels flabby and less likely to constrict the way they should, notes Jeanette Jacknin, M.D., a dermatologist in Scottsdale, Arizona. She suggests taking vitamin C along with bioflavonoids to help tone the blood vessels. As long as you don't have kidney or stomach problems, check your local drugstore or health food store for combination formulas, then take 500 milligrams three times a day.

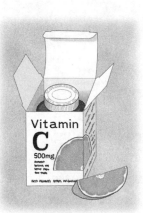

RUB IT IN. Try using herbal creams such as horse chestnut cream, which improves the tone of vein walls and is used to help shrink varicose veins, or rose wax cream (both of which are available at health food stores). Applying either cream twice a day may minimize rosacea, says Dr. Jacknin.

REDUCE INFLAMMATION. Grapeseed extract is an excellent natural anti-inflammatory that also shores up collagen. Dr. Jacknin recommends taking 50 milligrams in capsule form three times a day. Look for it at your local health food store.

Horse Chestnut

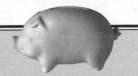
BREATHE DEEP. Surely you've heard the advice "Slow down and take a deep breath" when you're stressed or nervous. Well, according to a survey of National Rosacea Society members, it also applies to halting the crimson tide. When you're feeling overwhelmed, inhale and count to 10, then exhale for 10 more counts. Repeat this exercise several times, and you'll be less likely to flush.

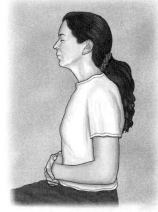

TRY HYPNOSIS. A step beyond deep, measured breathing, hypnosis teaches guided imagery and progressive muscle relaxation techniques to help you actually prevent your blood vessels from dilating, says Phillip Shenefelt, M.D., associate professor in the division of dermatology and cutaneous surgery at the University of South Florida in Tampa. You're getting very… intrigued? Ask your dermatologist about hypnosis and a referral to a trained clinician near you.

SLIP ON A SKI MASK. You're wise to avoid the midday sun and stay in air conditioning on humid summer days, but you should also take steps to keep cold air off your face in winter. The more you cover up when you're chilled (which makes the blood vessels overconstrict to conserve heat), the less your vessels will dilate as they throw off heat when you come inside, says Dr. Jacknin.

SEXUALLY TRANSMITTED DISEASES

Speed Sexual Healing

———————◆◇◆◇◆———————

If you have weird bumps, burning, or discharge in your genital area, you may not mention it to your friends—but don't keep it a secret from your doctor. Mustering up the courage to get yourself (and your partner) tested for a sexually transmitted disease (STD) can save you a lot of mortification and discomfort, preserve your reproductive organs, and possibly save your life.

WHY ME?

Frankly, this is a question for your partner, but I can help

FREEZE!

When you first feel the burning that signals a herpes outbreak on the horizon, get out the ice tray. Wrap some cubes in a small towel and apply it to the area for 10 minutes at a time several times a day. Not only will the burning subside, says Tori Hudson, N.D., you may even keep lesions from appearing.

---

fill in the blanks when it comes to the more common STDs.

If you're infected with the herpes simplex-2 virus (HSV), as one in five Americans now are, you'll feel itching, burning, or pain on or around your genitals, followed by redness and tiny, open blisters that will eventually scab over and disappear. Because HSV is with you for life, you may have repeat performances—usually triggered by illness, stress, or sunburn—four to six times a year.

If you have genital warts, which are caused by one of the 80-plus forms of the human papillomavirus (HPV), you may or may not be aware of these tiny, sometimes itchy, cauliflower-like growths that can crop up on the vulva, anus, and penis. In fact, the warts may not even show up for months or years after you've been exposed to the virus. Like HSV, however, HPV hangs around forever, and the warts have a tendency to reappear.

Gonorrhea, which is caused by bacteria, causes symptoms in only half of people who have it; in women, genital itching and burning urination may be mistaken for symptoms of a bladder infection. Gonorrhea is contagious until you've been treated, and a new exposure to the bacteria causes reinfection, even if you were previously cured.

Finally, if you're infected with chlamydia, which is caused by sneaky bacteria that leave few, if any, clues—especially in women—painful intercourse and abdominal pain should send you to your doctor for a test, pronto, before it spreads elsewhere and *really* causes trouble.

ON-THE-SPOT RELIEF

Smear on E

To stop the sting of herpes lesions, dry the area (using a hair dryer if you must), then use a cotton swab to apply vitamin E oil, which you can find at any drugstore or health food store. Your pain should vanish within 15 minutes, says Melody Wong, N.D.

MINIMIZING FLARE-UPS

No matter what your bug, treatment is never a do-it-yourself job. You need a powerful antiviral or antibiotic medication or, in the case of warts, a strong chemical to remove any growths that are bothersome. But that isn't to say there's nothing you can do. On the contrary, you can use natural methods to help your medications work better and faster, to ease discomfort, and to keep flare-ups of lesions and warts, for instance, to a minimum. Here's what they are.

GET CULTURED. If you're taking an antibiotic for chlamydia or gonorrhea, you can offset the side effects—namely, an overgrowth of yeast—by eating a cup of yogurt that contains live cultures of the "good" bacteria acidophilus daily. Check your supermarket or health food store for live-culture yogurt.

TRY ECHINACEA. This herb boosts production of T cells that fight viruses and of phagocytes that battle bacteria, says Tori Hudson, N.D., a naturopathic physician and director of A Woman's Time clinic in Portland, Oregon. To treat chlamydia, she suggests taking ¹/₂ teaspoon of liquid extract (available in any health food store) every 2 hours for two days, then taking ¹/₂ teaspoon

---

A HONEY OF A REMEDY

An active herpes eruption can last a heartbreaking week or two, but researchers in the Ukraine found that using a topical ointment containing propolis, a nutrient-rich substance made by honeybees that contains antiviral flavonoids, can cut lesion time to just three days. That's almost half the time it took for lesions to heal with standard medication. Check at health food stores or on the Internet for products that contain propolis.

✳ ✳ ✳

---

three times daily for the next two weeks. Don't use echinacea if you have lupus, rheumatoid arthritis, or multiple sclerosis, or if you are pregnant or nursing.

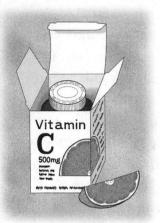

TAKE C FOR HERPES. As long as you don't have stomach or kidney problems, downing 600 milligrams each of vitamin C and bioflavonoids (available in drugstores and health food stores) three times daily for three days from the moment you detect tingling could cut your outbreak short, says Dr. Hudson.

TRY THIS DYNAMIC DUO. To help combat chlamydia and gonorrhea, Melody Wong, N.D., a naturopathic physician in Sausalito and Palo Alto, California, suggests taking 500 milligrams of vitamin C every 2 hours for two days, then 1,000 milligrams for the next two weeks to power up your immune system during treatment. To help the immune cells in the mucosal lining fight more fiercely, you also need a good amount of vitamin A. This is a lot of C, so check with your doctor first, and ask about the dosage that's right for you.

AVOID ARGININE. Nuts, seeds, chocolate, coconuts, and sardines are packed with arginine, an amino acid that helps the herpesvirus replicate, says Judith Boice, N.D., a naturo-pathic physician in Portland, Oregon. Fill up instead on lentils, legumes, black beans, wheat germ, and seafood, all of which are loaded with lysine, another amino acid that seems to help discourage herpes outbreaks.

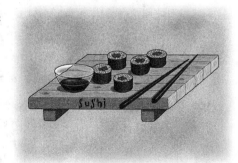

You can also take supplemental lysine (available at health food stores). Allan Warshowsky, M.D., director of the Women's

Health and Healing Program at Beth Israel Hospital in New York City, suggests taking 1,500 milligrams in capsule form three times a day during outbreaks.

GET LEMON AID. To help cut the healing time for genital herpes, Dr. Hudson recommends two antiviral herbs—lemon balm, also known as melissa (check your health food store for an ointment containing lemon balm and apply it two to four times a day) and licorice (apply a gel containing glycyrrhetinic acid, also available in health food stores—three times a day).

ZAP IT WITH ZINC. For milder, less frequent herpes outbreaks, take 25 milligrams of zinc and 250 milligrams of vitamin C twice daily for five weeks. If you start this regimen within 24 hours of the first telltale tingle, says Dr. Hudson, you may be able to completely suppress eruptions. Do not take this amount of zinc for longer than the recommended time.

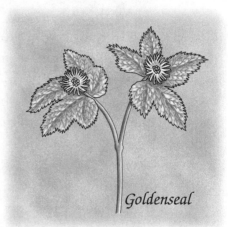

Goldenseal

PROCEED WISELY. To help heal herpes eruptions, rev up the immune cells in your mucous membranes with goldenseal and myrrh. Using a cotton swab, apply one to three drops of either tincture (available at health food stores) three times a day.

SHINGLES

Banish the Blisters

⟐

I find it ironic that despite comedian David Letterman's laid-back demeanor on-camera, off-camera he's had a number of stress-related conditions, including an outbreak of shingles (medically known as herpes zoster)—a vexing viral infection that's nothing to snicker at.

WHY ME?

Shingles usually hits people who are over 50 and under stress, but it can show up in any adult, since most of us harbor the herpesvirus that causes it. It's the same one we caught as kids that gave us chickenpox, and it's lain dormant in the nerve cells along our spines ever since. Stress of any kind, physical (such as getting the flu) as well as emotional, can cause the virus to "come alive" and multiply, as can taking immune-suppressant drugs such as corticosteroids or simply having a weakened immune system as a result of aging or chronic illness.

Once the bug is reactivated, it travels along the nerve pathways, causing burning and extreme sensitivity—usually on one side of the body—in the torso, arms, legs, or face, where it eventually erupts as a stinging, spotty rash that turns into blisters. A week or so later, the blisters crust, scab, and eventually disappear. For some people, the pain lingers, producing an offshoot condition called postherpetic neuralgia (PHN).

OUTLAST THE OUTBREAK

Antiviral medication such as famciclovar (Famvir) can quash the shingles bug if taken in the earliest stages of the attack—within 72 hours of when the rash first appears. But the following methods can keep you from wincing in pain or scratching at those blisters to the point where you invite infection. In fact, some remedies may even cut your outbreak short. Here's what to try.

COOL DOWN. "A number of cooled herbal teas can calm inflammation and itchy skin, but my favorite is chamomile," says Bradley Bongiovanni, N.D., a naturopathic physician in Atlanta. Buy some chamomile tea at a supermarket or health food store and steep a few tea bags in hot water. Let it cool, then soak a clean cloth in the solution and apply it to your blisters several times daily.

LICK IT. Sweet-tasting licorice root can help keep the virus from spreading as well as fight inflammation in a manner similar to cortisone—but minus the side effects. To use it

DON'T GO NUTS

Just as going nuts emotionally can trigger a shingles outbreak, eating nuts during an outbreak can encourage the spread of the virus. Almonds and peanuts (and chocolate) contain arginine, an amino acid that's "fuel" for the herpes zoster virus. Another amino acid—lysine, which is abundant in milk and whole wheat bread—however, can stop the virus in its tracks. The next time you have an attack, limit foods with arginine and supplement with lysine (available in health food stores). About 1,000 milligrams a day is ideal.

HOMEGROWN SOLUTION

◆ ◆ ◆

Backyard Balm

Just as lemon balm exudes a heavenly scent in your garden, when you use the moist leaves wrapped in a damp cloth as a salve for your shingles blisters, you can get heavenly relief from the itching—and perhaps even heal more quickly. You can also drink lemon balm tea, made by steeping 1 to 2 teaspoons of dried leaves in a cup of hot water for 10 to 15 minutes. Strain out the herb and sip three cups of tea a day.

topically, make a compress by simmering 1 teaspoon of dried licorice root (available in health food stores) in 2 cups of boiling water for 15 minutes, then soaking a clean cloth in the cooled solution and applying it to your blisters.

GO FOR ALOE. When your blisters begin to crust, your best defense is the anti-inflammatory gel you can drip straight out of an aloe vera leaf, says Dr. Bongiovanni. Use about a teaspoon on the lesions two or three times a day. If you opt for commercial aloe vera, check your health food store for the straight stuff, made without artificial colorings or preservatives.

SLATHER WITH E. Vitamin E oil will help any lesion heal more quickly, says Dr. Bongiovanni. Break open a capsule and apply the contents to your sores several times a day.

OPT FOR OLIVE. To hasten healing, Dr. Bongiovanni recommends taking olive leaf extract, which you can find at any health food store. The suggested dose is two 500-milligram capsules three times a day.

BET ON BIOFLAVONOIDS. Studies show that when combined with vitamin C, immunity-boosting bioflavonoids appear to prevent the viral growth and spread of shingles—especially if you take them in the early stages of a flare-up. Look for a commercial formulation that includes both, then follow the label directions.

FIGHT FIRE WITH FIRE. For pain that lingers after your blisters heal, try smearing on a paste made by blending a smidgen of red pepper with 1 tablespoon of aloe vera gel (or more, if the mixture feels too hot). The capsaicin in the pepper helps reduce substance P, a pain-producing chemical that your body releases during shingles outbreaks. Note that it may take about six weeks to work, and be sure to apply the mixture with a cotton swab so you don't burn your fingers.

A BLEND FOR PHN. To reduce residual nerve pain, Dr. Bongiovanni recommends adding three drops each of extracts of astragalus (an immune booster), St. John's wort (a wound healer), Jamaican dogwood (a nerve sedative), and licorice (an antiviral) to a glass of water, then drinking three glasses a day for up to 20 days. The extracts are available at health food stores. People with high blood pressure should avoid licorice.

TRY BIOFEEDBACK. One of the best stress-management techniques for beating the pain of shingles, biofeedback is really just a way of teaching relaxation. Electrodes are attached to your skin, and a computer "feeds" you information about your pulse, breathing rate, skin temperature, and muscle tension while you're practicing relaxation techniques. You then use that information to achieve the same results on your own. As a result, studies show, you can have less pain as well as improved immune function.

SINUSITIS

Unclog the Cavities

Not long ago, sinusitis seemed to rule our household. If my husband wasn't battling stuffiness, gobs of discharge, and crushing pain behind his eyes, it was our daughter's turn. In both cases, the triggering factors were allergens—pollen, dust, dander, milk, you name it. Those irksome irritants spark an inflammatory reaction in the lining of the nose and cause an increase in molasses-thick mucus.

When this gunk backs up, it causes so much painful pressure in the sinus cavities around the eyes that you wish a Roto-Rooter guy could drill through the congestion. This mucus buildup also deactivates the cilia, the tiny nasal hairs that normally serve as mini-propellers to whisk irritants and bacte-

---

HOMEGROWN SOLUTION

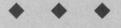

Thyme to Breathe Easier

You may have an effective mucus mover right under your nose—in your herb garden. Thyme has strong antiseptic properties and has long been used to treat clogged sinuses. Simply steep 1 to 2 teaspoons in a cup of boiling water for 10 minutes, strain, and drink a cup three times a day.

---

ria from the nose. If the cilia stop working and bacteria breed in the backed-up mucus, sinusitis can turn into a nasty sinus infection—and sinusitis by itself is nasty enough.

WHY ME?

My husband and daughter often have "chronic" sinusitis, which can spring from allergies or be caused by the body's overreaction to the fungi that normally reside in the nasal passages. An "acute" episode can be sparked by a cold virus, breathing too much smog, or even swimming in a highly chlorinated pool. In neither case, however, do drugstore remedies offer much help.

Nasal decongestants, for instance, can shrink swollen membranes in a jiffy, but if you use them for more than three days, they can cause rebound swelling. Plus, they make you jittery and keep you up all night. Antihistamines can actually thicken mucus. And if you're prone to sinus infections, repeated use of antibiotics can give rise to an infection that's resistant to all medications!

CLEARING CONGESTION

If your symptoms worsen, your mucus turns green, or you develop a fever, you need to see a doctor. In most cases, however, the following home remedies can clear your sinuses gently while clobbering pain, warding off infection, and, best of all, coaxing those cilia back to work.

FLUSH IT OUT. Using saline (saltwater) nose drops is the

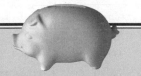

SAVE YOUR MONEY!

Don't Get Steamed

Your congestion will only worsen if you use a steam inhaler device or sit in a commercial sauna, since the activity of the cilia slows down at temperatures of 104°F and above. In fact, you're better off breathing the steam from a bowl of boiled water (which isn't as hot as the steam in a sauna) laced with a few drops of an aromatic antiseptic herb such as eucalyptus.

best way to loosen mucus, relieve both acute and chronic sinusitis, and get the cilia back on the job. Simply mix 1/2 teaspoon of table salt into a glass of warm water. Put the solution in a spray bottle, an ear syringe, or an Ayurvedic neti pot (an Aladdin's lamp–like container with a small spout, which you can find at health food stores) or any similar spouted container. Lean over a sink and turn your head so your left nostril is lower than your right, keeping your head tilted so your nose is higher than your mouth. Spray or pour the solution into your right nostril, allowing the water to drain from your left nostril and your mouth. Gently blow your nose, then repeat with the other nostril.

UNPLUG WITH A PULSE. For severe sinusitis, there are nasal irrigation attachments available for Water Pik–type devices that direct a pulsating stream of water into the nostrils. This can help repair damaged cilia, clear up congestion, and ward off infection, says Murray Grossan, M.D., a consultant in the department of otolaryngology at Cedars-Sinai Hospital in Los Angeles. Ask your doctor which device is best for you.

BET ON BROMELAIN. This enzyme present in pineapple reduces inflammation and fluid retention and helps shrink swollen sinuses, notes Dr. Grossan. You can find bromelain in capsule form at drugstores and health food stores; follow the label directions. Don't take bromelain if you take aspirin or prescription blood thinners.

GO FOR THE GOLD. Goldenseal, beloved by the Plains Indians as a remedy to help ward off infections of the mucous membranes, makes an ideal

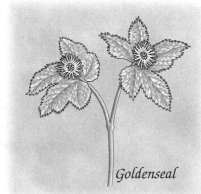

Goldenseal

addition to modern-day irrigation solutions. Add 1 teaspoon of liquid extract (available in health food stores) to your saltwater wash, suggests Nick Nonas, M.D., an otolaryngologist in Denver.

FIGHT BACK HERBALLY. If an infection has taken hold, fight back with a trio of powerful infection fighters (all available at health food stores): echinacea (200 milligrams twice daily), goldenseal (200 milligrams three times a day), and grapefruit seed extract (100 milligrams three times a day), suggests Robert Ivker, D.O., assistant clinical professor of otolaryngology at the University of Colorado School of Medicine in Denver. Skip the grapefruit seed extract if you're taking cholesterol-lowering medication, and don't take echinacea if you have an autoimmune disease such as lupus, rheumatoid arthritis, or multiple sclerosis, or if you're pregnant or nursing.

WRAP IT UP. Draping your face with a hot, moist towel helps increase blood flow to the sinuses and activates the cilia, says Dr. Grossan.

BRING ON THE HEAT. Hot condiments such as horseradish, wasabi, and chile peppers are all excellent mucus-moving agents that can stimulate the cilia and help open up a stuffy nose in seconds.

WAKE UP TO TEA

People who have chronic sinusitis often have body thermostats that don't easily adjust to the cool morning air upon arising, says Murray Grossan, M.D. As a result, they often wake up to stuffiness and endless throat clearing as their sinuses try to drain. To nip that icky concert in the bud, drink hot tea before you get out of bed. It will warm your body and activate the cilia, which will go a long way toward eliminating morning sniffling and hacking.

SNORING

Get Rid of the Racket

———◆◆◆———

I once slept at the home of a family member (who will remain nameless) and was kept awake by the most horrific snoring I'd ever heard coming from not one but two floors up. And lest you think the jumbo-jet-on-takeoff racket was coming from the stereotypical "old guy" depicted in comedies, this nocturnal noisemaker was barely taller than my kneecaps.

No matter what your age or gender, if you have any factor that narrows, relaxes, or irritates your airways, it's possible that your breathing during sleep has taken on a rumbling, buzzing quality. Not sure? Just ask your fellow sleepers.

WHY ME?

Fluctuating hormones at menopause or during pregnancy increase mucus production and nasal congestion—a prime cause of snoring. The extra effort required to draw air through a stuffy nose creates a vacuum in the throat, pulling on the slackened tissues and creating that distinctive rumble. Allergies, asthma, and the common cold can have the same effect.

Other causes of snoring include sleeping on your back (which makes your tongue flop backward) and having a deviated septum, large tonsils, and/or a prominent tongue—all of which can obstruct airflow. Drinking alcohol, taking sedatives, and being extremely fatigued can also cause snoring by over-relaxing the airways.

At the very top of the list of snoring culprits, however, are obesity and poor muscle tone. The fatter you are, the thicker your neck and the flabbier your throat tissue. The excess tissue can vibrate, creating a loud buzzing sound each time you inhale. That little piece of flesh hanging at the back of your throat—the uvula—can do the same thing.

SCALE DOWN SNORING

Do opera singers snore? Who knows? According to a British study, though, this much is clear: Performing vocal exercises for 20 minutes three times a day for three months helps to reduce snoring, perhaps because singing tones the flabby throat muscles that can cause snoring. A singing teacher may be able to help you with the correct exercises, but try belting out a Broadway tune each day on your own to see if, say, a little Sondheim can squelch your nighttime noisemaking.

In most cases, snoring is simply a nuisance—primarily to other people in the vicinity. For about 15 percent of habitual snorers (about a quarter of the population), however, throat tissue can become so flabby that it blocks airflow for as long as a minute hundreds of times each night. This condition—called sleep apnea—is much more than a nuisance. Air stoppage, however brief, deprives you of oxygen and can lead to memory loss, high blood pressure, depression, and even a heart attack. All of the factors that contribute to snoring play a role in sleep apnea, but again, being overweight heads the list.

STOP SAWING LOGS

If your snorting, gasping, whistling, and wheezing are punctuated by recurrent moments of dead silence, constant mouth breathing, or fitful sleep (ask your partner if you toss and turn), consult an ear, nose, and throat specialist (otolaryngologist) for a diagnosis, since you may have sleep apnea, which needs to be treated to prevent potential heart problems. If you do—or even

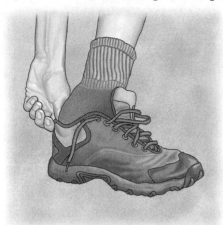

if you're simply an occasional, garden-variety snorer—your first priority should be to lose weight. In fact, if you lose 15 to 20 percent of your body fat, you could stop snoring permanently.

If you don't drop weight, warns Derek S. Lipman, M.D., an otolaryngologist and snoring expert in Portland, Oregon, none of the conventional—and, incidentally, pricey—treatments for apnea and snoring (such as wearing a cumbersome mask that delivers pressurized air to the throat or undergoing laser surgery to trim off slackened tissue) are likely to help. At best, you'll snore more silently, but you'll still snore, he says.

To stop the buzzing even as you're trying to drop a few, try these low-cost yet often highly effective self-help measures.

SLEEP ON YOUR SIDE. Look for a special pillow with an indented center that forces your head and shoulders to remain in a side-sleeping position. Or use the tried-and-true method of sewing a tennis ball into a pocket on the back of your pajama top to keep you from rolling onto your back and staying there while you sleep. It may look odd, but it's cheap—and word of mouth confirms its success for some snorers, says Dr. Lipman.

DOWN NATURAL ANTIHISTAMINES. For allergies, a good alternative to drugstore or prescription antihistamines that can dry out and thicken secretions is to take the anti-allergenic herb stinging nettle, suggests Robert Ivker, D.O., assistant clinical professor of otolaryngology at the University of Colorado School of Medicine in Denver. You can find it at a health food store, then take 300 milligrams in capsule form three times daily.

GIVE YOURSELF A WEDGIE. These pillows raise your upper body and create a slight incline that prevents your tongue from retracting into the back of your throat and impeding airflow. (FYI: Propping your head on a stack of pillows is counterproductive and may only hurt your neck and impede airflow.)

SLIP ON A STRIP. In one study, those commercial strips that attach like adhesive bandages to the bridge of the nose and open nasal passages were shown to reduce snoring by more than 70 percent.

TRY STEAM. Inhaling steam from water laced with a mucus-moving herbal oil can help shrink swollen throat and nasal tissues and stop the log sawing. Boil a pot of water to which you've added a few drops of any of the following oils, all of which you can find at health food stores: eucalyptus (it clears congestion), peppermint (its menthol will give you the sensation of free-flowing air), or thyme (a natural antiseptic and respiratory tonic). Put the pot on a table or counter and lean over it (but not so close that you burn your skin). Drape a towel over your head and shoulders to make a tent to capture the steam and inhale deeply through your mouth and nose.

SAVE YOUR MONEY!

Don't Sound the Alarm

Snorers (or their partners) desperate for a cure have spawned hundreds of devices, but most of them "work" by jarring you awake with an alarm or vibration when buzz sawing begins. You stop snoring, but you also stop sleeping soundly. As for the growing number of antisnoring nose and throat sprays made with "lubricating" oils, take a deep breath before you plunk down your hard-earned cash. None are backed by conclusive studies or approved by the FDA.

SORE THROAT

Swallow with Ease

⊰⦿⦿⊱

I got a doozy of a sore throat after a long flight to visit a friend on the West Coast recently, and I didn't have the heart to tell her that eating the tasty sushi she had made for me felt as if I were swallowing big chunks of broken glass. That's the thing about a sore throat: It can ruin an exquisite dinner, everyday conversation, and even your immediate outlook on life—just like that.

WHY ME?

A sore throat is usually a harbinger of worse things to come—a full-blown cold, for instance, or a bout with the flu. The characteristic redness

---

TRY OLD MAN'S BEARD

That's the folk name for usnea, a lichen that fights the strep bacteria, possibly as powerfully as penicillin, says Skye Weintraub, N.D., a naturopathic physician in Eugene, Oregon. Her Rx for strep throat: Add a dropper of usnea (available at health food stores) to a glass of water and gargle several times a day.

and swelling of tissues in your throat and the glands in your neck are part of your body's way of fighting off the virus. Your throat could also be scratchy and sore as a result of shouting; inhaling smog, paint fumes, or other pollutants; a backwash of stomach acid; post-nasal drip from sinusitis; or simply being exposed to dry air—as in my case, from being in an arid airplane cabin for 6 hours.

SOOTHE THE SORENESS

If you have sudden, excruciating soreness, with a pus-like discharge in the back of your throat and a fever, consult your doctor for a test to see if you have strep throat—a highly contagious infection caused by streptococcus bacteria that may require an antibiotic. For run-of-the-mill soreness, however, there are plenty of natural therapies—many based on time-honored remedies—that may help speed recovery instead of simply masking the pain, as conventional drugstore potions do. Here's what to try first.

ZAP IT WITH ZINC. If your sore throat is related to a cold virus, studies show that sucking on zinc gluconate lozenges (which you can find at drugstores and supermarkets) can cut its duration in half—if you start treatment within 24 hours of the first hint of scratchiness. The reason: Zinc blocks viruses from entering the cells in the respiratory tract.

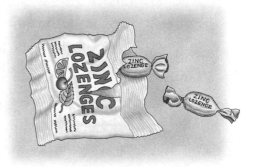

> ## A WRAP FOR THE SCRATCHIES
>
> Steam a small towel over water just as you would steam veggies (or heat it in the microwave) and fold it in a cotton cloth, then drape it around your neck and cover with plastic wrap. According to healing lore, if you wear this "fomentation" all night, your sore throat will vanish by morning.
>
> ✳ ✳ ✳

SIP A SLUSHIE

Drinking piping-hot liquids will swell the uvula—the soft structure that hangs at the back of your throat—and increase your discomfort, notes Murray Grossan, M.D., an oto-laryngologist in Los Angeles. Better to drink a cool or even icy drink to help curb both swelling and pain. Crush some ice in a blender, add your favorite juice, and sip it throughout the day. "That's my simple recipe," Dr. Grossan says.

Or you may want to try zinc acetate, which tastes better than zinc gluconate and is also effective. Follow the package directions for either type.

USE SLIPPERY ELM. Traditionally, slippery elm bark was chewed into a mushy paste to soothe a sore throat. Today, you can get the benefits of this root, which both helps you salivate and turns into gummy mucilage that coats inflamed membranes in your throat, by taking it in any of three forms—as a lozenge, tea, or spray. Visit your health food store and buy the formulation of your choice, then follow the label directions.

USE A CIDER SOOTHER. Gargling with apple cider vinegar may not sound very appetizing, but it's worth it, promises Jamison Starbuck, N.D., a naturopathic physician in Missoula, Montana. Add 2 tablespoons to a glass of warm water, gargle and spit until you finish the glass, then repeat the sequence. Your soreness should vanish within 3 to 4 hours, she says.

TRY TURMERIC. This Indian spice contains curcumin, one of Mother Nature's strongest antibacterials. Simply mix 1/2 teaspoon of turmeric and 1/2 teaspoon of salt in a cup of hot water, let it cool slightly, and gargle with it morning and evening until your pain fades, suggests Vasant Lad, M.A.Sc., director of the Ayurvedic Institute in Albuquerque.

SWALLOW MARSHMALLOW. Keeping throat tissues moist is vital, but you'll sabotage your efforts if you drink caffeine and alcohol—two notorious dehydrators. A good plan is to alternate drinking water and an herbal drink throughout the day. A top choice for the latter is a glass of warm water to which you've added 1 teaspoon of extract of marshmallow, a well-known type of mucilage that coats irritated membranes. Look for the extract at health food stores and drink up to three glasses daily.

SPRITZ IT. Echinacea—a renowned mucous membrane healer—numbs on contact and may kill off any virus that may be causing your misery. You can put 60 drops of tincture and some water in a small spray bottle and spritz your throat several times a day. Or take echinacea in capsule form (check the label for dosage directions) until your symptoms disappear. Both tincture and capsules are available at health food stores. Don't use echinacea if you have an autoimmune disease such as lupus, rheumatoid arthritis, or multiple sclerosis, or if you're pregnant or nursing.

DOSE WITH WILLOW. Willow bark contains salicin, which has the same chemical makeup as aspirin. Check your health food store for willow bark tincture and follow the label directions. Just be sure to steer clear if you're allergic to aspirin, and never use it with alcohol.

Sprains
and Strains

Sore No More

————◦◦◦◦◦————

In the past year, I've had almost as many sprained and strained muscles as a major league athlete—yet I haven't been anywhere near a playing field. In a single week, I sprained my ankle when I stepped off a curb and strained my shoulder by sitting for many hours at the keyboard. I was as stiff and sore that week as I would have been if I had played Serena Williams at Wimbledon—and all I'd done to get that way was to walk and type.

WHY ME?

No matter what you're doing, if you repeat the same movement over and over or overuse muscles that haven't

GO AHEAD, HORSE AROUND

You can keep a sprain from turning black-and-blue by applying a gel that contains horse chestnut extract (available in health food stores). The herb's aescin helps keep blood from seeping out of damaged blood vessels, thus minimizing discoloration.

been warmed up sufficiently, you can wind up straining a muscle—that is, causing tiny tears within the muscle fiber. Worse, if you move the joints of your ankles or knees the wrong way, as I did when I stepped off the curb, you can wind up with a sprain, an injury that occurs when you twist the ligaments that connect the bones to a joint or tendons. In both cases, when muscle damage occurs, the result is pain, swelling, and stiffness. In the case of sprains, you may also have purplish bruising.

ON-THE-SPOT RELIEF

No More Keyboard Shoulder

If you feel as if you need a can of WD-40 to lubricate your sore, stiff shoulders after long stints at the keyboard, try this: Head for an open doorway, grasp the jambs on both sides, and lean through the doorway with your upper torso while tilting your head toward the ceiling, suggests Eugene Zampieron, N.D. Do this every hour, and you'll release any tension in your shoulders and keep lactic acid from building up in your muscles.

Most mild strains and sprains respond to a little TLC and that lesser known acronym, RICE, which stands for rest (anywhere from a few minutes to a few days, depending on the injury), ice (wrap an ice pack in cloth and apply it to your injury for 20 minutes on, 20 minutes off), compression (wrap the injury snugly with an elastic sports bandage), and elevation (raise the injured area above the level of your heart to minimize swelling).

ERASING THE PAIN

RICE helps reduce swelling so healing can take place. As for easing the hurt, aspirin and ibuprofen are far from your only options. There are several herbs and supplements that rival drugstore remedies and may be gentler on your GI tract, including white willow bark—dubbed "Mother Nature's aspirin" because it contains salicin, which is similar to the salicylic acid

PULSE THERAPY

If you have a spray attachment in the shower, aim a shot of hot water on your strain for 3 minutes, then switch to cool water for 10 seconds, and finally, give it a 10-second icy-cold blast. Repeat three times three times a day, and you'll flush out dead cells and lactic acid and infuse your sore muscle with healing oxygen and nutrients.

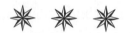

in aspirin. As long as you're not allergic to aspirin, check your health food store for white willow bark and follow the label directions. But don't stop there; follow these steps and you'll be back in the game (or at your keyboard) in no time.

Just one caveat: Skip the self-care and consult your doctor if you have severe pain or limited range of motion, if you hear a popping or ripping noise in your muscle or joint, or if your knee or ankle is wobbly when you put weight on it the next day.

FIRE IT UP. After applying ice to your injury on and off for 24 hours to reduce any swelling, switch to heat in the form of a warm bath, whirlpool, or heating pad. Using heat four times a day for 20 minutes at a time helps dilate blood vessels and promote healing, says Eugene Zampieron, N.D., a naturopathic physician and professor of botanical medicine at the University of Bridgeport in Connecticut.

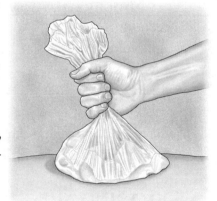

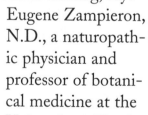

TRY TURMERIC. The same spice that gives curry its distinctive flavor makes an excellent pain reliever, in part because it breaks down bits of

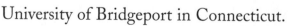

pain-causing protein that circulate in damaged tissue. Mix 1/2 teaspoon of turmeric with enough water to make a paste and apply it to the painful spot, suggests Vasant Lad, M.A.Sc., director of the Ayurvedic Institute in Albuquerque. Or down 250 to 500 milligrams of turmeric in capsule form three times daily, along with 1 teaspoon of flaxseed oil, which is an anti-inflammatory and may boost absorption. You can find both at supermarkets and health food stores.

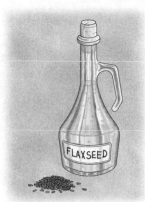

SLATHER ON A SALVE. For a pulled hamstring or tendinitis (strained tendons), Dr. Zampieron suggests using the commercial salve Botanogesic. It contains oils of wintergreen, cinnamon, and cloves (counterirritants that offset the sting of pain) combined with boswellia and ginger—two of the best natural anti-inflammatories around, he says. The salve is available at health food stores and from Internet sources.

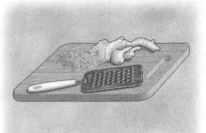

TREAT IT GINGERLY. Bet you didn't know that ginger contains zingibain, an aspirin-like substance that blocks the formation of pain-causing prostaglandins as well as the transmission of pain signals to the brain. Mix a bit of powdered ginger with coconut oil (available at health food stores), and rub it on the injured area. Your swelling, pain, and stiffness should melt away.

BET ON BROMELAIN. Studies show that this anti-inflammatory pineapple enzyme promotes circulation, cleans up the cellular debris in inflamed tissue, and may help you heal twice as fast. At the very least, you'll have less pain, swelling, and bruising,

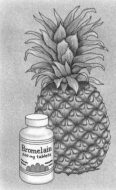

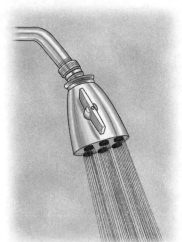

says Dr. Zampieron. Look for bromelain capsules at a health food store and follow the label directions, but talk to your doctor first if you're taking a blood-thinning medication.

OIL UP. To soothe a strain, take a warm shower using a shower gel mixed with a few drops of muscle-soothing oils such as birch bark, eucalyptus, rosemary, clove, or St. Johns wort (all available at health food stores), which help to block pain signals to the brain. Rub the oils into your strained muscle, pressing the meat of the muscle, not the bone, and stroke upward toward your heart.

ARM YOURSELF WITH ARNICA. Many naturally oriented doctors consider extracts of this wildflower to be effective for controlling bruising and swelling from a sprain. Look for it in gel form or add 1 tablespoon of tincture to 2 cups of water, soak a clean cloth in the solution, and apply it directly to your sore spot. Both gels and tinctures are available in health food stores.

STINKY BREATH

Sweeten Your Mouth

———◆◇◆———

I once worked with a woman who was so afraid of offensive breath that she shunned smelly onions or garlic when dining out, capped each meal with a stick of gum, and obsessively spritzed her mouth before every close encounter. Her purse reeked of peppermint.

While my colleague's behavior was a bit extreme, almost everyone dreads bad breath, or halitosis. You'll be interested to know, then, that the best way to combat it isn't with mints but simply with a few good habits.

WHY ME?

Smelly breath is caused by sulfurous waste products pro-

DON'T SUCK ON CITRUS

Lemon-flavored drops may seem like they'd be good breath fresheners, but they're actually highly acidic and create a haven for halitosis, says Ana Diaz-Arnold, D.D.S., professor of family dentistry at the University of Iowa in Iowa City.

Party Favor

At the buffet table, head for the apples, celery, carrots, and sparkling water, bypassing the fruity cocktails and protein-rich fare such as cheese and skewered chicken. Protein, citrus, and alcohol invite odor-causing bacteria in, while crunchy crudités can cleanse your breath. If you spy a sprig of parsley, by all means scarf it up! It's one of the best sources of chlorophyll, which will help turn your sour breath sweet.

duced by anaerobic (oxygen-hating) bacteria in the mouth. These stinkers tend to hang out in the nooks and crannies in the hard-to-reach rear of the tongue, so the best way to flush them out is by scraping the back of your tongue. Studies that show daily tongue cleansing with a toothbrush helps to reduce key odor-causing bacteria by 25 to 75 percent. And although brushing and flossing thoroughly every day—the classic good habit— also helps minimize halitosis, there are other effective strategies. Drinking lots of water is a good habit to acquire, especially if you're short on saliva—dubbed "Mother Nature's mouthwash"—which naturally washes away the odor-causing compounds. Saliva flow ceases when you sleep (which is why you wake up with "morning breath"), but other saliva stealers include drying agents such as antihistamines and antidepressants, alcoholic and caffeinated beverages, mouth-breathing, and even stress. (Remember how your mouth went bone-dry before that big date or crucial presentation at work?)

FRESHEN YOUR BREATH NATURALLY

Unfortunately, those minty/medicinal remedies—TicTacs, Altoids, Listerine, and the rest—can't save us. They contain either sugar (a veritable feast for bacteria) or alcohol (again, creating a drying atmosphere so odor causers linger). Plus, they merely mask the odor, and after an hour or so, "dragon breath" rears again.

Fresh breath starts with regular dental care to check for gum disease and cavities that may be trapping bacteria, proper brushing (after each meal) and flossing (at least once daily), drinking plenty of water, and eating less protein and more fibrous fruits and vegetables. Plus, there are dozens of natural, unsweetened, nondrying remedies that can actually deodorize your mouth and tame the bad-breath beast. Here's where to start.

GO GREEN. Chlorophyll—the substance that makes plants green—can make your breath as fresh as a daisy. One of the best sources is alfalfa, says Flora Parsa Stay, D.D.S., a dentist in Oxnard, California. She recommends drinking up to three cups of alfalfa tea (available at health food stores) daily or taking alfalfa tablets (check at the health food store, then follow the label directions). As a bonus, alfalfa helps clear up constipation, which some doctors believe may contribute to bad breath, since the toxins from waste build up and are exhaled through the lungs and mouth.

BRUSH WISELY WITH MYRRH

The same astringent herb linked to the Wise Men in the Bible is a treasure trove for mouth care, since it fights inflammation and infection and tightens gum tissue so plaque can't become trapped there. After regular brushing, simply dip your toothbrush into powdered myrrh (which you can find at health food stores) and brush again, suggests Flora Parsa Stay, D.D.S. Use only about 1/8 teaspoon (the taste is strong), and remember to brush your tongue.

STIMULATE SALIVA. Check your drugstore or health food store for mouthwashes, toothpastes, and gums containing betaine, an enzyme that has been shown to jump-start saliva flow. Avoid products that contain sodium lauryl sulfate—a foaming agent—which worsens dryness.

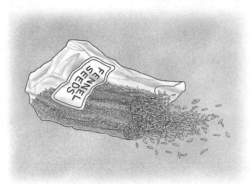

CHEW ON IT. You can chomp on a whole clove, which contains eugenol, a highly aromatic antibacterial. After crushing it with your teeth, move it around your tongue, then spit it out. A third option is to chew on a few cardamom seeds, which are rich in cineole, an antiseptic that fights bacteria.

THIN THE DRIP. Regular spritzing with a saline nasal spray helps thin out mucus from postnasal drip and keep it from collecting on the back of your tongue. Bacteria use this protein-rich gunk to make smelly sulfur molecules and leave a sour taste in your mouth. You can buy a spray at a drugstore or supermarket or make your own by dissolving 1/2 teaspoon of table salt in a glass of warm water and placing it in a bulb syringe.

ZAP IT WITH ZINC. Zinc-containing compounds interfere with bacteria's ability to produce sulfur compounds. Check your health food store for breath-freshening products that contain zinc gluconate and peppermint oil, one of nature's best neutralizers, and coenzyme Q_{10}, an antioxidant that tightens gum tissue so plaque can't become trapped there.

TRY XYLITOL. Another good odor eater is xylitol, a substance that comes from the bark of the birch tree and has been shown to suppress levels of oral bacteria. Look for gums and mouthwashes that contain xylitol at drugstores and health food stores, then follow the label directions.

STINKY FEET

Stamp Out the Stench

My friend's husband is a great guy. Despite the fact that he's extremely meticulous, though, the foul, ripe-cheese odor that arises when he removes his work boots is enough to make your eyes water.

In fact, it's not lack of hygiene that causes feet to reek (although failure to bathe regularly can make the odor worse). Rather, it's trapped sweat produced by the gobs of glands in your soles (approximately 3,000 per square inch) that pump out perspiration—about a gallon of it weekly.

WHY ME?

Normally, all that wetness simply evaporates, but if you

HEAD TO THE VEGGIE BIN

To absorb odor, you can always sprinkle baking soda between your freshly washed toes and in your socks and shoes. If you're fresh out of this handy powder, root around in your vegetable bin for radishes and turnips. Folklore holds that when rubbed on your feet, the juice from these natural deodorant root veggies can decrease smelliness.

A TEA FOR TOOTSIES

Many people are switching to cancer-fighting green tea, but when fighting odor is your aim, black tea rules. It contains tannic acid that helps close the sweat glands, thus starving odor-causing bacteria. Simply brew two tea bags in 1 pint of boiling water for 15 minutes, add the tea to 2 quarts of cool water, and soak your feet for 20 to 30 minutes. Do this for 10 days straight, and your feet will turn out sweet.

enclose your toes in sneakers, work boots, or panty hose that don't "breathe" and where temperatures can easily reach a scorching 102°F, you've got yourself a breeding ground for bacteria. Trapped in the damp, these bugs feed off components in your sweat and leave behind waste products that stink to high heaven.

Some people's feet just naturally sweat more than others' and therefore may be more prone to smelliness. But you may also have bromhidrosis, an inherited tendency toward excess perspiration and smelly feet. It affects twice as many men as women and may be influenced by metabolism, especially if your diet includes lots of meat and other animal-based foods. Drinking coffee or other caffeinated beverages can intensify matters, as can stress, medications, and hormonal changes that increase the amount of perspiration your body pumps out.

GET THE STINK OUT

Trying to mask your problem with foot sprays won't cut it. It's like spraying perfume over a stagnant pond when what you really need to do is drain the pond. Likewise, the first step toward solving foot odor is keeping your feet dry. Here are some tips to help decrease sweat production and keep your dogs daisy-fresh all day.

SOCK IT TO ME. Never wear shoes without socks—ideally,

all-cotton socks or cotton-soled pantyhose (which are "breathable"), says Michael L. Ramsey, M.D., associate professor of dermatology at the Geisinger Medical Center in Danville, Pennsylvania. If you can, change those socks at least once during the day.

DUNK 'EM IN CIDER. Several times a week, soak your feet in 1/3 cup of apple cider vinegar added to a small basin of warm water. The cider's tannins will help dry up your pores, which are the source of your odor, says Jeanette Jacknin, M.D., a dermatologist in Scottsdale, Arizona.

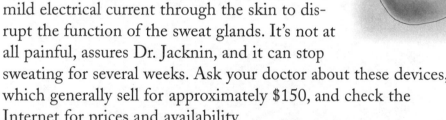

TRY A DRIONIC DEVICE. Drionic is the commercial name of a machine that uses a very mild electrical current through the skin to disrupt the function of the sweat glands. It's not at all painful, assures Dr. Jacknin, and it can stop sweating for several weeks. Ask your doctor about these devices, which generally sell for approximately $150, and check the Internet for prices and availability.

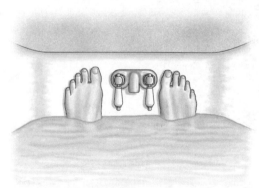

SOAK IN BUROW'S SOLUTION. Ask a pharmacist to point you toward this over-the-counter remedy, which slows the growth of bacteria. Soak your feet daily in a tub filled with 1 part Burow's solution to 40 parts water, says Dr. Jacknin.

BET ON BENZOYL PEROXIDE. The same stuff that fights the bacteria that feed zits also helps zap bacterial growth on the feet, says Martha A. Simpson, D.O., assistant professor of family medicine at Ohio University College of Osteopathic Medicine in Athens. Look for it in drugstores or supermarkets. Be careful when applying it, however, since it can bleach and discolor dark garments.

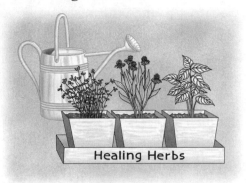

Healing Herbs

SPRITZ WITH SAGE. To banish body odor of any kind, Dr. Jacknin recommends combining five drops each of oil of sage (which dries perspiration), sweet-smelling coriander, and lovely lavender with 2 ounces of distilled witch hazel (a great source of tannic acid, which helps close the pores of the sweat glands so odor-causing bacteria are starved) in a spray bottle. Shake well, then spritz your feet. You can find all of these herbal oils at health food stores.

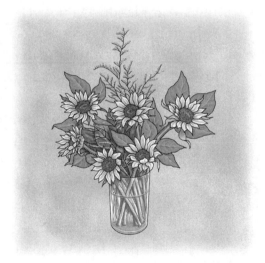

STOMACHACHE

Settle Your Belly

———⊰❋⊱———

I'll admit to occasions where I've slipped into Peter Rabbit mode and nibbled my way through a gourmet buffet, only to wind up with a cabbage patch–sized tummy ache at evening's end. But then, haven't we all?

WHY ME?

Overindulging is a leading cause of stomachaches, which are commonly attributed to indigestion—a term used to describe the general inability to properly digest food. Eating a platter's worth of rich hors d'oeuvres can painfully distend the stomach and prompt your body to amp up production of stomach acid in order to digest all those goodies. An excess of acid in your stomach just plain

BURP IT UP

Burping is not just for babies; it happens to be one of the best ways to relieve a stomachache caused by trapped gas, says Robert Pyke, M.D., Ph.D. To burp properly, stand up straight and swallow a little air slowly so the valve between your esophagus and stomach relaxes and opens. This allows the gas to come up and escape instead of going down and becoming painfully trapped.

hurts, and if this caustic stuff migrates upward from your stomach and seeps through the valve at the end of your esophagus, then you have the added misery of heartburn. Ouch!

Gobbling is another trigger for a stomachache. "When you don't thoroughly chew your food, you lose out on saliva, which contains digestive enzymes that help break down food before it hits your digestive tract," says Robert Pyke, M.D., Ph.D., a physician and pharmacologist specializing in digestive diseases in Ridgefield, Connecticut. The undigested food then ferments, and the result can be painful gas and bloating.

Of course, even if you chew your food as thoroughly as a Guernsey, you may get gassiness, achiness, and bloating in a number of ways. These include eating certain gas-producing foods such as beans, cauliflower, and my alter ego Peter Rabbit's beloved cabbage; from consuming ice cream and other milk products if you're lactose intolerant (meaning that you're unable to digest the lactose, or sugar, in milk); and from taking some medications and even vitamins. The B vitamins are particularly hard for some people to digest.

ALLEVIATE THE ACHE

If your stomach pain is severe or worsening, or if you have chronic stomach pain, see your doctor immediately. You may have an ulcer, gallstones, a bowel obstruction, a ruptured appendix, or some other problem that requires immediate attention.

For the occasional, mild stomachache, on the other hand, passing gas, belching, moving your bowels, and simply waiting it out usually do the trick, says Dr. Pyke. There are several herbs and nondrug remedies that you can use to ease your tummy troubles while you're waiting for Mother Nature to take her course. For instance, Peter Rabbit's mom's advice— skip the bread, milk, and blackberries and drink a little chamomile tea—still stands. This most gentle of all herbs contains an oil that relaxes the smooth muscles of the stomach, dispels gas, and generally helps food get to its final destination (but it may cause a reaction in people who are allergic to ragweed). For additional gentle stomach soothers, read on.

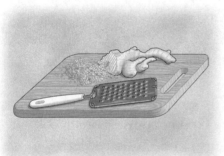

GET GINGER. This pungent root is the jack-of-all-trades for stomach ailments, but it's especially good for relieving pain, since the gingerol it contains helps stop intestinal contractions, says Dr. Pyke. You can take ginger in capsule form or drink it as a tea, but gnawing on a slice of raw ginger root also works. Check your supermarket or health food store for ginger in all its forms and follow the label directions.

EASE THE ACHE WITH LEMON BALM. This sweet-smelling herb, also known as melissa, can help relax muscles and calm a roiling digestive tract. Add 6 to 12 drops of lemon balm extract (available at health food stores) to a glass of water and drink it three times a day.

STICK WITH MARSHMALLOW. That's marshmallow root, not the gooey roasted treat. Marshmallow is an herb that helps coat and soothe the mucous membranes in the stomach. Try

taking up to six 400- to 500-milligram capsules per day or drink a cup or more of marshmallow root tea a day. You'll find both capsules and tea at health food stores.

GIVE IT THE SQUEEZE. For acute indigestion, try this old-time Ayurvedic remedy: Squeeze the juice from 1/4 of a lime into a cup of warm water and just before drinking it, add 1/2 teaspoon of baking soda. Then down it quickly, suggests Vasant Lad, M.A.ScD., director of the Ayurvedic

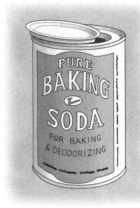

Institute in Albuquerque.

RUB AWAY YOUR BELLY-ACHIN'. To relax tense, constricted muscles and ease your pain, push gently into the lower left side of your belly or rub the area in circles for 30 seconds or more, says Dr. Pyke. You may even consider adding a few drops of antispasmodic fennel or peppermint oil (available at health food stores) to vegetable oil to boost the effects of the massage.

FUMIGATE THE AREA. Other people may not want to be around you when you use this remedy, but it works, says Dr. Lad. Mix 1/2 teaspoon of honey and 1/2 teaspoon of black pepper with 1/4 cup of fresh onion juice (an analgesic), then toss it back to ease stomach pain as well as any flatulence or bloating.

STRESS

Relax Naturally

———◦◦◦———

They say that merely sitting in the presence of the Dalai Lama, a man who has dedicated his life to meditation and peaceful pursuits, calms your body and your mind, immediately lowering your stress level by several notches. Unfortunately, most Americans I know spend time daily in the presence of stress makers. For my husband, it's the grind of a bumper-to-bumper commute. For my sister, it's the constant threat of a staff cut. As common as these types of stressors are, we think little of them—but our bodies take note.

WHY ME?

As if these everyday pressures weren't enough, we've learned that how our bodies respond to stress—especially ongoing stress—can wreck our health. Stress triggers a flood of adrenaline and cortisol, the "fight-or-flight" hormones that quicken your breathing, speed your heart rate, and clench your muscles. All of these responses are useful when facing a short-term threat such as a near collision, but when the hormone deluge continues without a healthy discharge, the result can be markedly unhealthful. Unrelieved stress can contribute to accelerated aging, higher blood pressure, wider waistlines, foggier memories, bluer moods, and conditions ranging from arthritis to psoriasis. Heck, the overproduction of cortisol itself may even predispose us to disease because it weakens the immune system.

SHORT-CIRCUIT STRESS

You may already know that the best "vaccine" against stress is regular exercise, mind-body techniques such as yoga (a single 50-minute session can lower cortisol levels, studies show), and socializing with friends and loved ones. But even seemingly minor, quickie stress busters also offer protection. Researchers have discovered, for instance, that simply giving a surgical patient a room with a view of trees rather than of a brick wall lowers stress levels and minimizes pain and the need for pain medication. And while taking slow, deep breaths and focusing on the sensation (called mindful breathing) won't shrink that long bank line, this easy-to-do technique can lower your heart rate and reduce other harmful effects of stress hormones.

The idea behind all stress-management tips and techniques is to help you gain a sense of control, and when you feel more in control, you're more immune to future

SMELL THE ROSES

Misting the air and inhaling aromatic herbs provides "a quick ride back to your center of calm," says herbalist Rosemary Gladstar, cofounder of Sage Mountain Retreat Center in East Barre, Vermont. She suggests a filling a spray bottle with 1 teaspoon of salt mixed with five drops each of oil of lavender, chamomile, bergamot, rose, geranium, lemon balm, and clary sage—all of which are calming and stimulating herbs that you can find at health food stores.

stress, says Paul. J. Rosch, Ph.D., director of the American Institute of Stress in Yonkers, New York. Here are a few easy ways to manage stress and maximize your sense of control.

SHARE A MOMENT WITH FIDO. If you can't sit with the Dalai Lama, being in the room with your golden retriever may be the next best thing. Pets serve as a buffer against acute stress and make you feel less hassled—even more so than being in the presence of a spouse or close friend, according to studies headed by Karen Allen, Ph.D., assistant professor of medicine at the State University of New York in Buffalo. One reason: Pets neither judge nor evaluate.

COMMUNE WITH NATURE. Any time spent reveling in the great outdoors can help stem the tide of stress hormones, possibly because biochemical pathways in the brain may respond positively to contact with nature, says Howard Frumkin, M.D., chair of environmental and occupational health at Emory University School of Medicine in Atlanta. The interesting part is, you don't even have to be outside: Strolling through a warm, aromatic greenhouse or simply admiring your neighbor's lawn or the park across the street through the nearest window will do.

PLAY AT YOUR DESK. The major source of stress for adults is workplace pressure, experts say, and we may do well to revive certain kindergarten pastimes. Stock your pencil holder with

ON-THE-SPOT RELIEF

Pinch Yourself

Once or twice daily, press firmly on the fibrous spot between your thumb and index finger, about an inch from the edge of the web. This acupressure point corresponds to the large intestine, and pinching it may help tone your exhausted adrenals and improve your ability to handle stress, says Jamison Starbuck, N.D.

Survivors of auto accidents, sexual abuse, and other traumatic events are understandably less stress-hardy later in life. A simple method called EMDR (eye movement desensitization and reprocessing), developed by a clinical psychologist, seems to help lower stress and anxiety in just two or three sessions. In a nutshell, the patient recalls the stressful event while following a therapist's finger moving rapidly back and forth in front of her eyes. For information, contact the international EMDR association at (512) 451-5200 or visit their Web site at www.emdria.org.

✳ ✳ ✳

colored pens, for instance, and when you're jotting down notes or thoughts, do it in, say, purple—and keep scribbling/coloring if you have the time and the privacy. Even this little throwback to childhood can help release tension and have a deeply calming effect, says Lois Levy, an organizational development consultant in Fort Worth, Florida.

MUNCH ON SCHISANDRA. Ongoing stress can wear out your adrenal glands. Schisandra, an herb available at health food stores, can help perk them up like a jolt of java, but without the jittery side effects, says David Hoffman, assistant professor of health studies at the California Institute of Integral Studies in Santa Rosa. Chew 1 teaspoon of berries twice daily, sip two cups of tea per day, or add 15 to 25 drops of tincture to a glass of water and drink it daily. Don't use schisandra if you're pregnant, however.

GET YOUR Bs. If your life is in overdrive, it's vital to include fish, milk, beans, peas, whole grains, broccoli, cauliflower, and kale in your diet. These foods all provide a bushel of pantothenic acid, which is critical for keeping your adrenal glands up to snuff when they may

be maxed out, says Jamison Starbuck, N.D., a naturopathic physician in Missoula, Montana. To be on the safe side, supplement daily with a B-complex vitamin that contains 50 milligrams of pantothenic acid, she says.

CUT THE CATASTROPHIC THOUGHTS. What you tell yourself can absolutely add to your stress level, says Richard Carlson, Ph.D., a psychotherapist and stress expert based in northern California. For instance, the next time you hear yourself saying, "I can't handle this," take a deep, calming breath and swiftly replace that thought with this one: "I am strong, I am in control, and I am handling this."

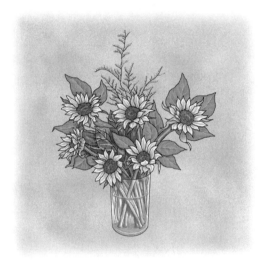

Sunburn

Put Out the Fire

———◦◦◦◦———

Despite my best efforts, I've had more than my share of sunburns—and not simply when I've neglected to slather on sunscreen with the appropriate sun protection factor (SPF). I've gotten seared, for instance, when I've stopped to chat with a friend during the peak burning hours of 11:00 A.M. to 2:00 P.M. without giving my dutifully applied sunscreen time to kick in. Did you know that it takes 20 minutes?

WHY ME?

More surprising sun-related facts: Wearing cosmetics containing citrus oils, such as bergamot, or taking various photosensitizing substances, such as antihistamines, antibiotics, antidepressants, and even St. John's wort, can pre-

---

SLURP SOME SPAGHETTI SAUCE

Tomatoes are brimming with lycopene, a substance that can stop free radical damage to cells caused by overexposure to the sun. Eating these scarlet veggies cooked with oil—in other words, eating foods made with prepared tomato paste—has been shown to help protect the skin from sun damage and redness. Apparently, the oil helps boost the uptake of lycopene in the body.

---

dispose you to sunburn. Plus, facial lotions containing lactic acid that are designed to minimize fine lines can actually prompt burning—which, ironically, can encourage wrinkles.

Of course, there's more to worry about than wrinkles, brown spots, or sagging skin as a result of sunburn. The ultraviolet rays (both UVA and UVB) can actually harm the DNA material inside skin cells and predispose you to skin cancer. Fair-skinned folks like me, who have less of the skin pigment melanin that helps block UV penetration, are more likely to burn and thus more likely to incur damage down the road.

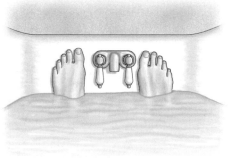

ON-THE-SPOT RELIEF

Got Sunburn? Get Milk

Whole milk dabbed on sunburn for 15 minutes every 2 to 4 hours can be ultra-soothing, says Jeanette Jacknin, M.D. It's the fat content that does the trick, but don't try it until the heat has gone out of the burn, or you'll feel as though you've jumped into a fire. For a soother with a more appealing aroma, try dripping lavender oil directly onto your sunburn.

SOOTHE THE SINGE

See a doctor if your burn is severe and accompanied by fever, chills, upset stomach, or confusion. For milder sunburn, though, here are a few natural remedies to assuage your pain and suffering.

SOAK YOUR SKIN. As quickly as you can, hop into a cool bath spiked with a heaping tablespoon of either baking soda or colloidal oatmeal (available at health food stores) to reduce inflammation and pain and moisturize your skin. Nowhere near a tub? Keep your skin moistened with a wet cloth, advises Sharol Tilgner, N.D., a naturopathic physician and director of the Wise Acres Herbal Education Center in Eugene, Oregon. Whatever you do, avoid applying any type of oil-based preparation. Oil will hold in the heat and cook your skin, doing more damage.

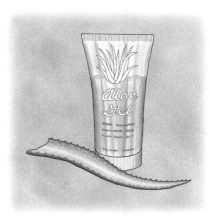

GO FOR ALOE. Aloe vera is an amazing healer for all burns, including sunburns, says Dr. Tilgner. The thick liquid inside the leaves contains enzymes that reduce pain and redness and speed healing by urging new skin cells to grow. You can scoop the gel straight out of a slit leaf or purchase aloe at a health food store. If you opt for the latter, look for "pure" aloe without colorings or other added ingredients.

MIX IT WITH C.

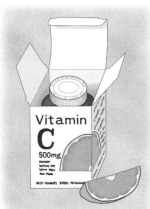

Vitamin C is an anti-inflammatory that can boost the soothing effects of aloe, notes Jeanette Jacknin, M.D., a dermatologist in Scottsdale, Arizona. Mix 2 tablespoons of vitamin C powder (which you can find at drugstores and health food stores) into 1/2 cup of commercial aloe juice, pour the mixture into a small spray bottle, and spritz your skin twice a day until it's healed.

GET GOTU KOLA. This Indian herb fights infection and speeds healing, as does vitamin C. Dr. Jacknin suggests taking 200 milligrams of gotu kola (available at health food stores) twice a day and—as long as you don't have stomach or kidney problems—1,000 milligrams of vitamin C three times a day until your sunburn heals.

BAG IT. Black tea contains tannins that help change the skin's protein structure and assuage burning, says Dr. Tilgner.

Brew two tea bags in a cup of water for 5 minutes. Chill them and wring them out, then place them on your sunburn. Strawberry leaves and witch hazel, both of which are also rich in tannins, are also effective, she notes.

TRY VINEGAR. Apple cider vinegar is

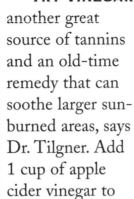

another great source of tannins and an old-time remedy that can soothe larger sunburned areas, says Dr. Tilgner. Add 1 cup of apple cider vinegar to your bathwater and soak for 15 minutes.

TAKE COMFORT IN COMFREY AND CALENDULA. Comfrey—a staple in Native American medicine kits—contains allantoin, which boosts tissue growth and promotes healing. Soak a clean cloth in cooled comfrey tea (which you can find at health food stores) and use it as a compress on your sunburn for 15 minutes twice daily. Calendula cream staves off pain and prevents scarring from blistering burns; look for it at health food stores.

SMEAR ON SOME E. To speed healing and possibly prevent deep cellular damage, keep your blisters

TEA FOR TENDER EYELIDS

When green tea is applied topically, it may help prevent sunburn and skin cancer, according to one report. If you're already burned, it may help stave off cellular damage and ease pain. Cooled tea bags are especially helpful for sunburned eyelids, notes Jeanette Jacknin, M.D. She recommends steeping four tea bags in a quart of boiling water for a several minutes, then letting them cool until they're lukewarm. Squeeze the liquid from the tea bags and apply them to your eyelids, then soak a small towel in the tea and place it over other sunburned areas. Reapply every 30 minutes until the pain fades.

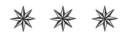

intact (they help shield burned skin) and smear vitamin E oil (available in drugstores and health food stores) over the affected area, suggests Dr. Tilgner.

ST. JOHN'S STIMULATION. Famous for boosting low moods, St. John's wort can also heal burns by stimulating tissue repair. Mix 1 part tincture (available in health food stores) with 9 parts water, then pat it on your burn for at least 15 minutes. Just be sure to wash off the solution if you're heading into the sun.

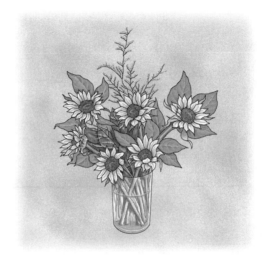

SWEATING

Control the Glow

———◆———

On muggy days, when I'm attending a dress-up affair and my face is glistening, my hair is matted to my head, and my hands are wringing wet, I often forget that my body isn't sabotaging my efforts to look calm, cool, and collected. Instead, it's keeping me upright—which, when you think about it, is absolutely key to looking all three.

On scorching days; during strenuous activity; when you're eating spicy foods, are nervous or angry, or have a fever; or when your hormones are fluctuating, your body temperature rises. The hypothalamus (the body's built-in thermostat) alerts the nervous system that controls the sweat glands—located mainly in your palms, the soles of your feet, and your armpits, forehead, and groin—to start the waterworks. The perspiration then evaporates on your skin to cool you down—and keep you standing. If you couldn't sweat off excess heat in this way,

GOBBLE THE GARNISH

Does your sweat stink? Simply munch on parsley, an excellent source of chlorophyll and a natural odor eater that works from the inside out!

INVITE YOUR FEET TO TEA

The age-old practice of soaking sweaty feet and hands in tea is also an excellent modern approach. The tannins in the tea help close your pores, thus shutting off the waterworks. To try it, steep five tea bags in a quart of hot water, let it cool, and soak your feet or hands for 30 minutes every other night for a week, suggests Andrew Weil, M.D., director of the Program in Integrative Medicine and clinical professor of internal medicine at the University of Arizona in Tucson.

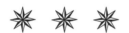

your body functions would simply shut down.

WHY ME?

Why are you sweating like mad when your companion has barely a trace of dew on her chin? Well, it may be a matter of quantity and/or quality. You may simply have more sweat glands than she does. She may be fitter (the more body fat you have, the higher your core body temperature), so her body may have learned to sweat more efficiently. Or, if you're a super soaker and sweat routinely soaks through your clothes, you may have hyperhydrosis, which is really just a fancy word for excessive sweating. It's often a family trait and may be caused by a dysfunction in the sweat glands, a hyped-up nervous system, diabetes, or an overactive thyroid.

WAYS TO STAY DRY

Whether you perspire a bit or produce buckets, sweating the sweat only makes it worse. Consult your doctor if you're bothered by profuse perspiration—or simply try these at-home sweat stoppers. Unlike super-strength prescription antiperspirants, which pack megadoses of aluminum salts that thicken sweat and plug sweat ducts, these gentle remedies stop the sweat before it even appears.

SAGE IS SUPER. In one study, researchers found that severe perspirers can reduce sweating by 50 percent by drinking tea made from dried sage, which seems to help suppress the perspiration-prompting nerve fibers. The effects don't kick in for a couple of hours, but they do last for several days. To try the tea, simmer 4 tablespoons (about 20 leaves) of dried sage (available at health food stores) in a quart of water for 10 to 15 minutes, then strain, let cool, and sip. Don't use sage if you are pregnant or breastfeeding.

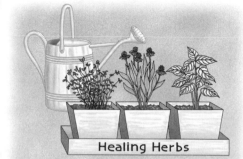

Healing Herbs

TRY WHITE PEONY. The root of this beautiful flowering plant helps stabilize the yin (active, fiery) energy in the body and inhibits spontaneous sweating and night sweating, says Subhuti Dharmananda, Ph.D., director of the Institute for Traditional Medicine in Portland, Oregon. In fact, it's traditionally used to discourage hot flashes and night sweats in menopausal women. Check your health food store for products containing white peony, then follow the label directions.

OIL YOUR MITTS. For excessively sweaty hands, coat your palms with astringent oils to close the pores and stop the sweat. Margaret Stearn, M.D., an internist in Oxford, England, recommends fragrant cypress and geranium oils, both of which are available at health food stores.

DE-STINK. Normally, sweat is odor-free because it's composed primarily of electrolytes and salts. The odor comes when perspiration mixes with the bacteria, yeast, and fungi that thrive in the damper, hairier regions of your body. If you've washed these areas with a mild antibacterial soap and you still smell funky, you may have a zinc deficiency or excess protein in your diet, says Dr. Jacknin. Try limiting foods such as fish, garlic, cumin, and curry, which contain protein oils that linger in the body's secretions.

TENDER BREASTS

Give Them Some TLC

———————◄◦●◦►———————

My friend Lily used to go about her days fairly oblivious to her breasts, until, for no discernible reason, they became excruciatingly tender; then they were on her mind 24/7. The pain, which was considerable, wasn't Lily's only concern. She also worried about what might be causing it and whether something—even the "big C"—might be seriously wrong.

As it turned out, she was 100 percent disease-free—and in that regard, she wasn't at all unusual. What breast tenderness usually indicates, as it did with Lily, isn't disease but simply hormonal flux.

WHY ME?

The most common type of breast tenderness is associated with run-of-the-mill menstruation, and the time of greatest hormonal change—in the decade or so leading to menopause—is also the time of greatest breast pain for many women. "During this period, some women may have either too little or too much progesterone or estrogen, and this may overstimulate the breasts," explains Dixie Mills, M.D., cofounder of the Breast Cancer High-Risk Clinic at the Dana Farber Cancer Institute in Boston and a gynecologist in Yarmouth, Maine.

EASING THE ACHE

Although many doctors prescribe tamoxifen or other heavy-duty medication, not all cases of hormone-related breast pain require medication. For those that don't, frequently all you have to do is minimize swelling (hormone-related and otherwise) and maximize pain control. Here's how to do both—no drugs required.

CURB CAFFEINE. Caffeine, which is present in coffee, tea, colas, and some pain medications, causes blood vessels to dilate—and that can contribute to breast swelling. To reduce your pain, simply reduce your consumption of caffeine as well as peanuts, chocolate, and peanut butter, all of which contain theophylline and theobromine, which are caffeine-like substances.

BRA BASICS

Forget those ill-fitting turquoise numbers you tend to find on the sale rack. If you have chronically tender breasts, you really need to invest in a custom-fitted bra, says Pat Abbott, owner of CustomFit bras in Dallas. Or you can purchase a ready-made bra that fits like it's made just for you. Here's what to look for.

"A bra that provides a healthy environment for your breasts should have a suspension system that evenly distributes the weight, taking 80 percent of the strain off your shoulders," says Abbott. Your bust should be positioned in front, and no breast tissue should spill over the top or sides of the bra. Your breasts should not bounce at all when you move, and you should be able to comfortably use the middle hooks. "If your bra doesn't do all these things," warns Abbott, "it's only a cover and not a support. And your breasts could be suffering."

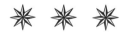

PACK AWAY THE PAIN

Placing a pad soaked with castor oil on your breasts can help break up tissue congestion and move pain-causing fluids. "But perhaps the best benefit is that it forces you to take at least 20 minutes to be calm and nurture yourself," says Dixie Mills, M.D. "We know that stress can add to breast pain, and using a castor-oil pack may help relieve stress hormone buildup." Simply saturate a wool flannel cloth with cold-pressed castor oil (available at health food stores) and place it on your breasts. Cover it with plastic wrap, then a heating pad set on low. Leave the pack on for an hour, if you can.

STARVE YOUR SWEET TOOTH. Too much sugar can block a substance that helps the kidneys flush out excess fluids, says Gloria Bachmann, M.D., associate dean of women's health at the Robert Wood Johnson University Hospital in Newark, New Jersey. Minimizing sweets can help minimize fluid buildup and reduce breast swelling and soreness.

HOLD THE DAIRY. "If your breasts are sore, you may be allergic to dairy foods or be reacting to either the animal hormones in them or what the animals ate," says Dr. Mills. See if cutting back on milk-based foods prior to your period eases the pain.

SAY SAYONARA TO FAT. Saturated fat may be at the root of some breast pain, says John Sunyecz, M.D., an obstetrician and gynecologist in Uniontown, Pennsylvania. Your breasts may be oversensitive to the estrogen spike that occurs from indulging in the saturated fat found in butter, burgers, and fries. Or saturated fats may be blocking your body's ability to convert the essential fatty acids (EFAs) found in cold-water fish (such as salmon and tuna) into gamma-linolenic

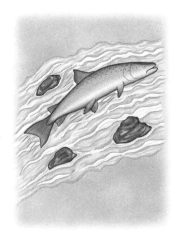

acid (GLA), which gives rise to substances that moderate pain. Whatever the case, your best bet may be to limit fat from land animals and eat more fish.

OIL UP WITH EVENING PRIMROSE. This enchanting-sounding oil is one of the richest herbal sources of GLA and is therefore a pain moderator. In fact, some studies show that evening primrose oil reduces tenderness in more than half of women with breast pain and may rival the effects of prescription hormone treatments, notes Dr. Sunyecz. Check with your own doctor first, but the suggested dose is 1 gram (1,000 milligrams) of oil or gel capsules three times a day with meals. You can find them at health food stores and some drugstores.

Evening Primrose

TRY VITEX. Also known as chasteberry, vitex was once thought to reduce sexual desire. Now we know it simply regulates female hormones and thereby relieves some breast tenderness. To get the full effect, take two 225-milligram capsules (available in health food stores) for three full menstrual cycles, then let your body take over, suggests Beverly Yates, N.D., a naturopathic physician with the Natural Health Care Group in Portland, Oregon. But don't take vitex if you're pregnant.

SAVOR FLAXSEED. In one study, women with severe cyclical breast tenderness who ate muffins containing 25 grams of ground flaxseed every day for three months had less breast pain than those who ate muffins without the flaxseed. This may be because flaxseed is rich in EFAs and phytoestrogenic compounds that may reduce the impact of estradiol, a form of estrogen. Be patient, though: The pain may not ease for two months. Not up to

baking? Some experts suggest taking 3¹/₂ tablespoons of flaxseed oil
(like flaxseed, it's available at
health food stores)
daily. Don't use
flaxseed oil if
you're taking
aspirin or pre-
scription blood
thinners, though.

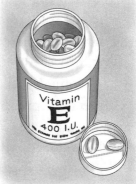

**UP VITAMIN
E.** This nutrient,
often in combina-
tion with evening
primrose oil, may help boost pro-
duction of substances that moderate pain. The usual dose is 400
IU a day.

GIVE FLUID A SHOVE. By gently massaging your breasts
upward, starting from the sides of the breast and moving to the
upper portion, you can help push any excess fluid there into circulation and ease congestion, says Judith Boice, N.D., a naturopathic physician in Portland, Oregon.

DITCH YOUR UNDERWIRE. The underwires in bras can
press into the lymph glands under your arms, "and when the
lymph nodes are constricted," says Dr. Boice, "fluid may not be
able to move freely from your breasts." That's a good reason to
revamp your lingerie wardrobe.

THYROID DISEASE

Get the Gland in Gear

———————◦◦◦———————

Most Americans can blame pudginess on the twin evils of humongous portions and habitual bench warming. But for my friend Nicole (and for one in five other Americans), the reason for her weight gain wasn't sluggish behavior but rather her sluggish thyroid gland, which was too pooped to rev up her metabolism to burn calories.

If you've piled on the pounds despite earnest efforts to lose or have other hard-to-explain symptoms, you could have a malfunction in the butterfly-shaped gland located just above the hollow notch in your neck. The thyroid produces hormones that regulate your metabolism as well as your heart rate. In Nicole's case, her underactive thyroid made her feel as if she were stuck in slo-mo. Besides the weight gain, she had no energy, was depressed and constipated, and had difficulty concentrating. Her skin was pale and dry, and her hands were always cold. When she finally consulted her doctor, a blood test revealed that her thyroid wasn't producing enough thyroid hormone, possibly

LIGHT A FLAME UNDER YOUR THYROID

Making your body resemble a candle, which is what you do when you perform the yoga pose called the shoulder stand, is believed to help stoke the thyroid gland. First, lie on your back with your knees bent and your feet on the floor. Inhale slowly as you raise your legs and spine, supporting your back by placing your hands on your lower back and resting your elbows on the floor. Raise your legs until they're straight up, with your toes pointing skyward—as straight as a candle's flame—and your weight is resting on your upper shoulders, with your chin tucked in. Hold the pose for about 2 minutes, then slowly bend your knees and curve your spine gradually back down to the floor.

because her immune system was attacking the gland and the onslaught had squelched the hormone output.

WHY ME?

Indeed, the root of an underactive thyroid (formally called hypothyroidism) is believed to be an autoimmune disease, frequently one called Hashimoto's disease. Doctors believe an underactive thyroid may also follow an infection such as Lyme disease, which somehow keeps the immune system on hyperalert so it mistakenly attacks the thyroid.

If blood tests show that you're producing anti-thyroid antibodies or that your levels of thyroid hormone are low, you'll need to replace the missing hormone. Some naturally oriented doctors prefer a natural thyroid product that's made from the glands of pigs and contains a range of thyroid hormones (see "Save Your Money" on page 426). The conventional synthetic thyroid replacement drug levothyroxine (Synthroid) contains just one hormone.

This is not a do-it-yourself disease, though, warns Susan

Marra, N.D., a naturopathic physician in Westport, Connecticut. It's tough to control the amount of hormone replaced, and too much can trigger an overactive thyroid. This is a less common form of thyroid disease known as hyperthyroidism, which can make you feel jittery and nervous. An overactive thyroid can also accelerate bone loss, so you can wind up with brittle bones. Once you have this form, the treatment calls for powerful drugs that squelch the thyroid. The message here is that you can't fiddle on your own with taking herbs, supplements, or nutrients that act on the thyroid.

TURN UP YOUR THYROID

If you have symptoms that may signal an underactive thyroid—that is, you're gaining weight and feel sluggish, depressed, and cold—and a blood test indicates low levels of thyroid hormone, follow your doctor's orders, which may include taking a high-potency multivitamin that contains 800 IU of vitamin D (necessary for thyroid hormone production). Also consider trying these nondrug helpers—but only after discussing them with your doctor.

TRY TYROSINE. The thyroid gland uses tyrosine, an amino acid available in supplement form at health food stores, to produce thyroid hormone. Ask your doctor about adding it to your regimen, advises Dr. Marra.

CHECK YOUR TEMP

If you suspect that you may have thyroid disease, check your morning temperature by inserting a thermometer under your armpit for 10 minutes while you're still lying down, advises Stephen E. Langer, M.D., a preventive medicine specialist in Berkeley, California. A chronically low temp (below 96°F) may indicate a problem with your thyroid. If it's low for two days in a row, tell your doctor, who may give you further tests. Note that your body temperature naturally dips when you're menstruating.

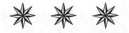

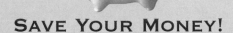
ADD IODINE. The thyroid also requires iodine, so crumbling some iodine-rich dried sea vegetables into your salad may be useful. Just don't go overboard. A thyroid deficiency isn't caused by lack of iodine, so loading up on salty foods such as bladderwrack—a type of brown seaweed once considered a remedy for an underactive thyroid—isn't likely to be much help.

MOVE IT WITH ALOE. Topically, this herb is used to soothe burns, but taken internally, aloe can help stimulate a bowel that's sluggish due to an underactive thyroid, says Dr. Marra. Check your health food store for dried aloe in capsule form and take two 500-milligram capsules with warm water before bed.

SUPPLEMENT SELENIUM AND ZINC. The minerals most crucial for production of thyroid hormone are selenium and zinc, which help convert the hormone into a more active form. Ask your doctor about helpful dosages of both.

GET YOUR OMEGA 3's. To combat dry skin as a result of thyroid disease, supplement with either black currant oil, borage oil, or flaxseed oil, all of which are packed with omega-3 essential fatty acids and are available at health food stores. As long as you're not taking blood thinners, try 800 to 1,200 milligrams a day, suggests Dr. Marra.

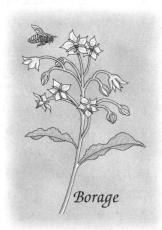

Borage

TMD

Muzzle Jaw Pain

———◦◦◦◦◦———

If your jaws ache when you awake, or if they pop, click, or lock up when you're chewing your Cheerios, chances are your jaw joint is working overtime—even when you're not. One woman I know, totally stressed while planning her daughter's wedding, developed such tender jaws from grinding her teeth in her sleep that tasting the wedding cake she and her daughter had agonized over was excruciating. Her diagnosis (you could call it her own wedding present) was temporomandibular disorder, or TMD (also called TMJ for its site of origin—the temporomandibular joint).

WHY ME?

Stress-induced tooth grinding or clenching (bruxism) is a leading cause of TMD, an umbrella term that covers any pain, stiffness, or related symptoms involving the bone, muscles, and nerves in the hinge-like temporo-

LIFT JAW PAIN

Ever grunt when you lift weights or do strength training? You may also be gritting your teeth and killing your jaws, says Stacy Cole, D.D.S. If so, consider wearing a mouth guard (available at sporting goods stores) during your workouts.

mandibular joint, where the lower jaw joins the skull.

TMD can also be caused by yelling, chomping gum, wearing braces, or even sitting in front of the computer for hours with your head thrust forward. All of these factors place stress on the hard-working joint and can throw the jaws off-kilter, causing the muscles to tense up and the surrounding tissue to become painfully inflamed. The result? A throbbing jaw, sometimes accompanied by aching that extends to your head, neck, and back. You may also hear popping or clicking when you talk or have ringing in your ears.

TMD can also stem from arthritis, a head injury, tooth loss, or a crooked bite that prompts the jaws to try to compensate for the abnormality and shift just enough that they don't quite fit. A severe bite problem or pain may require braces or jaw wiring to help align the teeth and rebalance the musculature of the jaw, but the vast majority of people with TMD (most of whom, by the way, are women) find relief with nonsurgical—and nondrug—remedies.

STOP THE POPS

In many cases, easing TMD is simply a matter of managing muscle tension and inflammation. Start by easing off on caffeine, which can make muscles contract and worsen jaw pain. Invest in a headset for your phone to avoid crooking your neck while holding the receiver, which can pull your jaws out of alignment. Cut your food into tiny bites and skip the caramel apples, gum, and other chewy fare that can tax the jaw muscles. Then give these tips a try. Each can bring noticeable pain relief within just six months.

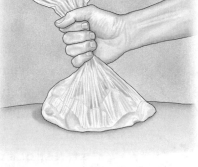

ICE IT. The quickest way to ease pain and stiffness in any joint—including the jaw joint—is to use an ice pack. Apply it to the area for 15 minutes, then remove it for 15 minutes, and repeat this sequence several times a day, says Stacy Cole, D.D.S., a holistic dentist in Fort Worth, Texas.

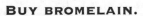

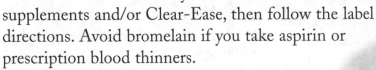

BUY BROMELAIN. This anti-inflammatory enzyme found in pineapple can reduce pain and swelling and allow you to talk and chew with greater ease. Murray Grossan, M.D., a consultant in the department of otolaryngology at Cedars-Sinai Hospital in Los Angeles, reports that his TMD patients find relief by taking Clear-Ease, a product that combines bromelain and papain, another natural anti-inflammatory. Check your health food store for bromelain supplements and/or Clear-Ease, then follow the label directions. Avoid bromelain if you take aspirin or prescription blood thinners.

HEAT THINGS UP. For added relief, smear your sore joint with capsaicin cream (available in drugstores). Capsaicin, the ingredient that gives hot peppers their zing, helps deplete the proliferation of pain-causing prostaglandins. Apply the cream with a cotton swab, and don't get it near your eyes.

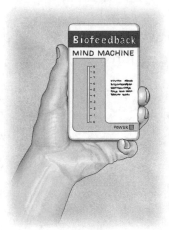

GET BETTER WITH BIOFEEDBACK. This technique will help you recognize when you clench your teeth and then teach you how to stop it. Here's how it works: First, a technician places sensors on your jaw that are connected to a monitor. While you're wired, you perform relaxation exercises, and the monitor shows you (feeds back) when you're clenching and when you're not. Eventually, you'll be able to recognize a clench for what it is right away and relax your jaw immediately. Ask your doctor about the technique and for a recommendation to a reputable biofeedback specialist.

GET NEEDLED. In one study, acupuncture helped more than half of the participants with TMD. What's more, they were still pain-free a full year following treatments. Ask your doctor to recommend a reputable acupuncturist.

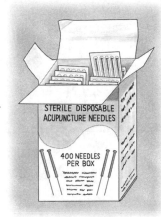

CLAMS BEAT IBUPROFEN!

Taking glucosamine sulfate, a compound derived from shellfish, works better than ibuprofen at reducing TMD pain, Canadian researchers found. The compound is a building block for cartilage and hyaluronic acid, the fluid that greases the joints. Unless you're allergic to shellfish, check your health food store or drugstore for glucosamine supplements, then follow the label directions.

TRY A MOUTH GUARD. Why not risk looking like a linebacker for a few nights by slipping in an athletic mouth guard before bed? If you wake up with less jaw pain, ask your dentist to custom-make a bite plate that may help your muscles relax and gently move your jaw back into its natural position.

RELAX YOUR BACK. "When my patients receive tension relief in the muscles from the neck down, jaw pain often disappears," says Dr. Cole. One of the most effective methods is craniosacral therapy, during which the practitioner makes very slight rhythmic movements in the bones at the back of your head and at the base of your spine (sacrum) and in the connective tissues. This helps your body release constriction that can radiate up to your jaws. To find out more and locate a practitioner, call (800) 233-5880 or visit www.upledger.com.

STAND LIKE A MOUNTAIN. This simple but effective yoga pose can help relax and align your spine and head to ease sore jaws, says Julie Gudmestad, a yoga instructor and physical therapist in Portland, Oregon. Simply stand with your feet slightly apart and firmly planted on the floor, keep your shoulders down and your head back so that it's positioned right in the center of your shoulders, and imagine that a string affixed to the top of your head is pulling you up toward the ceiling.

ULCERS

De-Bug Your Gut

———————

I have a harried relative who insists that her demanding boss and accident-prone son are giving her an ulcer—but she's fingering the wrong suspects. The truth is, everyday stressors are more likely to cause a hammering headache than an ulcer.

Ulcers typically announce themselves with gnawing, burning, or aching pain between your breastbone and belly button, either just before you eat or several hours afterward. They form when the mechanism that protects the walls of the stomach and intestines weakens, and caustic stomach acid literally eats into them. If the ulcer erodes your stomach wall, it's called a gastric ulcer; if it attacks your intestine, it's called a duodenal ulcer (for the duodenum, the

GIVE IT THE SLIP

When banana is dried and pulverized, it helps to fortify the mucosal lining of the stomach and promote healing of ulcers, according to researchers in India. The dose used in the study was two capsules of dried, raw banana powder (available in health food stores) taken four times a day for two months. Try it—you may go bananas over the results!

uppermost part of the small intestine, which connects to the stomach). Together, gastric and duodenal ulcers are referred to as peptic ulcers, a reference to the stomach enzyme pepsin.

The culprit in both cases isn't stress, as many people assume, but a microscopic bacterium called *Helicobacter pylori*, which is spread person to person via the oral/fecal route. The bug attacks your stomach's protective mucous lining and ratchets up acid production. The result—*sometimes*—is an ulcer.

WHY ME?

Not everyone infected with *H. pylori* gets erosions. Your chances are greater if someone in your family has ulcers or if you regularly use nonsteroidal anti-inflammatory drugs (NSAIDs), such as aspirin and ibuprofen. These painkillers block the enzymes that make prostaglandins, which protect the stomach lining.

If x-rays (called an upper GI series) confirm you have an ulcer or the beginning of one, the conventional cure—a triple-whammy regimen that includes two potent antibiotics plus an acid suppressor—can mend the damage. The downside is some nasty side effects, such as nausea, diarrhea, and an uprising of yeast when the "good" bacteria that check yeast are wiped out.

DE-STRESS WITH A SPOT OF TEA

Since the acid production caused by stress aggravates ulcers, you'll feel better if you manage stressful situations well, says Gary Gitnick, M.D., chief of digestive diseases at the University of California, Los Angeles, School of Medicine. Along with deep breathing and other calming techniques, Dr. Gitnick suggests regularly sipping chamomile tea, which may help decrease inflammation and ease the anxiety that could be fanning your ulcer. Unless you're allergic to ragweed, check your supermarket for chamomile tea, then follow the package directions.

HEALING THE HOLE

If your doctor tells you that your ulcer is severe, you won't be able to avoid the conventional cure, but you may be able to use the following gentler remedies (which may do the trick for a milder ulcer)—along with standard medications—to speed healing and keep side effects to a minimum.

TAKE IN THE WELCOME MAT. Start by making your stomach as inhospitable as possible to *H. pylori*. Stop taking all NSAIDs and opt instead for an aspirin-like herbal painkiller such as meadowsweet (check at a health food store for tea and sip three to six cups a day), which may even help heal gastric ulcers. Eat lots of fruits and veggies, since they contain bioflavonoids, which squelch the growth of bacteria. Load up on fiber (found to be effective against duodenal ulcers). Avoid tea, coffee (decaf, too), alcohol, citrus juices, and even milk, all of which promote acid and may make ulcers worse.

LICK IT. Studies show that licorice root stimulates mucus production in the stomach and may be as effective as acid blockers such as ranitidine (Zantac) for treating ulcers. Licorice also blocks acid output, beefs up normal protective mechanisms, gives the boot to *H. pylori*, and seems to work best for ulcers caused by NSAIDs, says Robert Pyke, M.D., Ph.D., a physician and pharmacologist specializing in digestive diseases in Ridgefield, Connecticut. Check your health food store for deglycyrrhizinated licorice (DGL)—the form that doesn't elevate blood pressure—and take two to four 380-milligram tablets before meals and at bedtime every day.

GET "GOOD" BACTERIA. Taking probiotics—that is, beneficial bacteria such as *Lactobacillus acidophilus*—can help standard antibiotics work faster and more thoroughly, keep the bad guys from spreading, and ensure that the yeast that normally resides in the gut doesn't take over and cause an infection. In fact, used alone, megadoses of acidophilus may be equivalent to using a standard antibiotic, says Skye Weintraub, N.D., a naturopathic physician in Eugene, Oregon—although it may take four to five months to do the job. Check your health food store for capsules or liquid products with at least 500 billion colony-forming units (cpu) as stipulated on the label, then follow the label directions for use. Be sure to refrigerate any product you purchase.

GUM UP THE WORKS. Mastica, taken from a Mediterranean-grown evergreen shrub, battles *H. pylori* in the gut and helps heal erosions. Check your health food store for mastica gum capsules and take 1 gram—four to eight capsules—with water before bed. You should feel relief in one week. After a month, reduce the dose to one capsule.

SEAL IT TIGHT. Glutamine is an amino acid available in health food stores that nourishes the protective cells in the stomach lining and helps speed the sealing of the holes, says Dr. Pyke. The suggested dose is 500 milligrams once a day.

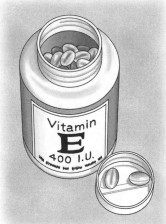

TAKE YOUR VITAMINS. Vitamin E helps heal ulcers, as does vitamin A, but you need to take high doses of the latter, so get your doctor's approval first, advises Dr. Pyke. (Never take vitamin A if you're pregnant.) Vitamin C can also beat back *H. pylori*, but look for the coated kind, such as Ester-C, that doesn't promote acid production.

QUAFF CABBAGE WATER. "This old-time remedy is rich in vitamin C and glutamine, so its reputation as an ulcer healer makes sense," says Dr. Pyke. In fact, studies show that drinking a quart per day of freshly made cabbage water can heal ulcers in about 10 days. Simply soak a whole head in water overnight, then drink four cups of the soaking water (flavored with carrot juice, if you like) throughout the day.

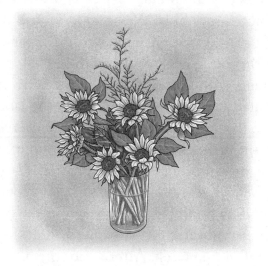

URINARY
TRACT
INFECTIONS

Stop the Sting

———◆◇◇◇◆———

In my view, a urinary tract infection (UTI) is one of Mother Nature's cruelest jokes. The bacteria that can strike any part of the plumbing system—the kidneys in the upper part or, more commonly, the bladder and urethra in the lower—create an absolutely urgent need to sprint to the ladies room, but *fast*. When you get there, though, the expected flood is more like a trickle, and it stings—big time.

One in five women goes through this urge-burn scenario at some time her life. Part of the reason, it seems, lies with the female plumbing system itself.

WHY ME?

A woman's urethra is shorter than a man's. As a result, bacteria from the rectum (typically *E. coli*) have a relatively short distance to travel to take up residence in the urethra and bladder walls. Simply wiping from back to front after using the toilet gives bacteria a free ride. Sexual activity can also escort them into the urethra, which is why women are advised to urinate before and after intercourse. Plus, if you tend to "hold it" until your bladder is nearly bursting, you give germs more time to multiply and affix to your bladder wall. Urine has antibacterial properties, and frequent urination is nature's best means of flushing the system.

Other factors that leave you prone to UTIs include anything that irritates the bladder, such as taking bubble baths, wearing a diaphragm, and even urinating while you have a tampon in place. The loss of estrogen during menopause can thin the bladder walls and allow bacteria to cling more easily. Finally, some women have defects in their bladder walls that prevent bacteria from being flushed out, so they often have recurrent UTIs.

BEAT THE BUGS

The moment urination stings, start using the following measures. If you've reached that critical stage where the bacteria have migrated north, a prescription antibiotic is probably a must. On the other hand, if you're able to act quickly at the first hint of burning, you may be able to flush out the bad guys with a number of these "natural antibiotics" before they can take up residence and spoil the neighborhood.

CHUG CRANBERRY JUICE. Turkey Day's star fruit harbors a

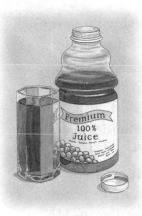

bacteria-fighting weapon: proantho-cyanidins, condensed tannins that have been shown to keep UTI-causing bacteria from attaching to the urinary tract—even in people who have strains that resist standard antibiotics. Drink 2 cups of unsweetened cranberry juice every hour at the first hint of burning, or pop one 400-milligram capsule (available at health food stores) four times a day.

SAVOR BLUE, TOO. Blueberries provide the same anti-infection protection as their crimson cousins when it comes to keeping bacteria from binding to the bladder wall.

DRINK GOBS OF GOLDENSEAL. The idea is to drink at least 2 liters of the plant world's leading antibiotic a day. You'll be running to the bathroom a lot, which is the key to flushing out bacteria. Check for goldenseal tea at health food stores, then make it according to the label directions and drink as much as you can manage.

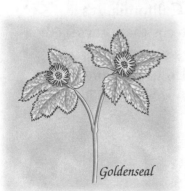

Goldenseal

SIP CORNSILK TEA. Any of the time-honored diuretic teas—those made from nettle, bucchu, cleavers, or cornsilk (all available at health food stores)—will get you running to the

WHEN TO DIAL THE DOC

• • • • • • • • • • •

If you try these remedies and don't get relief within 24 to 36 hours, or if you have a fever, chills, or blood in your urine, see your physician immediately. You need a culture test to identify the bacteria strain and medication to prevent it from traveling to your kidneys, or worse, into your bloodstream, where it can cause bigger problems. You should also consult a doctor if you have repeated infections—more than five a year—to determine if you have any underlying problems.

POP AN OLIVE

An olive branch may stand for peace, but for the bacteria that cause UTIs, olive leaf capsules (four daily) could mean death, says Skye Weintraub, N.D., a naturopathic physician in Eugene, Oregon. Check your local health food store for capsules made from the species grown in Italy (the label should say "olea europa") to ensure that you get the calcium elenolate that stimulates white blood cells to gobble up bacteria. Follow the label directions.

bathroom so you'll flush your system. Cornsilk tea does double duty, though, because it also soothes the mucous membranes in the urinary tract, says Christine Matheson, N.D., a naturopathic physician at the Women's Pelvic Health Center at Sunnybrook Health Sciences Center in Toronto. To make your own, steep a handful of the strands of silk from fresh corn in a cup of hot water for 15 minutes, strain, and sip.

ADD EMERGEN-C. Some experts believe that taking vitamin C helps acidify the urine, which prevents bacteria from clinging; others say the supplement's biggest benefit is as a powerful antioxidant that helps fight infection. Either way, the best form to take is Emergen-C, says Melody Wong, N.D., a naturopathic physician in Sausalito, California. It's a powdered formula available in health food stores that provides 1,000 milligrams of C along with electrolytes such as potassium, which may easily be flushed away if you're also using diuretics. As long as you don't have stomach or kdney problems, follow the package directions.

VAGINAL DRYNESS

Lubricate Naturally

———✦———

Hot flashes are now discussed as freely as tummy tucks, while the most vexing of all menopausal discomforts—vaginal dryness—remains in the closet, despite being incredibly common. In fact, lack of lubrication is the leading reason that "women of a certain age" turn to their gynecologists for help.

When estrogen ebbs during menopause, the vaginal and urethral tissues thin, and mucus in the vaginal tract can dry up. And here's the rub: Without ample lubrication, the friction of sexual intercourse can be painful, which can put a damper on

GET SLIPPERY

As its name implies, when tissue-soothing slippery elm is moistened, it becomes slick. Simply mix 2 tablespoons of slippery elm powder (available at health food stores) with enough water to make a paste and add a dab of pure aloe gel (you can either purchase it at your local health food store or scoop it straight out of a leaf). Use clean hands to spread the slick stuff over your vulva and inside your vagina.

COME ON OVER TO RED CLOVER

Like soy, red clover is brimming with phytoestrogens. In fact, red clover has twice as many of these plant estrogens (which mimic human estrogen) as soy and may be six times more potent. In one study, women who took one tablet of Promensil—the leading red clover supplement—daily for two months had less vaginal dryness. There's just one caveat: Red clover may stimulate breast tissue, so you shouldn't take it if you're at risk for estrogen-fueled cancers. Be sure to ask your doctor about Promensil before trying it.

desire. Lack of sexual activity can lead to even less lubrication, and, as one expert put it, vaginal dryness becomes a self-fulfilling prophecy.

WHY ME?

Vaginal dryness can also occur after childbirth, during breastfeeding, or if you take birth control pills or use drying medications such as antihistamines on a regular basis. (You can see why it's so prevalent.) Other than potent estrogen preparations, though, conventional medicine has little to offer.

Fortunately, many natural therapies can come to the rescue, and the sooner you seek out these remedies, the better. Lack of lubrication can leave the vagina more prone to infections and injury during intercourse.

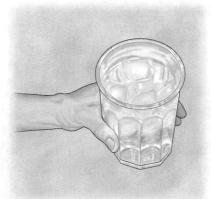

HOW TO GET WET

An excellent but exceedingly simple way to help increase lubrication is to drink water throughout the day. Think of it this way: What goes in comes out. Here are more equally simple but effective steps to ease dryness.

OIL UP. Simply swallowing 1 tablespoon of oil (canola, olive, sunflower, or soybean) daily may help add lubrication to all tissues, including vaginal tissues, notes Christine Matheson, N.D., a naturopathic physician with the Women's Pelvic Health Center at Sunnybrook Women's College of Health Sciences in Toronto.

CRUNCH NUTS. Holistic gynecologist Christiane Northrup, M.D., director of the Women to Women clinic in Yarmouth, Maine, says that many women find that vaginal resiliency and moisture are restored when they start eating whole soy foods regularly—and the higher the daily dose of isoflavones (natural plant estrogens abundant in soy), the better, she says. A quarter-cup of soy nuts, for instance, has more than twice the amount in a cup of soy milk.

REACH FOR FLAX. You may get the same moisturizing effect by

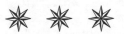

eating 2 to 3 tablespoons of flaxseed (available at health food stores) every day, says women's health herbalist Susun Weed of the Wise Woman Center in Woodstock, New York. You may notice a change in lubrication in just a few weeks. If you stop eating the seeds, however, dryness may return.

INSERT E. "I recommend using vitamin E capsules as vaginal suppositories, because it's both simple and

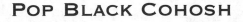

POP BLACK COHOSH

In studies comparing it with estrogen, this old-time favorite of Native Americans proved to be a worthy rival in reducing vaginal dryness and boosting tissue tone and elasticity. "Start with two 40-milligram capsules twice a day," says Tori Hudson, N.D., a naturopathic physician and director of A Woman's Time clinic in Portland, Oregon. "You should see results in two to four weeks." You may be able to reduce the dose in the future, she adds, and you can feel free to experiment with dosages since there doesn't seem to be any long-term harm from taking this herb.

✳ ✳ ✳

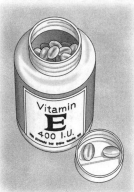

cheap," says Melody Wong, N.D., a naturopathic physician specializing in women's health in Sausalito, California. You don't even have to break open the capsule—the outer coating will dissolve naturally. Insert one capsule daily for a week, then once or twice a week. Or take vitamin E capsules orally in doses of 100 to 400 IU a day. In four to six weeks, studies indicate, dryness could disappear.

MOISTURIZE. Head for the drugstore and plunk down $13 for Replens, a lubricant that contains polycarbophil, an ingredient that prompts vaginal tissue to soak up water and become thicker. When used daily, it's as effective as estrogen for restoring vaginal moisture, studies show. Plus, it can be used as a lubricant during sex.

SITZ IT. Some herbalists recommend taking a sitz bath—basically, sitting in a tub filled to hip level—in water to which 2

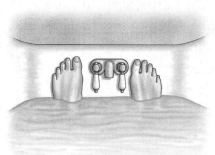

quarts of healing comfrey tea (look for it at health food stores) have been added. Remain in the bath for 5 to 10 minutes, and repeat several times weekly.

PERFORM PELVIC PUSHUPS. Kegel exercises (the equivalent of pelvic floor pushups) are designed to whip your pelvic floor muscles into shape—and in the process, they enhance blood flow and increase vaginal wall thickness as well as moisture. Here's what to do: First, to identify the right muscles, imagine holding back gas or squeezing around a penis; the muscles you use to do both are the muscles in your pelvic floor. To begin, squeeze those muscles, pulling up toward your head while keeping your buttocks and inner thigh muscles relaxed. Hold for a count of 10, then release for a count of 10. Repeat several times daily.

VAGINAL INFECTIONS

Tackle Trouble Down Below

———⊰∘∘∘∘⊱———

In my college days, the campus infirmary dispensed antibiotics like M&Ms, even for run-of-the-mill colds caused by viruses. Too often, the rampant use of antibiotics led to rampant vaginal yeast infections, because the drugs wiped out the "good" bacteria that normally check the "bad" bacteria (yeast, or *Candida albicans*) that reside in the body. Candida thrives in warm, dark environments, and with nothing stopping their growth, they can literally take over like a campus sit-in—only itchier.

WHY ME?

You don't have to be a coed—or take antibiotics—to wind up with a vaginal infection (also called vaginitis) from yeast gone wild. If you routinely wear panty hose, tight jeans, or any other garment that seals in moisture, for instance, you're at increased risk. You're also more prone to yeast-based vaginitis if you eat a sugary diet (the equivalent of Miracle Gro for these organisms), take birth control pills, or are pregnant or menopausal. If you're

MAKE A GARLIC TAMPON

Before you turn up your nose at the idea, consider this: The allicin in garlic is an excellent antifungal and antibacterial that can stop candida in its tracks. Tori Hudson, N.D., recommends carefully peeling a clove so that you don't nick it, slathering it with olive oil, and inserting it into your vagina for no more than 6 hours. (The oils in garlic are potent, so if you feel any burning, remove the clove immediately.) You can also thread the clove for easy removal, insert it in the morning, and remove it 6 hours later, then insert an acidophilus capsule in the evening. The approach provides a powerful one-two punch—killing the bad bugs (candida) and repopulating the vagina with the good bugs (acidophilus).

plagued by repeated infections, you may also have an underlying problem such as diabetes or a thyroid disorder.

Unfortunately, yeast infections are just the most common form of vaginitis—not the only one. Gardnerella, the second most likely culprit, is best treated with a potent prescription antibiotic. If left untreated, this microscopic menace can easily infect the uterus and fallopian tubes and lead to dangerous pelvic inflammatory disease.

Finally, a third type of infection is caused by a parasite called trichomonas. "Trich" can inflame the urethra and bladder and cause extreme burning upon urination.

Vaginal infections are sexually transmitted, so if your partner isn't treated along with you, you can end up passing the organisms back and forth between you like a football.

WIPE OUT VAGINITIS

A foul or fishy odor and/or a grayish-green discharge are tip-offs that the culprit is bacteria or trich—and that you should see your doctor for treatment. When you see the white, cottage cheese–like discharge that signals a yeast infection, however, it's tempting to simply pop by the drugstore and pick up an anti-yeast product such as Monistat right away, but you should really hold off until you see a doctor. For one thing, repeated use of anti-yeast products may create a drug-resistant strain of yeast. For another, it's always possible that your particular problem may be caused by one of the nonyeast bugs mentioned earlier.

Once you're diagnosed, help your medications (which include both OTC antifungals and prescription antibiotics) complete their mission by wearing cotton underwear and breathable workout wear. Avoid sugary snacks, white bread and other refined carbohydrates, fruit, and alcohol to starve the bad bugs. And wipe out vaginitis for good with the following steps. (If you're pregnant, don't use a treatment that involves inserting anything into your vagina.)

THE BEST WAY TO BEAT VAGINITIS

Boric acid suppositories boast an impressive 98 percent cure rate against yeast infections. In fact, studies show that inserting two 600-milligram boric acid suppositories, one in the morning and one at night, can do the job in as little as three to seven days. Here's what you do: Buy "size zero" gelatin capsules at the drugstore and fill them with boric acid powder, which you can find at health food stores. Finally, smear the capsule with vitamin E oil or olive oil to offset any burning sensation as it melts, then insert it in your vagina.

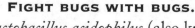

FIGHT BUGS WITH BUGS.
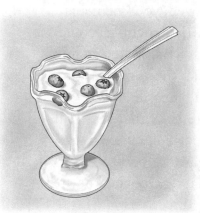
Lactobacillus acidophilus (also known as simply lactobacillus or acidophilus) crowds out the bad bugs that cause vaginitis and restores the acid-alkaline balance (pH) of the vagina so fewer infections can occur in the future. In fact, simply eating 8 ounces of yogurt containing live, active cultures of this beneficial bacteria can result in a three-

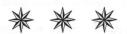
fold decrease in infections, says Tori Hudson, N.D., a naturopathic physician and director of A Woman's Time clinic in Portland, Oregon. If you opt for acidophilus capsules or liquids (available in health food stores), look for products that contain 6 to 10 billion organisms per dose, then follow the package directions.

TRY SUPPOSITORIES. You can place those good bugs exactly where they're needed most by using acidophilus capsules as suppositories and inserting them into your vagina, points out Christine Matheson, N.D., a naturopathic physician at the Women's Pelvic Health Center at Sunnybrook Health Sciences Center in Toronto. The recommended dose is two capsules once or twice daily for a few days to several weeks, depending on the severity of your vaginitis.

DOUCHE WITH VINEGAR. Like your oven, your vagina is self-cleaning. In fact, washing it regularly (by douching) could remove the normal bacteria that fight infections. When vaginitis rears up, however, you may need to establish the proper pH to discourage the takeover and help the good bacteria grow. Douching with vinegar is an old standby remedy that may still help, says Susan W. Ryan, D.O., an osteopathic physician in Denver. Simply add 1 tablespoon of vinegar to a pint of water and douche twice a day for two or three days. (Douche kits are available at drugstores; follow the package directions.)

BEAT IT WITH BERBERINE. Berberine is the active constituent in goldenseal and Oregon graperoot, two well-known antibacterial/immune-enhancing herbs that target microbes that invade mucous membranes—including those in the vagina. Health food stores carry both as teas, capsules, and liquids, but the best way to use them is as a douche, says Melody Wong, N.D., a naturopathic physician in Sausalito, California. Simply make two cups of tea from tea bags, let it cool, and use a drugstore kit to douche twice daily for no more than one week. Avoid douching and any herbs that contain berberine if you're pregnant.

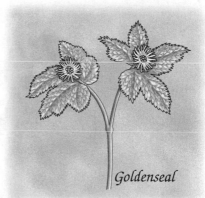

Goldenseal

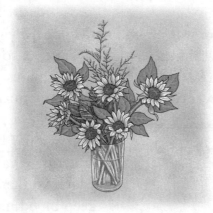

VARICOSE VEINS

Banish the Bulges

My mom was blessed with shapely legs, but she's cursed with snaky, bluish veins from kneecap to ankle—so many, in fact, that they resemble major thoroughfares on a Rand McNally map. Seventy-five percent of Americans (most of them, like my mom, women over age 65) have the same affliction—varicose veins, in which weakened valves fail to keep blood moving back to the heart, so it pools in the large veins, usually in the legs and feet. The stagnated blood gives the veins a purple or dark blue appearance.

WHY ME?

A tendency toward varicose veins may be inherited.

BARK UP A PINE TREE

Studies show that taking 100 milligrams of Pycnogenol (an extract from grapeseed and the bark of a French pine tree that's loaded with flavonoids) three times a day helps reduce bulging, blueness, and discomfort within just two months. Check your health food store specifically for brands that use the capital P.

Beyond that little twist of fate, however, women may be more likely than men to develop them because the hormones estrogen and progesterone weaken vein walls. In fact, hormone overload during pregnancy or with the use of birth control pills can make the walls more fragile long before the age at which veins walls naturally begin to weaken.

Besides creating unsightly highways of purple or dark blue, varicose veins can cause nighttime cramping, heaviness, and itching, and your feet can swell so much that you need a crowbar to get into your shoes. And speaking of shoes, if you favor high heels, you may be making matters worse. High heels keep your calf muscles clenched, putting extra strain on the veins. Weight gain, chronic constipation, and prolonged sitting or standing can do the same thing.

For some people, the veins are barely noticeable yet cause extreme discomfort. For others, like my mom, the blue bulges may look pronounced and painful, but they're merely a mild nuisance. No matter what your symptoms, however, self-care measures are a must, since they can keep your veins from worsening and prevent clots and even ulcers (sores or ulcers can form when skin tissue sur-

ENCOURAGE THE PUMP

Placing hot, then cold compresses soaked in circulation-boosting herbs on your problem veins expands and then contracts them, providing a soothing pumping action, says Jeanette Jacknin, M.D. To give it a try, soak a cloth in a solution made by mixing 10 drops each of cypress, geranium, ginger, juniper, lavender, and rosemary oils (all available at health food stores) with 1 quart of hot water. Press the cloth to your leg for 15 minutes, then soak another cloth in a second batch of solution made with the oils and cold water and apply it for 15 minutes. Follow up with a gentle leg massage (aided by a few of those aromatic, circulation-boosting oils), being sure to stroke upward toward your heart.

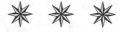

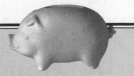
rounding varicose veins doesn't get enough nourishment).

KICKIN' SOLUTIONS

See your doctor if you have extreme pain or sudden swelling, especially if it's in only one leg. Otherwise, here's how to keep the blood pumping and ease the strain on your veins even as you shore up their walls—all without resorting to pricey and sometimes painful procedures such as sclerotherapy (destroying the vein with saline or lasers) or vein-stripping surgery, which provide only temporary results anyway.

GIVE YOUR GAMS A HUG. It's true that wearing skin-tight slacks or banded knee socks can cut off blood circulation. On the other hand, donning graduated compression stockings (which you can find at surgical or medical supply stores) that exert pressure on the legs can actually help return blood to your heart and minimize pooling. Worn during pregnancy, compression hose can even help prevent varicose veins. Ask your doctor to prescribe stockings that provide the appropriate amount of pressure, says Lisa Meserole, N.D., a naturopathic physician in Seattle. If the compression is too strong, you may aggravate your problem.

TRY BIOFLAVONOIDS. These little blood vessel builders strengthen the vein walls and the connective tissue that helps hold up the vessels, explains Jeanette Jacknin, M.D., a dermatologist in Scottsdale, Arizona. As long as you don't have stomach or kidney problems, she recommends taking 300 milligrams of bioflavonoids combined with 1,000 milligrams of vitamin C three times a day (look for individual or combination supplements at drugstores and health food stores). Add 200 IU of vitamin E twice daily to help thin the blood and boost circulation.

SAVOR ONION SKINS. That's right: Onion skin is one of the best sources of quercetin, a hardworking bioflavonoid that reduces capillary fragility, says Dr. Jacknin. Toss an onion—skin and all—into soup or stew so the helpful bioflavonoids leach into the liquid, then discard the skin before digging in.

FIRM 'EM UP HERBALLY. Herbal formulas that include the classic vessel strengtheners butcher's broom, horse chestnut, yarrow, and stoneroot may help reduce leaking from veins and decrease inflammation inside them, says Dr. Meserole. The only catch is, you may need to stay on these herbals forever if you're prone to varicose veins to make sure the veins don't return to make their mark. Check your health food store for vessel-shoring formulas. One caveat: Don't take formulas containing horse chestnut if you're pregnant or breastfeeding.

APPLY HORSE CHESTNUT SOLO. The seeds of the stately horse chestnut tree, once used to treat horse ailments, have been shown to improve circulation in the legs, decrease inflammation and swelling, and strengthen the capillaries and veins, says Dr. Jacknin. Combine 1 part horse chestnut tincture (check your health food store for a tincture that packs 50 milligrams of aescin per dose) with 10 parts distilled witch hazel (a vessel strengthener in its own right) and apply the solution to your problem veins once a day. Patience is key, though, since it could take three months to see an effect.

Horse Chestnut

YELLOW TEETH

Brighten Your Smile

A friend of mine once asked her dentist to recommend the best way to brighten dingy teeth naturally. His reply: Wear a brown shirt—the contrast of the dark color will make your teeth appear as white as Chiclets chewing gum! My friend wasn't the least bit amused.

In our beauty-worshiping culture, having dull, gray, or yellowing teeth is no joke—especially when dental-office bleaching procedures typically carry price tags of $500 or more. It's even less amusing when you consider that in most cases, our own eating and drinking habits are what got us into trouble in the first place.

WHY ME?

Coffee, cola, cabernet, and blueberries are just a few of the deeply pigmented substances that set off a chemical reaction in the plaque on our teeth and turn our pearly whites into an off-putting yellow. Tobacco smoke, water fluoridation, high doses of iron supplements, and taking a tetracycline antibiotic in childhood, when tooth enamel was forming, can all turn teeth gray. For the most part, however, dinginess is just a normal aspect of aging. As we get older, tiny fissures form in the teeth and collect stains. In addition, tooth enamel can thin to the point where the naturally yellow dentin beneath it begins to show through. No wonder professional whitening procedures and over-the-counter whiteners and stain removers have become big business—but they're an expensive solution in more ways than one.

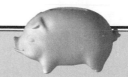

SAVE YOUR MONEY!

It's All Hype!

Whitening toothpastes that don't contain bleach simply can't deliver on their promise, and those that do contain peroxide are quickly washed off the teeth by saliva. You can expect whitening toothpastes to make your teeth shinier (thanks to the wax and polishing molecules these products contain), but they won't necessarily be whiter.

Dental-office bleaches, which are based on hydrogen peroxide, can make your teeth sensitive to heat and cold, while "power bleaching"—involving lasers that bond the bleaching agent and speed up whitening—may damage the pulp. At-home bleaching products carry risks, too: Bleach from those one-size-fits-all dental trays and bleach-impregnated whitening strips can leach onto your gums or, worse, be swallowed. Over-the-counter stain-removing toothpastes can be so abrasive that they can leave your teeth looking duller than they did before you began using the stuff.

In addition to all that, after all your time and trouble, you may not even get the results you're after, says Fred Siemens, D.D.S., formerly a cosmetic dentist in Milpitas, California. Even if you do, you'll have to repeat the bleaching within a few months.

WHITEN GENTLY

Experts say that whitening procedures may not do the trick for grayish-hued teeth, so you may need caps or veneers to cover them. If you have slightly yellowish or brownish teeth, however, give the following nondrug remedies a try. Also, be sure to sip dark drinks through a straw whenever possible, and brush immediately after eating berries, soy sauce, and other staining foods.

BET ON BAKING SODA. Toothpastes made with baking soda can help lighten tea, coffee, and other surface stains, says Flora Parsa Stay, D.D.S., a dentist in Oxnard, California, but you can also use the stuff straight out the box. Just pour a little in your hand, add a drop or two of water, and dip your wet toothbrush into the powdery paste.

TRY HYDROGEN PEROXIDE. Brushing with a 3 percent solution of drugstore hydrogen peroxide combined with 1/4 teaspoon of baking soda may be just as effective as any of the over-the-counter whitening products, says Dr. Siemans. Just be careful not to swallow it, and use it only once a week at most. If you have sensitive teeth or are pregnant, skip it entirely.

ON-THE-SPOT RELIEF

Lipstick Magic

It's Revlon to the rescue! Red, orangey, or brown-tinted lipstick can instantly make yellowish teeth appear whiter, while shades with bluish undertones, such as pinks and magentas, can do the same for gray-tinted teeth. Not sure whether your teeth are yellow or gray? Stand in front of a mirror, hold a piece of printer paper next to your teeth, and compare.

BANISH STAINS WITH BERRIES. An old-time remedy for removing fresh coffee stains and the like calls for rubbing the teeth with crushed slices of fresh strawberries. Let the pulp sit on your choppers for 5 minutes, then rinse thoroughly.

SCRUB WITH CRUDITÉS. Celery, carrots, apples, and other crunchy fruits can help sand away stains safely, says Robert Henry, D.M.D., associate professor at the University of Kentucky School of Dentistry in Lexington. So give 'em a try!

USE AN IONIC TOOTHBRUSH. Reid Laurence Winick, D.D.S., a holistic dentist in New York City, suggests trying an ionic toothbrush (available in drugstores), which safely breaks the bonds of plaque with an electronic charge, instead of using abrasive brushing or toothpastes that use friction to scrub away yellowing matter. Users have reported brighter, lighter teeth, he says.

PAIR IT WITH ECO-DENT. To enhance an ionic toothbrush's effect, use it with an effervescent tooth powder such as Eco-Dent (available in health food stores and from the Internet). These bubbling products break up stains with less abrasion than other stain lifters, so they're less likely to damage tooth enamel.

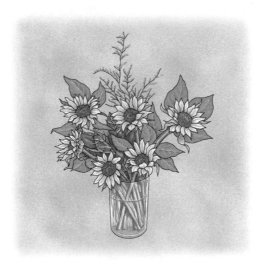

INDEX

Bikini line, shaving, 351
Biofeedback treatments, for
    bladder leaks, 89
    shingles, 375
    temporomandibular disorder, 430
Bioflavonoids, for
    allergies, 15
    shingles, 374
    varicose veins, 452–53
Biotin, for
    brittle nails, 109
    hair care, 76–77
Birch bark, for sprains and strains, 392
Bitter melon, for diabetes, 189
Bitters, for
    gas, 229
    heartburn, 259–60
Blackberries, for allergies, 15
Blackberry root, for diarrhea,
        192
Black cohosh, for
    back pain, 70
    hot flashes, 277
    vaginal dryness, 443
Black currant oil, for thyroid
        disease, 426
Black elderberry, for colds and flu, 159
Black pepper, for stomachaches, 404
Black tea
    effect on iron absorption,
        22
    as treatment for
        bleeding gums, 95
        canker or cold sores, 138
        foot odor, 398
        itchy skin, 298
        osteoporosis, 336
        sinusitis, 379
        sunburn, 412–13
        sweating, 416
Black walnut tincture, for nail fungus,
        328
Bladder leaks
    causes, 87
    treatments, 87–90
Bleeding gums
    causes, 92–93
    treatments, 93–96
    when to call a doctor, 95

Bloating
    causes, 97–98
    treatments, 97–101, 404
    when to call a doctor, 100
Blood sugar levels
    cold medications and, 159
    effect on
        headaches, 250
        memory loss, 312–13
        sleep, 189
    specific foods and, 183, 186, 187
Blueberries, for
    allergies, 15
    athlete's foot, 57
    memory loss, 314
    urinary tract infections, 439
Body fat. See Belly fat; Body weight
Body odor
    causes, 102–3
    treatments, 103–7, 415
Body temperature, thyroid function and, 425
Body weight. See also Weight loss
    effect on
        asthma, 50–51
        bladder leaks, 90
        knee pain, 42
        snoring, 381–82
Bok choy, for
    endometriosis, 212
    high blood pressure, 268
Bone scans, for osteoporosis diagnosis, 335
Borage, for
    allergies, 14–15
    angina, 28
    asthma, 50
    Raynaud's disease, 157
    thyroid disease, 426
Boric acid, for
    earaches, 206
    yeast infections, 447
Boron, for
    arthritis, 43
    back pain, 70
Botanogesic, for sprains and strains, 391
Bottlebrush. See Horsetail
BPPV, 196
Brahmi. See Gotu kola
Brandt-Daroff maneuver, for dizziness, 197
Bras, tender breasts and, 419, 422